Endoscopic Sinus Surgery

Anatomy, Three-Dimensional Reconstruction, and Surgical Technique

Second Edition

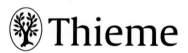

Endoscopic Sinus Surgery

Anatomy, Three-Dimensional Reconstruction, and Surgical Technique

Second Edition

Peter-John Wormald, M.D., F.R.A.C.S., F.C.S.(S.A.), F.R.C.S. (Ed.), M.B.Ch.B.
Professor and Chairman
Department of Otolaryngology
University of Adelaide
Adelaide, Australia

Thieme
New York • Stuttgart

Thieme Medical Publishers, Inc.
333 Seventh Ave.
New York, NY 10001

Editor: Esther Bumpert
Managing Editor: J. Owen Zurhellen
Vice President, Production and Electronic Publishing: Anne T. Vinnicombe
Production Editor: Heidi Pongratz, Dovetail Content Solutions
Vice President, International Marketing: Cornelia Schulze
Sales Director: Ross Lumpkin
Chief Financial Officer: Peter van Woerden
President: Brian D. Scanlan
Compositor: Compset
Printer: Everbest Printing Co.

Library of Congress Cataloging-in-Publication Data

Wormald, P. J.
Endoscopic sinus surgery / Peter-John Wormald. — 2nd ed.
   p. ; cm.
  Includes bibliographical references and index.
  ISBN 978-1-58890-603-8 (Americas) — ISBN 978-3-13-139422-4 (Rest of World)
    1. Paranasal sinuses—Endoscopic surgery. I. Title.
    [DNLM: 1. Paranasal Sinuses—surgery. 2. Endoscopy—methods. 3. Paranasal Sinus Diseases—surgery. 4. Paranasal Sinuses—anatomy &
histology. 5. Video-Assisted Surgery. WV 340 W928e 2007]
  RF421.W67 2007
  617.5'230597—dc22

                                        2007022759

Important note: Medical knowledge is ever-changing. As new research and clinical experience broaden our knowledge, changes in treatment and drug therapy may be required. The authors and editors of the material herein have consulted sources believed to be reliable in their efforts to provide information that is complete and in accord with the standards accepted at the time of publication. However, in view of the possibility of human error by the authors, editors, or publisher of the work herein or changes in medical knowledge, neither the authors, editors, nor publisher, nor any other party who has been involved in the preparation of this work, warrants that the information contained herein is in every respect accurate or complete, and they are not responsible for any errors or omissions or for the results obtained from use of such information. Readers are encouraged to confirm the information contained herein with other sources. For example, readers are advised to check the product information sheet included in the package of each drug they plan to administer to be certain that the information contained in this publication is accurate and that changes have not been made in the recommended dose or in the contraindications for administration. This recommendation is of particular importance in connection with new or infrequently used drugs.

Some of the product names, patents, and registered designs referred to in this book are in fact registered trademarks or proprietary names even though specific reference to this fact is not always made in the text. Therefore, the appearance of a name without designation as proprietary is not to be construed as a representation by the publisher that it is in the public domain.

Printed in China

5 4 3 2

The Americas ISBN: 978-1-58890-603-8

Rest of World ISBN: 978-3-13-139422-4

Dedicated with love to Fiona, my wife, without whom this book would not have been possible and to Nicholas and Sarah, my children, who provide my inspiration.

Contents

Contents

DVD Contents

Foreword

The first edition of Professor Wormald's book on endoscopic sinus surgery was a great success internationally and was named "Best ENT Book of 2005" by the British Medical Association, among other recognitions. In this second edition, Professor Wormald has significantly expanded upon the original book in its breadth and its depth while also remaining focused on careful and detailed teaching of the indications and techniques of endoscopic sinus surgery, for inflammatory sinus disease as well as the more recent extended endoscopic orbital and skull base procedures. The book uses a detailed step-by-step approach to clearly demonstrate Professor Wormald's techniques and richly illustrates the text with color endoscopic photographs, drawings, and radiographic images. The result is a book that clearly elucidates both the surgical anatomy and the surgical steps, making conceptualization and learning easy. This second edition is accompanied with an expanded DVD containing videos of the key points of surgical procedures, thereby providing an excellent learning adjunct to the text. As with the first edition, the book is authored entirely by Professor Wormald and draws heavily on his extensive teaching experience and upon his own personal techniques and cases.

This book will be of particular value to residents as well as to practicing otolaryngologists who wish to further advance their knowledge within the field of sinus surgery, improve their surgical techniques, or improve their understanding of the surgical anatomy. The clear, concise illustrations bring the key points across clearly and in a manner that makes them easy to remember. This second edition will also be of particular value to surgeons who wish to increase their knowledge of the newly expanded endoscopic techniques and should enhance the endoscopic surgical finesse significantly for those who review it.

David W. Kennedy, M.D., F.R.C.S.I.
Rhinology Professor and Vice Dean
University of Pennsylvania
Philadelphia, Pennsylvania

Preface

There are two reasons why this second edition so closely follows the first edition. First, the recent rapid progress in the development of transnasal techniques for intracranial, infratemporal, and parapharyngeal surgery has necessitated that the anatomy of and surgical approaches to these regions be described from an endoscopic perspective. Second, the concepts guiding the surgical approach to the maxillary and frontal sinuses have been significantly refined over the 4 years that have elapsed since the manuscript for the first edition was submitted. In the first edition, the technique of reading sinus computed tomography (CT) scans in three planes then reconstructing these into a three-dimensional image was outlined. This process enables the surgeon to create a detailed operative plan before surgery begins and allows him or her to know exactly which sinus cell is being dissected at any time throughout the entire procedure. At any time, the surgeon should be able to turn to the CT scans and identify the cell on the scans. This concept of creating a three-dimensional picture and, subsequently, a detailed surgical plan has been expanded considerably in the second edition by the presentation and explanation of most of the multiple variations of the anatomy of the sinuses. In addition, each step needed to develop a three-dimensional picture is outlined in this text, and the value and importance of the axial CT scans for determining the drainage pathways is presented. In the accompanying DVD, these variations are illustrated both with CT scans and operative videos, which allows the reader to check to see if the three-dimensional picture and surgical plan he or she created was similar to that actually seen during surgery.

This text differs from many others on this subject in that its scope is purely anatomic and operative. No attempt is made to cover the pathology or medical treatment of any of the conditions discussed. This information can be found in several excellent texts currently available. Many of the operative techniques presented in this book are novel, but the results achieved with them have been carefully audited and published in peer-reviewed journals. It is hoped that the description of the relevant anatomy and surgical techniques in this text are sufficiently clear so that the reader will be able to apply them in his or her everyday practice. The concepts are presented with extensive use of illustrations, CT and magnetic resonance imaging scans, and intraoperative and postoperative photographs. In addition, the accompanying DVD has exercises allowing the reader to perform three-dimensional reconstruction of the anatomy and subsequently develop a surgical plan. Each of these is followed by an edited video clip of the surgery, where the reader can confirm that the reconstructions he or she created reflect the anatomy seen during surgery. This combination of text and DVD video clips should reinforce understanding of sinus anatomy and give the surgeon confidence to tackle the many anatomic variations and technical challenges that can occur during sinus surgery.

Acknowledgments

A book of this nature is an accumulation of all knowledge gleaned from many teachers over a number of years. However, I would like to single out the late Mike McDonogh as the teacher who had the greatest influence on my career as a rhinologist. Mike was an exceptional person who was highly innovative and his humor, wit, and intelligence will be greatly missed. His ideas led to the development of the "swing-door" uncinectomy and the "bath-plug" closure of cerebrospinal leaks. I will remain forever indebted to him for his teaching, mentoring, and friendship.

I would also like to thank Simon Robinson, Richard Douglas, and Suresh Rajapaksa for reading the manuscript and making helpful suggestions on how it could be improved and Erik Weitzel for his valued help in the compilation of the accompanying DVD.

Andrew van Hasselt deserves a special mention for his support over many years. In addition, I would like to thank the Australian ENT Society members for making me welcome in Australia and for their support of the development of academic ENT.

Peter-John Wormald

1

Setup and Ergonomics of Endoscopic Sinus Surgery

In the past two decades, there has been a significant shift from external and headlight sinus surgery to endoscopic sinus surgery (ESS). This dramatic change was initiated by the pioneering studies of Messerklinger in which he demonstrated that each sinus has a predetermined mucociliary clearance pattern draining toward its natural ostium irrespective of additional openings that may have been created into the sinuses.[1] This philosophy of opening the natural ostium of the diseased sinus was then popularized by Stammberger[2] and Kennedy.[3] ESS is now accepted as the surgical management of choice for chronic sinusitis. In addition, as our knowledge of the anatomy of the sinuses has improved, other ancillary techniques such as endoscopic lacrimal surgery[4] and orbital decompression[5] have been developed. The development of specialized instruments has facilitated the endoscopic management of benign endonasal tumors[6,7] and more recently the endoscopic management of malignant tumors[8] of the nose and sinuses. Endoscopic sinus surgery, ancillary nasal and sinus procedures, and, more recently, endoscopic transnasal intracranial surgery require a broad range of specially designed endoscopic surgical instruments.

◆ INSTRUMENTS

Disclaimer: Several instruments presented in this book are manufactured and sold by Medtronic ENT. Those that are identified by an asterisk (*) have been designed by the author, and he receives a royalty from the sale of these instruments. There are no undeclared financial incentives associated with any other instruments.

A complete list of endoscopic sinus surgery instruments used by the author is presented in **Table 1–1**. If the instrument is produced by several companies, no manufacturer is named. If a particular instrument is produced by only one company, then the manufacturer is named. Of the instruments in the table, the following are the most important for basic sinus surgery:

- Small rotating back-biting forceps
- Sickle knife

- Small (2.5 mm) straight and 45-degree upturned Blakesley forceps
- Small (2.5 mm) straight and 45-degree upturned through-biting (cutting) Blakesley forceps, endoscopic scissors
- Double right-angled ball probe
- 45-degree and 90-degree giraffe cup forceps, 45-degree and 90-degree through-biting giraffe forceps
- Hajek Koeffler forward-biting punch
- Suction Freer elevator
- Curettes (straight, 45-degree, and 90-degree curettes)
- Malleable suction Freer elevator* (Medtronic ENT, Jacksonville, FL, USA)
- Malleable suction curette* (Medtronic ENT)
- Malleable frontal sinus probe* (Medtronic ENT)

Powered Microdebriders

Powered microdebriders now form an essential part of the instrumentation required to perform endoscopic sinus surgery. These instruments allow the surgeon to remove blood from the operating field with the gate open, and then with considerable precision the tissue can be cut by the rotating inner blade of the microdebrider. This precision cutting of mucosa minimizes the potential for stripping of the mucosa and helps to achieve maximum mucosal preservation, which should improve postoperative healing and consequently the results of the surgery. These instruments are very effective at removing tissue and if placed in the wrong area, such as the orbit, can create significant damage to the orbital contents in a very short space of time.[9,10] Because of its soft consistency, orbital fat can be sucked into the blade opening and cut by the rotating inner blade at a frightening rate. If the surgeon is unaware of having penetrated the orbital periosteum with a microdebrider, significant damage can occur within a few seconds. There are numerous case reports in the literature, unfortunately, in which powered microdebriders have caused inadvertent injury to the orbital contents and to the medial rectus muscle.[9,10]

Table 1–1 Full List of Operating Instruments

Quantity	Instrument	Quantity	Instrument
	Jacobson angled 7-inch needle holder		**Wormald Sucker Bipolar* (Medtronic ENT)**
	6-inch fine needle holder		Wormald suction bipolar forceps*
	Small Luc forceps		Sterilization case
	Angled Heyman turbinectomy scissors		Bipolar cable
	Tilley Henkel forceps		Bipolar diathermy 22.2 cm, 0.5 fine tip (upturned)
2	Tilley packing forceps		**Medtronic ENT Frontal Trephine Set**
2	Mosquito curved artery clips		Medtronic frontal trephine set
5	Backhaus towel clips		Drill guide
	Sponge holder		Drill pin
	McIndoe forceps		Irrigation cannula (reusable; keep six in stock)
	Adson toothed OR Adson Brown forceps		Sterilizing tray
	Adson plain OR tungsten tip forceps		**Wormald Malleable Frontal Sinus Instruments***
2	Suture scissors		**(Medtronic ENT)**
	Iris curved scissors		Wormald malleable frontal sinus probe
	No. 7 scalpel blade handle		Wormald malleable frontal sinus suction
	Freer dissector		Wormald malleable elevator blunt
	Frazier 9-French gauge sucker and stilette		Wormald malleable frontal sinus curette
	Frazier 10-French gauge sucker and stilette		Sterilization tray
	Dental syringe		**Wormald Dacryocystorhinostomy Set* (Medtronic ENT)**
	Heath mallet		Sickle knife
	Small Killian speculum		Spear knife
	Medium Killian speculum		Lusk microbite forceps
	Large Killian speculum		**Wormald Skull Base Instrument Set* (Medtronic ENT)**
			3-mm soft tissue scissors: left, right, and straight
	Sinoscopy Instruments		5-mm soft tissue and thin bone scissors: left, right,
	Medium straight Blakesley forceps		and straight
	Medium upcutting Blakesley forceps		7-mm thin bone scissors: left, right, and straight
	Blakesley forceps straight through-cut		Malleable probe, straight
	Blakesley forceps upturned through-cut		Malleable probe, right-angled hook
	Right ostrum punch downcut		Malleable dissector
	Left ostrum punch downcut		Malleable suction
	Sinus short sucker		Malleable suction cage
	Sinus long sucker		Malleable small and large 45-degree ring curettes
	Sickle knife		Malleable small and large 90-degree ring curettes
	Freer dissector		**Equipment**
	Double-ended probe		**Camera System**
	Kuhn Bolger frontal ostium seeker		STORZ IMAGE 1 digital camera
	Kuhn Bolger frontal sinus curette,		0-degree endoscope (4 × 11 mm Hopkins)
	55 degrees		30-degree endoscope
	Antrum curette		45-degree endoscope
	90-degree curette		70-degree endoscope
	Sucker Freer and stiletto		**Lens Washer**
	Rotating microbite backbiter		Medtronic Endoscrub II
	Hajek Koffler sphenoid punch, 90-degree		**Consumables**
	upcut forward		0-degree Endoscrub II sheath
			30-degree Endoscrub sheath
	Special Instruments (Singles)		**Microdebrider**
	Sinoscopy scissors, straight		XPS 3000
	Sinoscopy scissors, curved left		M4 handpiece
	Sinoscopy scissors, curved right		**Topical Solutions**
	Kuhn Bolger giraffe forceps, horizontal		Cocaine solution (10% × 2 mL)
	Kuhn Bolger giraffe forceps, vertical		Adrenaline (1:1000 × 1 mL)
	Kuhn Bolger forceps, 60 degrees		Normal saline (0.9 × 3 mL)
	Kuhn Bolger forceps, 90 degrees		
	Kuhn Bolger forceps, 90 degrees right-angled		
	Kuhn Bolger forceps, 90 degrees left-angled		
	Ligature clip carrier		

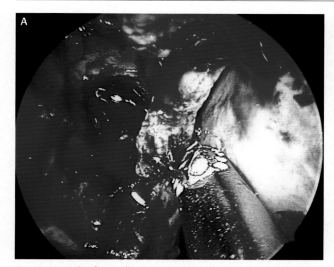
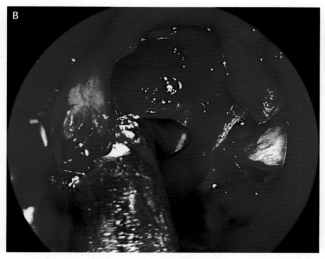

Figure 1–1 The figure illustrates (**A**) the blade open and (**B**) with tissue being sucked into the blade prior to rotation of the inner blade and severing of the tissue.

The blade is used in oscillate mode for the majority of the surgery. Most of the instruments will have a default setting that will allow the blade to oscillate at 3000 rpm. The foot pedal will also usually have a switch that allows the surgeon to select either variable or full speed when the pedal is depressed. Variable mode allows the surgeon to slow the speed, whereas full speed will result in the blade turning at 3000 rpm immediately when the pedal is depressed. It is important to understand that the speed at which the blade turns determines the amount of tissue that is cut. The higher the speed, the less time the port is open and the less tissue is able to be sucked into the blade before the turning blade cuts the tissue. Conversely, the slower the speed, the more tissue is sucked in and the more aggressively the blade cuts. **Figure 1–1A** shows the blade in open mode and **Fig. 1–1B** shows tissue being sucked into the port of the blade before rotation of the blade cuts the tissue.

In forward and reverse modes, the revolutions may vary from 3000 to 15,000 rpm and consequently the blade is open for only a very short period of time. Tissue cutting in these modes is thus severely limited. Forward mode is usually used for the various burr attachments that can be used in place of the blade.

Endoscope Cleaners

A large number of companies manufacture endoscope cleaners or scrubbers. These are designed to wash the lens of the endoscope should it become obscured with blood. If the surgical field is bloody, the endoscope cleaner keeps the scope lens clear of blood and allows the operation to proceed without the need to remove the endoscope from the nose and manually clean it. The endoscope cleaner speeds up the operation, improves the safety of the surgery by maintaining visibility, and decreases the surgeon's frustration level by allowing the surgery to progress more rapidly.

Cameras and Monitors

Surgery can be performed either through the eyepiece of the endoscope (traditional technique) or by connecting a video camera to the endoscope enabling the surgeon to operate off the monitor. The traditional technique (viewing down the endoscope) may give some surgeons a degree of orientation and depth perception. Most surgeons nowadays, however, prefer to operate from the video monitor. A significant advantage of operating from the monitor is the ergonomic advantage this affords the surgeon as he or she can sit or stand next to the patient and not have to bend either his or her back or neck to obtain a view of the nasal cavity. This is especially valuable if the frontal recess is being operated on, because the surgeon viewing the procedure through the eyepiece may have to almost have his or her head on the patient's chest to obtain an adequate view. In addition, if a large instrument such as the microdebrider is being used at the same time, this instrument may touch the surgeon's head when it is being manipulated in tight spaces. The monitor provides a large magnified image that can be advantageous for delicate work (such as optic nerve, skull base, and intracranial surgery), and it allows two surgeons to operate together (pituitary, infratemporal fossa, and intracranial surgery).

Another major advantage of operating from the monitor is that it allows a senior surgeon to monitor the trainee's surgery and allows the trainee (and all in the operating room) to watch the senior surgeon operate. The nurse can anticipate the surgical instrument required for the next step, and the anesthetist can monitor the operating field and undertake anesthetic interventions to improve the surgical field as required. If the surgeon is operating from the monitor, a high-quality three-chip or digital camera is required with a powerful light source and medical grade monitor. Single-chip cameras generally do not cope well with blood in the surgical field, and depth perception and tissue contrasts can be lost. If inferior cameras are used, visibility and orientation become increasingly difficult for the surgeon, and the risk of complications rises.

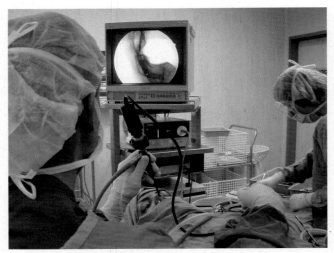

Figure 1–2 A picture of the operating setup with the surgeon, the patient's head, and the video monitor all in a straight line. The scrub nurse stands opposite the surgeon, which allows a view of the monitor and facilitates the handing of instruments to the surgeon.

◆ POSITION OF THE PATIENT AND THE SURGEON

My preference is to sit at the right-hand side of the patient. The surgeon may stand but if his or her elbow is not resting on the operating table, the monitor image tends to move excessively reflecting the instability of the hand holding the endoscope. The patient should be prone and the operating table tilted to 30 degrees anti-Trendelenburg. The patient's head should be in a neutral position (neither flexed or extended). This allows the surgeon to operate in a plane parallel to the skull base, which diminishes the risk to skull base by decreasing the angle of approach. The video monitor should be positioned so that the surgeon, the patient's head, and the monitor are in a straight line (**Fig. 1–2**).

A thin arm board is placed next to the patient's head to widen the upper part of the operating table so that the surgeon can comfortably rest his or her elbow on the arm board. If this position is too low and extra height is needed, sterile drapes folded into a square are placed to build this up. The patient's head can also be turned toward the surgeon, which decreases the height at which the elbow needs to be supported. The scrub nurse should position her instrument table so that the far edge of the table is parallel with the head of the operating table. This allows the monitor stack to be placed in a straight line with the patient's head and the surgeon (**Figs. 1–3**).

◆ PRINCIPLES OF ENDOSCOPE PLACEMENT AND INSTRUMENT PLACEMENT DURING ENDOSCOPIC SINUS SURGERY

With the surgeon's elbow resting on the added arm board, the endoscope is slid into the nose. The endoscope should then be pushed as far superiorly as possible. This should distort the nasal vestibule by placing the endoscope high in the nasal vestibule. This creates a space in the nasal vestibule below the endoscope through which all instruments are placed (**Fig. 1–4**).

The endoscope and the instruments should never cross during surgery. It is only very rarely when dissecting in the frontal sinus with a 70-degree endoscope that the endoscope needs to be placed below the instrument. When this is done, the surgeon loses sight of the tip of the instrument, and accurate and careful dissection is no longer possible. The 0-degree endoscope should be used whenever possible, and in the techniques described in the following chapters it is used unless otherwise stated. This makes the surgery as simple as possible and decreases the risk of unnecessary injury to the adjacent or surrounding mucosa during passage of the

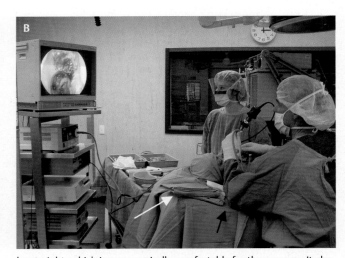

Figure 1–3 The arm board is placed on the operating table (**A**) (*white arrow*) to allow the surgeon to rest his or her elbow (**B**) (*black arrow*) to stabilize the camera. This allows the surgeon's forearm and wrist to be straight, which is ergonomically comfortable for the surgeon. It also ensures that the monitor picture is stable (**B**). The height of the elbow can be adjusted with sterile towels (*white arrow*) as required.

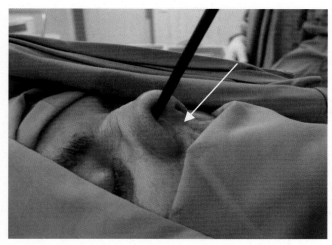

Figure 1–4 The scope is used to tent the nasal vestibule superiorly creating space below the endoscope (*white arrow*) through which the instrument is passed into the nose.

endoscope and instrument. It also limits the risk of disorientation that can occur when using angled endoscopes. If angled endoscopes are used, instruments need to be curved so that the tip of the instrument can be manipulated in the center of the endoscope view (see Chapter 7). The greater the angle of the endoscope, the longer the curve needs to be

on the instrument. The greater the angle of the endoscope and curve of the instrument, the greater the degree of difficulty of dissection, so it is best to use the angled endoscopes (especially the 70-degree endoscope) as infrequently as possible during surgery.

References

1. Messerklinger W. Endoscopy of the Nose. Munich: Urban and Scharzenberg; 1978:52–54
2. Stammberger H. Endoscopic endonasal surgery – concepts in treatment of recurring rhinosinusitis. Otolaryngol Head Neck Surg 1986;94:143–156
3. Kennedy DW. Functional endoscopic sinus surgery. Technique. Arch Otolaryngol 1985;111:643–649
4. Wee DT, Carney AS, Thorpe M, Wormald PJ. Endoscopic orbital decompression. J Laryngol Otol 2002;116:6–9
5. Wormald PJ. Powered endoscopic DCR. Laryngoscope 2002;112:69–72
6. Wormald PJ, Ooi Eng, van Hasselt A, Nair S. Endoscopic removal of sinonasal inverted papilloma including endoscopic medial maxillectomy. Laryngoscope 2003;113:867–873
7. Wormald PJ, van Hasselt CA. Endoscopic removal of juvenile angiofibromas. Otolaryngol Head Neck Surg 2003;129(6):684–691
8. Knegt PP, Ah-See K, vd Velden LA, Kerribijn J. Adenocarcinoma of the ethmoidal sinus complex. Surgical debulking and topical fluorouracil may be the optimal treatment. Arch Otolaryngol Head Neck Surg 2001;127:141–146
9. Graham SM, Nerad JA. Orbital complication in endoscopic sinus surgery using powered instrumentation. Laryngoscope 2003;113:874–878
10. Bhatti MT, Giannoni CM, Raynor E, Monshizadeh R, Levine LM. Ocular motility complications after endoscopic sinus surgery with powered cutting instruments. Otolaryngol Head Neck Surg 2001;125:501–509

2

The Surgical Field in Endoscopic Sinus Surgery

The presence of significant bleeding in the surgical field is a critical factor in the potential success or failure of endoscopic sinus surgery (ESS).[1-4] When significant bleeding is present, recognition of anatomical landmarks becomes difficult.[2-4] Bleeding obscures surgical planes and makes the identification of the drainage pathways of the sinuses difficult. Cell walls become difficult to distinguish from the lamina papyracea or skull base, and the risk of causing complications increases.[3,4] If the patient has significant inflammation of the sinuses from chronic infection or the presence of pus or fungal debris, increased vascularity will often contribute to more bleeding.[2,5] If the surgeon must manipulate an instrument in the surgical field after the discernible anatomy is covered in blood, the risk of a complication increases. In addition, greater surgical trauma may occur, cells may be left behind, and there is an increased likelihood of postoperative scarring and failure of the surgical procedure. It is therefore critical to optimize the surgical field and in so doing make the surgical dissection as easy as is possible.[2-4]

Our department has a special interest in this aspect of ESS and has conducted several double-blind, randomized controlled studies in an attempt to establish which maneuvers to reduce bleeding are worthwhile. To date, not all maneuvers have been scientifically evaluated, but where there is evidence for a specific maneuver, this will be presented. The first important issue to address is a grading system for bleeding in the surgical field. Boezaart et al described and validated a grading system of five grades presented in **Table 2–1**.[3]

Although this grading system is valuable, we have found that the majority of surgical fields are around grade 3 with some grade 2 and some grade 4.[2] Only on rare occasions are grade 1 and 5 fields seen. This tends to compress the grading system and makes differentiation of more subtle changes difficult. Grade 3 may need to be further divided to allow variation within grade 3 to be discerned.[2] We have recently developed and validated an endoscopic sinus surgical field score that separates the middle grades allowing more accurate grading of the surgical field (**Table 2–2**).

◆ LOCAL VERSUS GENERAL ANESTHETIC

Local anesthetic has the advantage of not inducing generalized vasodilation. Increased circulating catecholamines may also improve the surgical field by continuing to act on the prearteriolar and precapillary sphincters. However, there are several limitations to local anesthetic use:

- Patient anxiety and sudden patient movement during delicate surgery can be problematic.
- Surgery takes between 1 and 2 hours. Some patients (especially older patients) have difficulty remaining still for this length of time.
- Appropriate anesthesia needs to be achieved in all the sinuses and the nasal cavity.
- If the procedure is bloody, the patient may have difficulty dealing with the volume of blood trickling into the pharynx. If the patient is sedated, aspiration can occur.
- Water from the scope scrubber may add to the secretions in the pharynx that the patient needs to deal with.
- Teaching of residents can be more difficult when the patient is awake.

In our department, local anesthetic is offered to patients having limited ESS confined to the middle meatus. We prefer general anesthesia for ESS that involves the frontal recess and/or posterior ethmoids and/or sphenoids.

◆ STANDARD NASAL PREPARATION FOR ENDOSCOPIC SINUS SURGERY

Laryngeal Mask versus Endotracheal Intubation

It is our current practice to use laryngeal masks rather than endotracheal intubation for all our patients undergoing sinus surgery. The rationale for this is that it allows the patient to be kept under a lighter general anesthetic with less vasodilation and less intraoperative bleeding. In addition, the patient

Table 2–1 Boezaart and van der Merwe Grading System for Bleeding During Endoscopic Sinus Surgery

Grades	Surgical Field
Grade 1	Cadaveric conditions with minimal suction required.
Grade 2	Minimal bleeding with infrequent suction required.
Grade 3	Brisk bleeding with frequent suction required.
Grade 4	Bleeding covers surgical field after removal of suction before surgical instrument can perform maneuver.
Grade 5	Uncontrolled bleeding. Bleeding out of nostril on removal of suction.

Source: Data from Boezaart AP, van der Merwe J, Coetzee A. Comparison of sodium nitroprusside- and esmolol-induced controlled hypotension for functional endoscopic sinus surgery. Can J Anaesth 1995;42:373–376.

does not cough and strain on the endotracheal tube as he or she recovers from the anesthetic avoiding the venous congestion and subsequent hemorrhage often associated with such straining. One of the potential downsides of a laryngeal mask is the possibility of contamination of the upper airway by blood. This is prevented by the placement of a small throat pack above the laryngeal mask in the back of the throat to catch any blood from the nasal cavity. Another possible downside is the potential difficulty with ventilation of the patient during surgery. Our standard protocol is total intravenous anesthesia with a laryngeal mask in a nonparalyzed patient. The remifentanil infusion (part of total intravenous anesthesia [TIVA]) suppresses spontaneous ventilation and allows the patient to be ventilated through the laryngeal mask. The lack of paralysis provides additional safety against intraoperative

Table 2–2 The Wormald Grading System for Bleeding During Endoscopic Sinus Surgery (from Unpublished Data)

Grade	Surgical Field
0	No bleeding
1	1–2 points of ooze* (no blood in the sphenoid)
2	3–4 points of ooze (no blood in the sphenoid)
3	5–6 points of ooze (slight blood accumulation in the sphenoid)
4	7–8 points of ooze (moderate blood accumulation in sphenoid—fills after 90 seconds)
5	9–10 points of ooze (sphenoid fills after 60 seconds)
6	>10 points of ooze, obscuring surface (sphenoid fills between 40 and 60 seconds)
7	Mild bleeding/oozing from entire surgical surface with slow accumulation of blood in postnasal space (sphenoid fills by 40 seconds)
8	Moderate bleeding from entire surgical surface with moderate accumulation of blood in postnasal space (sphenoid fills by 30 seconds)
9	Moderately severe bleeding with rapid accumulation of blood in postnasal space (sphenoid fills by 20 seconds)
10	Severe bleeding with nasal cavity filling rapidly (sphenoid fills in <10 seconds)

*Points of ooze are bleeding points.

awareness because the patient should move if the level of anesthesia becomes too light.

Positioning the Patient

The positioning of the patient was described in Chapter 1. It is important to have the patient 30 degrees to 40 degrees head up so that the venous return from the head and neck is facilitated. This puts the patient's head above the chest, which lowers the arterial pressure and prevents venous congestion thereby improving the surgical field.[6]

Topical Vasoconstriction

In a study recently published, we showed that any packing material placed in the nasal cavity tends to cause damage to the nasal mucosa.[7] The more abrasive the packing, the worse the trauma.[6] Taking this into consideration, the least-abrasive packing material is used: namely, neurosurgical cottonoid patties. The anesthetist is consulted to ensure there is no contraindication to the use of cocaine. If there is a concern, then 1% oxymetazoline is used in place of cocaine. In an adult patient, a mixture of 2 mL 10% cocaine, 1 mL 1:1000 adrenaline, and 4 mL saline is divided with half used to soak six neuropatties. These six neuropatties are placed in the nose once the patient is anesthetized. The other half of the cocaine mixture and remaining four neuropatties are kept sterile on the instrument trolley for later use during surgery if required. Three neuropatties are placed on each side directly after intubation using a Freer elevator to manipulate them gently into place. The first neuropattie is placed in the spheno-ethmoidal recess, the second under the middle turbinate, with the third being placed over the axilla of the middle turbinate (**Fig. 2–1**). If there is a concha bullosa or significantly lateralized middle turbinate, the neuropattie is

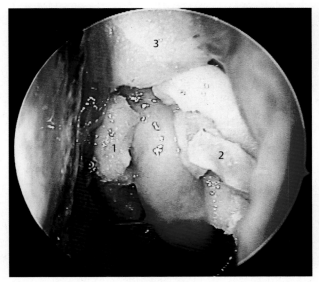

Figure 2–1 Placement of the neuropatties in the left nasal cavity prior to surgery. The no. 1 pattie is in the spheno-ethmoidal recess, no. 2 is in the middle meatus, and no. 3 is in the region of the axillary flap.

placed along the inferior margin of the middle turbinate. No force is used to place the neuropatties in the middle meatus.

As only half the solution is used at the beginning of surgery, the total dose of cocaine that the patient is exposed to is ~100 mg. The toxic dose of cocaine is 3 mg per kg without the simultaneous use of adrenaline. It has also been shown that the presence of adrenaline inhibits mucosal absorption and that a proportion of the solution will remain in the neuropattie. This decreases the amount of cocaine that the patient is exposed to, and the doses used are well below the toxic dose in adult patients. The dose needs to be appropriately adjusted in children.

Local Infiltration

A 2% solution of lidocaine (lignocaine in the United Kingdom and Australia) with either 1:80,000 or 1:100,000 is administered with a dental syringe and needle. The injections are given after the patient has been draped and the camera and endoscope are available. Under endoscopic guidance, the area above the middle turbinate is infiltrated. This is followed by infiltration into the anterior end of the middle turbinate. Note that the area anterior to the uncinate is not infiltrated as bleeding from an injection site can obscure the uncinate during its removal. In some patients where there is expected increased likelihood of bleeding, a third injection is given into the back end of the middle turbinate in the region of the sphenopalatine artery. A spinal needle is used because the dental needle is usually not long enough to reach this area. **Figure 2–2** illustrates the routine infiltration points used.

Preoperative Antibiotics and Steroids

Inflammation increases the vascularity of tissues, and when surgery is conducted on highly inflamed tissues, increased

bleeding results. Patients with acute sinusitis who have an infective complication requiring surgery will often have a very bloody surgical field. It therefore stands to reason that using antibiotics in patients with a significant infection preoperatively should improve the surgical field. However, most of our patients undergoing ESS have had extended medical therapy that normally includes numerous courses of antibiotics and often systemic steroids and therefore rarely have an acute infection present. The value of using antibiotics preoperatively in this elective patient group is unknown as there are no well-designed studies addressing this issue. The important questions that remain unanswered are the type of antibiotic, the length of time it should be used before surgery, and the patient group most likely to benefit from its preoperative use. Currently, the author does not routinely place patients on antibiotics preoperatively.

It has been suggested that patients with significant nasal polyposis may benefit from a course of preoperative steroids. The theory is that steroids should decrease the size of the polyps and the vascularity associated with these polyps. Although this argument seems logical, it is yet to be confirmed in properly designed and controlled studies. A recently published preliminary study evaluated the effect of preoperative steroids on the degree of bleeding during sinus surgery.[8] In this study, prednisone 30 mg daily was given for 5 days preoperatively and the results showed a significant improvement in a visual analogue grading of the surgical field during surgery.[8] However, it remains unclear what dose of steroids should be given, for how long, and to which patient groups. Empiric treatment regimes range from 30 mg[8] prednisolone to 50 mg daily for between 5 and 7 days preoperatively.

◆ ADDITIONAL MANEUVERS FOR OPTIMIZING THE SURGICAL FIELD IN ENDOSCOPIC SINUS SURGERY

Suction Bipolar Cautery* of Isolated Bleeding Areas

It is common to see isolated bleeding vessels in the surgical field during ESS. These result from the transection of small blood vessels, and these may continue to ooze into the surgical field and can significantly add to the volume of blood that may obscure the surgical field.[4] In addition, such an ooze may obscure the end of the endoscope requiring either the endoscope scrubber to be used or the endoscope to be removed from the nose to be cleaned. If the axillary flap approach to the frontal recess is used (see Chapter 7), the mucosal incision edge may bleed, and this can be controlled by use of the suction bipolar cautery. Other common areas where bleeding is seen are the posterior region of the maxillary sinus, the sphenopalatine regions of the lateral nasal wall, and the anterior wall of the sphenoid below its ostium. The suction bipolar allows the bleeding vessels to be accurately identified and cauterized. Not having to remove the instrument from the nose after the suction clears the blood to allow

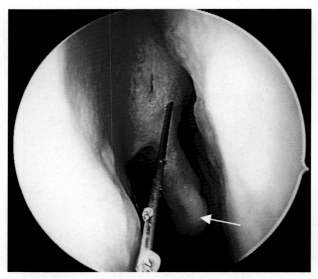

Figure 2–2 Injection sites in the right nasal cavity for local anesthetic prior to endoscopic sinus surgery. The needle is in the region of the axillary flap and the white arrow indicates the injection site on the anterior end of the middle turbinate.

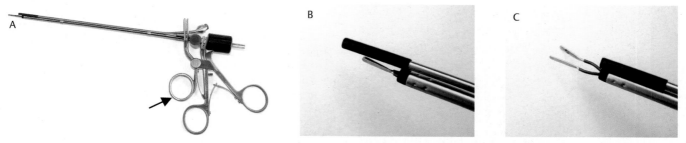

Figure 2–3 (**A**) The suction bipolar is in the normal position. (**B**) The suction bipolar is extended beyond the bipolar paddles. When the manipulating lever (*black arrow* in **A**) is relaxed, the suction retracts behind the bipolar paddles (**C**).

identification of the bleeding point is a significant advantage of this instrument (**Figs. 2–3**).

The Anatomy of the Greater Palatine Canal and Local Anesthetic Infiltration of the Pterygopalatine Fossa

Injection of local anesthetic into the pterygopalatine fossa does improve the surgical field.[9,10] The maxillary artery and its terminal branches make up the main blood supply for the nose. There are two approaches: the less reliable approach is direct infiltration into the region of the sphenopalatine foramen. The needle is introduced just under the posterior end of the middle turbinate. Sometimes the needle can be felt to slip into the sphenopalatine foramen, but in most cases location of the foramen is difficult and the injection is given into the general region of the foramen. This should cause vasospasm of the vessels exiting the foramen. Because the foramen is not easily located, however, the resulting vasoconstriction achieved may not be as great as injecting the pterygopalatine fossa through the greater palatine canal.

The second more reliable approach is to inject the pterygopalatine fossa through the greater palatine foramen and canal. First, the greater palatine foramen needs to be located on the hard palate (**Fig. 2–4**). The greater palatine foramen is located just anterior to the posterior edge of the hard palate opposite the second molar tooth.[11] It is usually half way between the tooth and the midline of the hard palate. The opening of the foramen into the canal is funnel-shaped and the canal is angled at ~45 degrees to the hard palate.

In a cadaver study performed at our department to evaluate the anatomy of the greater palatine canal, 20 cadaver heads were scanned by computed tomography (CT) in the axial plane at 0.5 mm.[12] Parasagittal reconstructions were performed in the plane of the greater palatine canal. The length of the canal and depth of the soft tissue overlying the canal were measured. In addition, needles were bent at 10, 20, and 30 mm and inserted into the greater palatine canal prior to CT scanning to demonstrate the degree of penetration into the pterygopalatine fossa in four cadavers (**Fig. 2–5**).

This was done to ascertain the likelihood of damage to the contents of the fossa (maxillary nerve and maxillary artery,

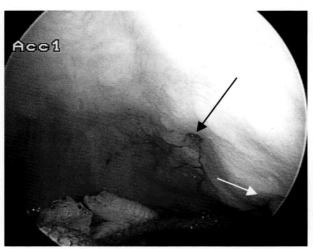

Figure 2–4 Blood staining can be seen from where the needle was introduced into the greater palatine canal (*black arrow*) of the left hard palate. The second molar tooth is marked with a white arrow.

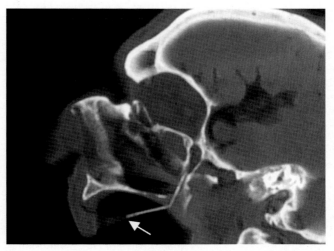

Figure 2–5 Cadaver with needle (*white arrow*) bent at 20 mm and inserted into the greater palatine canal after which the CT scan was performed. (From Douglas R, Wormald PJ. Pterygopalatine fossa infiltration through the greater palatine foramen: where to bend the needle. Laryngoscope 2006;116(7):1255–1257.)

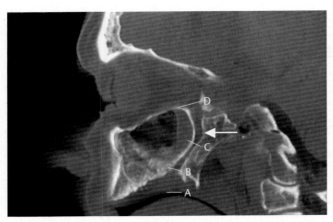

Figure 2–6 The soft tissue measurement was from *A* to *B*, the greater palatine canal from *B* to *C*, and the height of the pterygopalatine fossa from *C* to *D*. The funnel-shaped opening of the greater palatine canal into the pterygopalatine fossa is indicated with a white arrow. (From Douglas R, Wormald PJ. Pterygopalatine fossa infiltration through the greater palatine foramen: where to bend the needle. Laryngoscope 2006;116(7):1255–1257.)

pterygopalatine ganglion) and the orbit. Note the bend in the needle stops at the soft tissue overlying the hard palate and that this soft tissue had a mean thickness of 6.9 mm (95% CI = 6.2 to 7.6) (**Fig. 2–6**). The mean length of the greater palatine canal was 18.5 mm (95% CI = 17.9 to 19.1), and the mean height of the pterygopalatine fossa was 21.6 mm (95% CI = 20.7 to 22.5).[12] Therefore, to perform an effective infiltration of the pterygopalatine fossa, the needle should be bent at 25 mm from the tip at an angle of 45 degrees.[12] This will result in the tip of the needle just penetrating the pterygopalatine fossa without putting any of the contents of the fossa at risk.[12]

The greater palatine canal has an hourglass shape, dilating as it enters the pterygopalatine fossa. This funnel-shaped entrance into the greater palatine canal means that it can be difficult to determine exactly where the pterygopalatine fossa ends and the greater palatine canal begins (**Fig. 2–6**, white arrow).

The easiest way to locate the greater palatine foramen is by palpating the palate with the finger. This is performed by placing a tongue depressor in the mouth and holding down the tongue, then passing a finger and the endoscope into the mouth together. The finger first locates the posterior free edge of the hard palate and then slides anteriorly over this ridge onto the hard palate. The foramen should be felt as a depression directly anterior to the free edge about midway between the second molar tooth and the midline of the palate. Visualize the finger palpating the foramen on the monitor and identify the spot on the palate as the finger is withdrawn from the mouth. With the needle bent at 25 mm and at 45-degree angle, insert the needle into the spot that was visually marked on the palate. If the needle strikes bone, then a small amount of lidocaine is infiltrated, the needle is withdrawn, and an adjacent spot is tried. The assumption is that the needle had just missed the foramen and that a slight adjustment needs to be made before the foramen is located. If repeated attempts to introduce the needle fail, then the landmarks for the foramen (the midpoint between the second

molar tooth and midline of the palate) are reassessed, and the finger and endoscope are replaced into the mouth and the foramen relocated. The needle is reintroduced until the foramen is located by the needle advancing into the greater palatine canal without any resistance up to the bend in the needle. After aspirating (to ensure that the needle is not in a blood vessel), the pterygopalatine fossa is infiltrated with 2 mL of 2% lidocaine and 1:80,000 adrenaline.

Our department has conducted a double-blind, randomized controlled trial in which the effects of local anesthetic and adrenaline infiltration of the pterygopalatine fossa were assessed on the surgical field in 55 patients.[10] To be included in the study, the patient required bilateral ESS with similar procedures performed bilaterally. A surgeon not involved in the surgery randomly infiltrated one fossa transorally so that the operating surgeon would not be aware of which side had been infiltrated. The surgeon then alternated the surgery on the patient and assessed the surgical field on each side. Statistical analysis showed that the side that had received the pterygopalatine fossa injection had significantly better surgical field (mean surgical grade of 2.59) than the control side (mean surgical grade of 2.99; *P* < 0.01).[10]

Beta-Blockers

Inhalational agents given during general anesthesia result in relaxation of the prearteriolar muscle sphincters.[6] This produces significant peripheral vasodilation and usually mild hypotension.[3,4,6] This peripheral vasodilation with paralysis of the arteriolar and precapillary sphincters can result in significant bleeding if surgery is performed in the nose and sinuses.[3,4,6] In an attempt to compensate for this reduced venous return and low cardiac output, reflexes increase the heart rate in an attempt to improve the cardiac output.[3,4,6] In a seminal paper, Boezaart et al showed that vasodilation induced by sodium nitroprusside caused a significant worsening in the surgical field despite the lowered blood pressure.[3] What they also showed was that esmolol, a highly selective β1 beta-blocker, improved the surgical field with a much smaller drop in blood pressure.[3]

Esmolol is a short-acting cardioselective beta-adrenergic receptor–blocking drug that has a fast onset and short half-life. In contrast with a drug such as sodium nitroprusside, which while effectively lowering the blood pressure results in a compensatory increase in heart rate, esmolol is highly effective at depressing cardiac output and results in a slowing of the pulse rate despite a fall in blood pressure.[6] Esmolol is given by a constant intravenous infusion and has a very short half-life (around 3 minutes) so its effect can be closely controlled. Although this can be a very worthwhile maneuver, it is a very expensive drug and there is some resistance (based on cost) against using it as a regular or routine part of ESS anesthesia. The expense of this drug stimulated our department to conduct a double-blind, placebo-controlled, randomized prospective study on the effects of metoprolol taken orally 20 minutes before general anesthetic compared with a vitamin B placebo.[2] This study showed that the patients who received the beta-blocker (metoprolol) had a significantly lower pulse rate (mean of 59) than the placebo group (mean of 69). There was no significant difference in blood pressure or surgical fields in the two groups. However, what was interesting was the significant correlation between heart rate in the overall patient group with surgical grade.[2] Thus, irrespective of whether a beta-blocker is given to the patient or not, if the heart rate of the patient can be kept below 60 beats per minute, the surgical field was usually good.[2] Therefore, we recommend the use of a beta-blocker (atenolol, metoprolol, or esmolol) in patients who at induction of anesthesia have a pulse rate significantly above 60 beats per minute and who do not have a contraindication (such as asthma) as a worthwhile manipulation that can improve the surgical field. However, asthma is a common comorbidity in patients with chronic sinusitis and alternatives are needed. In this group of patients, we use clonidine.

Clonidine

Clonidine is a centrally active alpha-agonist that initially results in an elevation of blood pressure before depressing the cardiac output by inhibiting the central cardiac regulatory mechanism. It should be used with caution and should be given in small increments, as the effect is not easily reversible. It also results in mild postoperative sedation, and its effects on the blood pressure are usually seen in the initial few hours after surgery. This is beneficial for the majority of patients because this mild hypotension allows the small blood vessels in the nose to coagulate with a reduced chance of postoperative epistaxis. There are no properly designed and controlled studies that quantify the effect of clonidine on the surgical field in ESS.

Total Intravenous Anesthesia and Inhalational Agents

As can be seen from the above discussion, vasodilation is detrimental to the surgical field. General anesthesia results in vasodilation, and the extent of the vasodilation is to a certain extent dependent upon the type and quantity of inhalational agent used.[6] Halothane gives significant vasodilation and should not be used.[6] Isoflurane and sevoflurane produce less vasodilation, but if they are used to deepen the level of anesthesia with the intention of lowering the blood pressure, significant vasodilation can occur.[6] TIVA is usually given by using a constant infusion of propofol and remifentanyl. Propofol induces anesthesia by enhancing the action of GABA neurotransmitter on the GABA receptor, which allows the chloride channels to be opened causing hyperpolarization and reduced excitability of the cell.[13] Propofol is short-acting and needs to be administered as a constant infusion. Although it does depress the heart, this response is not dose dependent, and increasing the infusion rate of propofol will not result in an increasing suppression of pulse rate and cardiac output. It however does not affect the muscle tone of the prearteriolar and precapillary sphincters and does not cause vasodilation and increased bleeding. This allows inhalational agents to be avoided. If bleeding during ESS continues to be problematic despite the patient receiving TIVA, other drugs such as beta-blockers or clonidine can be added. In a recent study at our department, we performed a randomized, controlled single-blinded (to the surgeon) study using TIVA and isoflurane. This study showed that the surgical fields were better if TIVA was used.[14] All other factors were kept constant during the surgery. The pulse rate, when analyzed independently, again correlated with the surgical field emphasizing the importance of the pulse rate on the surgical field. Some anesthetists are uncomfortable using TIVA as it can be difficult to judge the depth of anesthesia, so it is a good idea to discuss the merits of use of TIVA with the anesthetist before surgery.

◆ GENERAL GUIDELINES FOR MANEUVERS FOR IMPROVING THE SURGICAL FIELD

The ideal surgical field is grade 2 on the Boezaart scale and grades 1 to 4 on the Wormald scale. However, the majority of our patients fluctuate between grades 2 and 3 on the Boezaart scale. Operating in more bloody conditions can be aided by the use of suction dissection instruments* (see Chapter 1) such as the suction curette* and suction Freer*. These instruments allow the blood to be cleared from the surgical field during the dissection and obviate the need to change from a dissecting instrument to a suction to clear the surgical field.

Surgical Field Change from Boezaart Grade 3 to Grade 4 or 5 (Note: Surgery Should Not Be Performed if the Surgical Field Is Grade 5)

- Check positioning of the patient.
- Check that you have properly infiltrated the lateral wall of the nose with lidocaine and adrenalin.
- Place neuropatties soaked with cocaine and adrenalin in the surgical field.
- Check the patient's pulse rate and if greater than 60, ask the anesthetist to adjust this to below 60 (using beta-blockers if not contraindicated).
- If the patient is hypertensive, ask the anesthetist to bring the mean blood pressure down to around a mean of 65 to 75 mm Hg without increasing the inhalational agent (consider the use of a beta-blocker or clonidine).

Recheck Your Surgical Field

- If there is a specific bleeder, cauterize it with the suction bipolar*.
- If the bleeding is emanating from the posterior region of the nasal cavity, consider replacing the neuropatties and performing a pterygopalatine fossa block.
- If bleeding still is not controlled or is coming from the anterior aspects of the nose, then consider asking the anesthetist to further lower the pulse rate with small incremental doses of clonidine. Remember to stay within

the safe range of mean blood pressure (>55 mm Hg[6]) especially when considering the age of the patient and the previous mean blood pressure of the patient. If the patient was known to suffer from hypertension, this figure should be higher.

◆ Consider changing the patient from inhalational anesthesia to TIVA.

References

1. Stankiewicz JA. Complications of endoscopic intranasal ethmoidectomy. Laryngoscope 1987;97:1270–1273
2. Nair S, Collins M, Hung P, Rees G, Close D, Wormald PJ. The effect of beta-blocker premedication on the surgical field during endoscopic sinus surgery. Laryngoscope 2004;114:1042–1046
3. Boezaart AP, van der Merwe J, Coetzee A. Comparison of sodium nitroprusside- and esmolol-induced controlled hypotension for functional endoscopic sinus surgery. Can J Anaesth 1995;42:373–376
4. Boezaart AP, van der Merwe J, Coetzee AR. Re: Moderate controlled hypotension with sodium nitroprusside does not improve surgical conditions or decrease blood loss in endoscopic sinus surgery. J Clin Anesth 2001;13:319–320
5. Mortimore S, Wormald PJ. Management of acute complicated sinusitis: a 5-year review. Otolaryngol Head Neck Surg 1999;121:639–642
6. van Aken H, Miller ED. Deliberate hypotension. In: Miller RD, ed. Anesthesia, vol. 2. New York, NY: Churchill Livingstone; 1994:1481–1503
7. Shaw CL, Dymock RB, Cowin A, Wormald PJ. Effect of packing on the nasal mucosa of sheep. J Laryngol Otol 2000;114:506–509
8. Sieskiewicz A, Olszewska E, Rogowski M, Grycz E. Preoperative corticosteroid oral therapy and intraoperative bleeding during functional endoscopic sinus surgery in patients with severe nasal polyposis: a preliminary investigation. Ann Otol Rhinol Laryngol 2006;115:490–494
9. Wormald PJ, Wee DTH, van Hasselt CA. Endoscopic ligation of the sphenopalatine artery for refractory posterior epistaxis. Am J Rhinol 2000;14(4):261–264
10. Wormald PJ, Ananasiadis T, Rees G, Robinson S. An evaluation of effect of pterygopalatine fossa injection with local anesthetic and adrenalin in the control of nasal bleeding during endoscopic sinus surgery. Am J Rhinol 2005;19:288–292
11. Mercuri LG. Intraoral second division nerve block. Oral Surg Oral Med Oral Pathol 1979;47(2):109–113
12. Douglas R, Wormald PJ. Pterygopalatine fossa infiltration through the greater palatine foramen: where to bend the needle. Laryngoscope 2006;116(7):1225–1227
13. Sonner JM, Zhang Y, Stabernack C, Abaigar W, Xing Y, Laster MJ. GABA(A) receptor blockade antagonizes the immobilizing action of propofol but not ketamine or isoflurane in a dose-related manner. Anesth Analg 2003;96:706–712
14. Wormald PJ, van Renen G, Perks J, Jones JA, Langton-Hewer CD. The effect of the total intravenous anesthesia compared to inhalational anesthesia on the surgical field during endoscopic sinus surgery. Am J Rhinol 2005;19(5):514–520

3

Radiology

It is fortunate that the development of endoscopic sinus surgery (ESS) has coincided with major advances in computed tomography (CT) scanning technology. Before CT scanning was available, the extent of sinus disease and anatomy of the nose and sinuses were assessed on plain x-ray films. Plain x-ray films are no longer used in this role, as they do not provide sufficient anatomical detail or accurate information on the extent of nasal and sinus pathology. The CT scan has allowed the detailed anatomy of the sinuses to be evaluated, and in this textbook CT scans are used extensively to reconstruct the anatomy of the sinuses enabling a surgical plan to be made before surgery begins. The surgical philosophy of this textbook is underpinned by the availability of high-quality CT scans in three planes.

◆ COMPUTED TOMOGRAPHY SCANS

The Value of Computed Tomography Scans in Three Planes

CT scans are used as an aid for both the diagnosis of chronic sinusitis and for the planning of the surgery. However, there is a significant incidence of mucosal abnormalities seen in completely asymptomatic patients.[1] Thus, it is important that the patient has had adequate medical treatment for the nasal and sinus condition before a CT scan of the sinuses is performed.[2] The coronal scan is the primary scan used to assess the anatomy of the sinuses.[3] These scans should be sufficiently close together so that an identified cell can be followed from one slice to the next. This allows a three-dimensional image of the anatomy to be reconstructed from the scans.[4–6] The axial scan is of particular value in determining the drainage pathway of the frontal

sinus. This is important when deciding where the curette or probe is going to be slid during the dissection of the frontal recess. Our department recently published a study evaluating the value of the parasagittal scan in assessing the frontal recess and in the understanding and planning of the surgery.[7] We found that the parasagittal scan significantly improved the surgeon's ability to assess the frontal recess and improved the understanding of the anatomy by a mean of 57% on a 10-point visual analogue scale. The parasagittal scan also altered the surgical plan for the patient in more than 50% of patients studied. We therefore recommend that all patients undergoing ESS should have a high-definition, helical multislice CT scan of the sinuses with the scans presented in all three planes. An example of the quality of the CT scans that should be expected using this protocol is shown in **Fig. 3–1**.

Scanning Protocol

Good-quality CT scans are critical to the ability of the surgeon to reconstruct the anatomy and drainage pathways of the sinuses. Ideally, images should be in the coronal, axial, and parasagittal planes and should be relatively close together so that a cell can be followed from one scan to the next. Our current CT scan imaging protocol on a multislice CT helical scanner requires scans to be performed in the axial plane at 0.5- to 1-mm intervals with coronal and parasagittal reconstruction. Images in all planes are printed for the surgeon. The windows of the scan are set between 1500 and 2000 with a center of +100 to +300 for highest bony definition. If there is a suspicion of fungal sinus disease, the window settings are changed to soft tissue settings. This allows the opacified sinuses to be assessed for double densities that are often present in chronic fungal sinus disease.

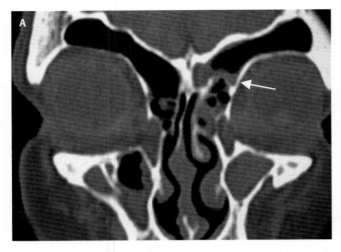

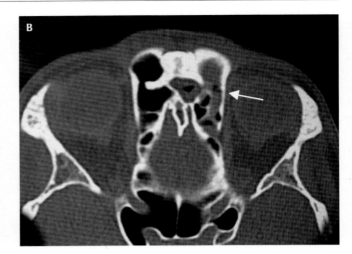

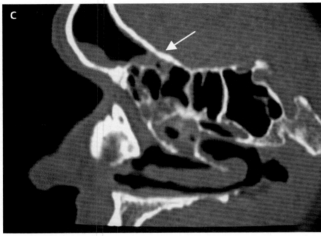

Figure 3–1 CT scans with slices in the (**A**) coronal, (**B**) axial, and (**C**) parasagittal planes. The disease in the left frontal recess (*white arrow*) can be evaluated and the cellular structure better understood if all three planes are available.

Three-Dimensional Computed Tomography Views and the Concept of Building Blocks

Some CT scanners have software in which cursors can be moved through a series of scans in one plane while at the same time the views of where the cursor is in the other planes are simultaneously displayed. Such software can be purchased independently if not available on the scanner (e.g., Voxar, Edinburgh, UK). Computer-aided surgical (CAS) systems also have this facility. With these systems, the CT scans can be scrolled in a particular plane and the other views change depending upon where the cursor is placed on the scan being viewed. If either the software is available or an image-guidance machine is going to be used for a particular patient, it is valuable to utilize this technology to try and get a better understanding of the three-dimensional anatomy of the patient before the patient is operated on. An example of a cursor placed in a position in one plane and then displayed by the computer in the other planes is shown in **Fig. 3–2**.

A central theme throughout this book is the use of high-quality CT scans in three different planes to build a three-dimensional picture of the anatomy of the sinuses. In general, the coronal scans are viewed first and cells identified and followed in an attempt to build up a three-dimensional picture of the anatomy. This is done in the frontal recess (see Chapter 6), and after completion of the frontal recess, the process is repeated in the posterior ethmoids and sphenoid (see Chapter 8). After the anatomy is reviewed on the coronal scans (**Fig. 3–2A**), the parasagittal scans are reviewed (**Fig. 3–2C**). This often helps with the anterior posterior placement of the cells. Finally, the axial view (**Fig. 3–2B**) is reviewed, as this is often helpful for establishing the drainage pathway of the frontal sinus. The building block concept is based around using a single building block for each cell identified in the frontal recess and in the posterior ethmoids. After placement or stacking of the building blocks, the drainage pathway of the frontal sinus is established. This is of vital importance as it allows curettes and probes to be passed along this drainage pathway and for the cells to be removed from the outflow tract of the frontal sinus and spheno-ethmoidal drainage pathway (see Chapter 6). The concept of three-dimensional anatomical reconstruction by using building blocks to re-create the

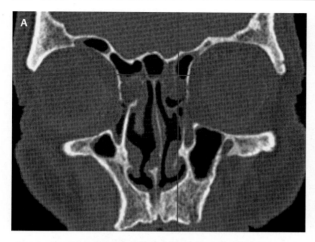

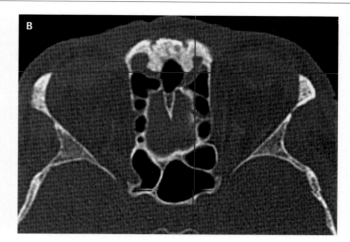

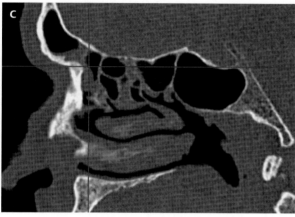

Figure 3–2 (A–C) The crosshairs are placed on one scan by the computer mouse. The position of the crosshairs is seen in other planes.

anatomical formation in the frontal recess and posterior ethmoids and then to surgically establish the drainage pathways is the central theme of this book.

◆ MAGNETIC RESONANCE IMAGING SCANS

Magnetic resonance imaging (MRI) scans are not routinely used for the assessment of patients undergoing ESS because they do not provide bony definition. In addition, MRI scans are very sensitive to mucosal thickening of the nasal or sinus mucosa (especially of a vascular region such as the inferior turbinate). Normal mucosa may be enhanced and in some patients even appear pathologic even though it is normal. The MRI scan can be very useful in several situations, however. We routinely request an MRI scan in patients who had previously undergone an osteoplastic flap with obliteration who have ongoing symptoms.[8,9] In these patients, it can differentiate sepsis or mucocele formation from those with healthy fat in their obliterated frontal sinuses. All patients who have an intranasal tumor are assessed with a MRI scan.[10] In these patients, we are primarily interested in whether an opacified sinus is filled with tumor or retained mucus and whether a breach or invasion of the dura or orbital periosteum has occurred.

An example of the usefulness of a MRI in surgical planning is shown in **Fig. 3–3**. This patient had an adenocarcinoma with opacified frontal sinuses and right maxillary sinus on CT scanning. In the MRI, it can clearly be seen that the left frontal sinus and right maxillary sinus are filled with mucus not tumor.

Our protocol to assess these patients is to perform a T1-weighted fat saturation gadolinium-enhanced scan and a T2-weighted scan. The tumor enhances on the T1 gadolinium-enhanced scan but the fluid in the sinuses does not. If the T2-weighted scan is reviewed, fluid (mucus) usually enhances significantly. In scans B and D, the lamina papyracea and skull base are eroded. However, it appears that the orbital contents have been pushed laterally by the tumor rather than the tumor invading into the orbit. In this patient, both orbits were preserved and there was a good surgical plane between the tumor and the orbital periosteum. The tumor also appears to push the dura superiorly rather than eroding through the dura. Again, we were able to establish a good surgical plane between the tumor and the dura and achieve a complete macroscopic resection of the tumor without resection of the dura. The patient had postoperative radiotherapy and continues to be tumor-free 3 years after the surgical procedure.

MRI scans are also useful in the assessment of complications of sinusitis particularly for orbital complications with

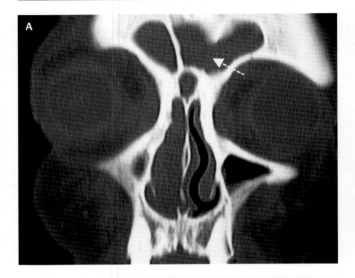

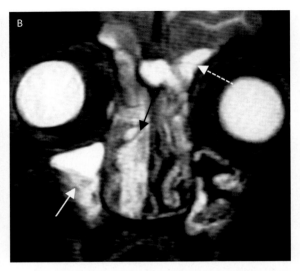

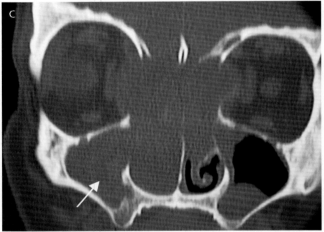

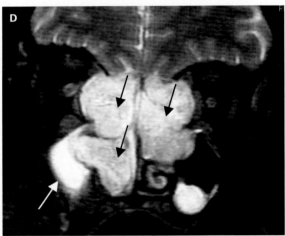

Figure 3–3 CT and MRI scans of a patient with adenocarcinoma. CT (**A**) and MRI scan (**B**) show opacification of the frontal sinuses (*broken white arrow*, **B**) and the right maxillary (*solid white arrow*, **B**). (**B, D**) T2-weighted MRI scans show that the left frontal sinus (*broken white arrow*, **B**) and that both maxillary sinuses (*solid white arrow* for right sinus) contain fluid and not tumor (right frontal unclear on this scan). The black arrows indicate the tumor.

subperiosteal abscess formation and intracranial complications.[11] MRI scans are used as first-line assessment for pituitary tumors and for extended skull base lesions such as clival tumors.

◆ ANGIOGRAPHY

Angiography is useful in patients who have a suspected vascular tumor and an attempt is to be made to remove this tumor endoscopically.[12] It is of great importance that the vascularity of the tumor be reduced as far as possible to facilitate endoscopic removal. Vascular tumors that have not been embolized can bleed so profusely during endoscopic resection that the procedure needs to be abandoned. Several tumors can benefit from preoperative embolization, and this intervention is of particular value in angiofibroma (**Fig. 3–4**).[12]

◆ DACRYOCYSTOGRAM AND LACRIMAL SCINTILLOGRAPHY

A dacryocystogram (DCG) can be very useful for assessing the anatomy of the nasolacrimal system.[13,14] It is important to identify patients with a significant stricture of the common canaliculus because these patients are not suitable for dacryocystorhinostomy.[13,14] In some patients with significant epiphora, a DCG reveals a free flow of dye from the canaliculus to the nose. A DCG is not a physiologic test as abnormally high pressures are generated in the nasolacrimal system during injection of the dye. In these patients, lacrimal scintillography can be very useful as the placement of a radioisotope in the tear lake with subsequent detection of its passage into the nasolacrimal system and nose provides important information regarding the function of the system (**Fig. 3–5**). These tests will be fully elaborated upon in Chapter 11.

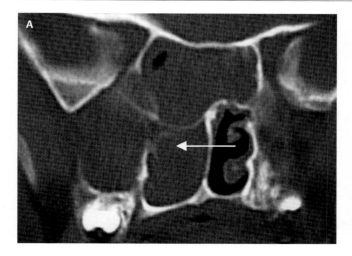

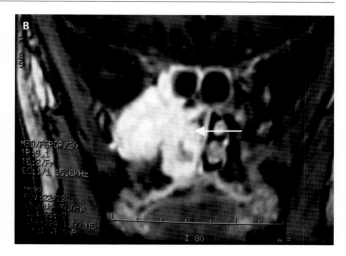

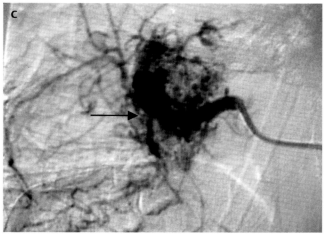

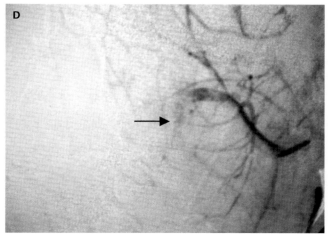

Figure 3–4 (**A**) The CT scan shows an angiofibroma (*white arrow*) filling the posterior nasal cavity with extension into the ptery-gopalatine and infratemporal fossae. (**B**) The tumor (*white arrow*) extent is better seen on the MRI. (**C**) The digital subtraction angiogram illustrates in the intense vascularity of the tumor (*black arrow*) before embolization, and the effectiveness of embolization is illustrated in (**D**) where no tumor blush can be seen (*black arrow*).

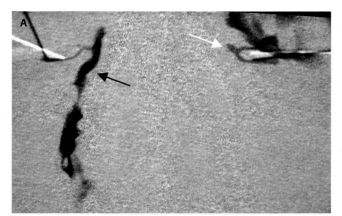

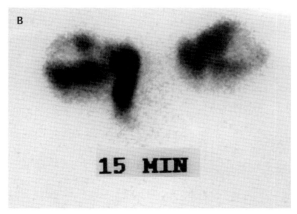

Figure 3–5 The DCG is presented in (**A**). The right side is normal with the normal lacrimal sac (*black arrow*) and canaliculi clearly seen. On the left side, the superior, inferior, and common canaliculi can be seen, but dye does not penetrate the lacrimal sac (*white arrow*) and there is no filling of the lacrimal sac. This represents a common canaliculus obstruction. Panel (**B**) represents the corresponding lacrimal scintillogram for the patient in (**A**). A normal scintillogram can be seen on the right. There is some isotope filling of the left lacrimal sac but no nasal penetration. This indicates probable kinking of the common canaliculus as it enters the sac.

References

1. Flinn J, Chapman ME, Wightman AJA, Maran AGD. A prospective analysis of incidental paranasal sinus abnormalities on CT head scans. Clin Otolaryngol 1994;19:287–289

2. Lusk RP, Muntz HR. Endoscopic sinus surgery in children with chronic sinusitis: a pilot study. Laryngoscope 1990;100:654–658

3. Kennedy DW, Zinreich SJ. The functional endoscopic approach to inflammatory sinus disease: current perspectives and technique modifications. Am J Rhinol 1988;2:89–96

4. Wormald PJ. The agger nasi cell: the key to understanding the anatomy of the frontal recess. Otolaryngol Head Neck Surg 2003;129:497–507

5. Wormald PJ. The axillary flap approach to the frontal recess. Laryngoscope 2002;112(3):494–499

6. Wormald PJ, Chan SZX. Surgical techniques for the removal of frontal recess cells obstructing the frontal ostium. Am J Rhinol 2003;17:221–226

7. Kew J, Rees G, Close D, Sdralis T, Sebben R, Wormald PJ. Multiplanar reconstructed CT images improves depiction and understanding of the anatomy of the frontal sinus and recess. Am J Rhinol 2002; 16(2):119–123

8. Wormald PJ, Ooi E, van Hasselt CA, Nair S. Endoscopic removal of sinonasal inverted papilloma including endoscopic medial maxillectomy. Laryngoscope 2003;113:867–873

9. Wormald PJ. Salvage frontal sinus surgery: the modified Lothrop procedure. Laryngoscope 2003;113:276–283

10. Wormald PJ, Ananda A, Nair S. The modified endoscopic Lothrop procedure in the treatment of complicated chronic frontal sinusitis. Clin Otolaryngol 2003;28:215–220

11. Mortimore S, Wormald PJ. Management of acute complicating sinusitis: a 5-year review. Otolaryngol Head Neck Surg 1999;121: 639–642

12. Wormald PJ, van Hasselt CA. Endoscopic removal of juvenile angiofibromas. Otolaryngol Head Neck Surg 2003;129(6):684–691

13. Tsirbas A, Wormald PJ. Endonasal dacryocystorhinostomy with mucosal flaps. Am J Ophthalmol 2003;135(1):76–83

14. Wormald PJ. Powered endoscopic DCR. Laryngoscope 2002;112:69–72

4

Powered Inferior Turbinoplasty and Endoscopic Septoplasty

◆ POWERED INFERIOR TURBINOPLASTY

Turbinectomy is seldom required in patients with chronic sinusitis because successful surgical management of the sinuses will in most cases result in normalization of the mucosa of the inferior turbinates. The inflammatory cytokines and cells contained within the mucus emanating from the diseased sinuses cause an inflammatory response from the mucosa of the inferior and middle turbinates. Once the sinuses are properly aerated and this inflammatory exudate resolves, the edema of the turbinate mucosa subsides. In the few patients who have intractable inferior turbinate hypertrophy (nonresponsive to treatment), however, reduction can improve the patient's nasal airway and quality of life. There have been many techniques described for inferior turbinate reduction, and these include submucous turbinoplasty, partial turbinectomy, complete turbinectomy, and diathermy (usually performed in the submucosal plane).[1-5] Arguments against complete removal of the inferior turbinates cite the risk of the patient developing atrophic rhinitis, especially in hot and dry climates.[1] In addition, amputation of the turbinate flush with the lateral nasal wall will inevitably result in a significant bleed at the time of surgery as the branch of the sphenopalatine artery to the inferior turbinate is cut.[6] This may require diathermy of the bleeder, and this again increases the amount of necrotic tissue and results in significant postoperative crusting. Partial turbinectomy may also result in significant bleeding and require diathermy for control. Submucosal turbinoplasty and diathermy, though initially effective, does not appear to have the same long-term success as partial or complete turbinectomy.[1,7] In addition, we are all aware of the patients who have had turbinectomy and have a capacious nasal airway but still have the sensation of nasal obstruction.[1] This may be due to the removal or destruction of airflow receptors on the medial and superior aspect of the inferior turbinate. However, this remains to be proved. The other significant problem patients suffer from after turbinectomy or diathermy (not submucous turbinoplasty) is crusting on the cut surface of turbinate.[6-8] This problem increases if diathermy has been used to control bleeding. These crusts can be uncomfortable and cause nasal obstruction. In addition, hemorrhage may occur when they either fall off or are removed.[1,3] In the group of patients undergoing submucosal diathermy and to a lesser extent submucosal turbinoplasty, they have significant postoperative swelling of the inferior turbinate that obliterates the nasal cavity and makes the first 3 weeks after surgery very uncomfortable for patients, who are usually unable to breathe through their noses.[7]

Powered inferior turbinoplasty was designed to preserve the medial wall of the inferior turbinate thereby preserving the airflow receptors. In addition, the technique allows the inferior turbinate to be reduced in size by ~50% without leaving a raw surface for crusts to form in the postoperative period.

Surgical Technique

Under general or local anesthetic, the anterior end of the inferior turbinate is infiltrated with lidocaine 2% and 1:80,000 or 1:100,000 adrenaline. A spinal needle attached to a 2-mL syringe is used to infiltrate along the posterior inferior border of the inferior turbinate. The turbinate is fractured medially allowing space for the endoscope (0 degree) and powered microdebrider to be placed. A 12-degree or straight blade is used in oscillate mode to remove the soft tissue from the lateral aspect of the vertical portion of the inferior turbinate (**Fig. 4–1**).

The debrider is then set on forward mode and the majority of the bone removed with the rotating blade. If the oscillate mode is used for bone removal, this may result in bone and portions of the medial surface of the turbinate being removed. If possible, this should be avoided, as the medial portion of the turbinate should be preserved so it

A

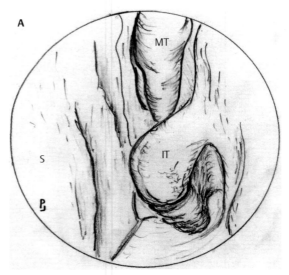

B

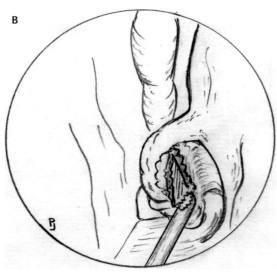

Figure 4–1 In (**A**), the inferior turbinate (IT) has been sufficiently mobilized to allow the microdebrider and endoscope to pass underneath it into the inferior meatus. The middle turbinate (MT) and septum (S) are seen. In (**B**), the microdebrider blade is used to remove the tissue and some of the vertical bone from the lateral aspect of the inferior turbinate.

can be rolled upon itself at the end of the procedure. Any residual bony fragments are dissected free with a ball probe (**Fig. 4–2**). The inferior turbinate bone often thickens considerably as the dissection is continued anteriorly. It is often useful to use the pediatric backbiter to facilitate the dissection of this bone. It is critical that this bone be removed because it is at this region that the nose is narrowest and where the greatest degree of benefit of the operation will be achieved.

Once all the lateral mucosa and bone has been removed, the remaining mucosa is rolled upon itself covering the raw area. The Freer elevator is used to roll the mucosa and if necessary fracture the horizontal portion of the remaining inferior turbinate laterally. This reduces the size of the turbinate by ~50% (**Fig. 4–3**).

The before-and-after pictures taken during surgery are presented in **Fig. 4–4**. It can clearly be seen that the size of the inferior turbinate is reduced by around 50%. A rectangular

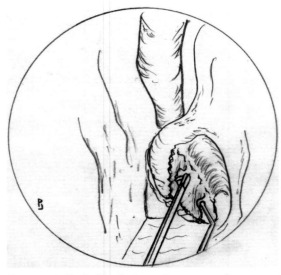

Figure 4–2 The ball probe is used to remove the more posterior bony fragments and the backbiter used for the thicker more anterior bone.

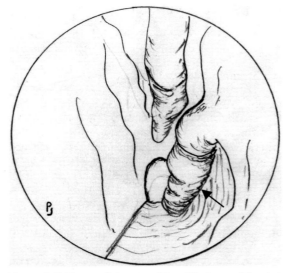

Figure 4–3 The medial mucosal flap (*black arrow*) is rotated on itself reforming the turbinate without any exposed mucosa. Note the turbinate is about half its original size.

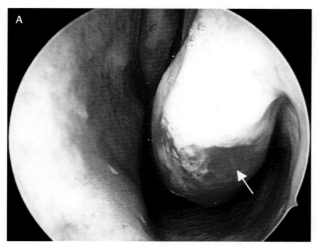

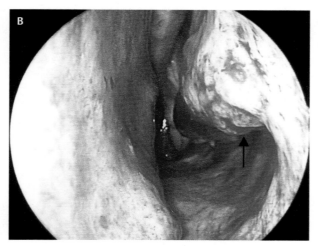

Figure 4–4 (**A**) The left inferior turbinate (*white arrow*) is seen. (**B**) After inferior turbinoplasty, the much smaller turbinate is seen with the mucosal flap (*black arrow*) rolled on itself reforming the turbinate without exposed raw surfaces.

sheet of Surgicel is placed over the rolled turbinate to keep it in place and to prevent the mucosa from unrolling (**Fig. 4–5**). It also provides a degree of hemostasis. No other packing is placed in the nose.

Alternative Surgical Technique

This technique published by Dr. Ray Sacks follows the same principles as the technique described above but modifies the technique for removal of the vertical portion of the inferior turbinate bone. Infiltration of the inferior turbinate with local anesthetic remains unchanged. To gain access to the inferior turbinate, however, the anterior head of the inferior turbinate is shaved. This is done so that the endoscope and microdebrider blade can both be placed under the inferior turbinate without causing a fracture of the inferior turbinate bone. In addition, shaving the head of the

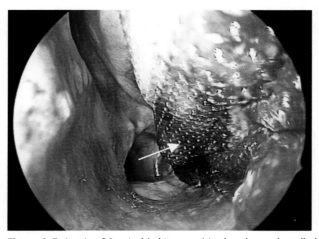

Figure 4–5 A strip of Surgicel (*white arrow*) is placed over the rolled mucosal flap to keep it in place and to prevent it from unrolling.

turbinate exposes the vertical anterior end of the inferior turbinate bone. The removal of the lateral aspect of the inferior turbinate is performed as above without any attempt to remove the underlying turbinate bone. The bone is removed by creating a surgical plane between the exposed anterior end of the inferior turbinate bone and the medial vascular portion of the turbinate (**Fig. 4–6**). The malleable suction curette* (Medtronic ENT, Jacksonville, FL, USA) is used as it provides suction and also has a relatively sharp anterior end that facilitates the dissection of the subperiosteal plane. After the bone has been dissected free from the turbinate, the residual tissue is rolled on itself in the same manner as the previously described technique and supported with a strip of Surgicel.

Postoperative Care

The patient starts saline nasal douche within a few hours of the surgery. This is continued for a month postoperatively. After a day, the patient is allowed to very gently blow his or her nose after saline wash. Systemic antibiotics are given for 5 days. The patient is reviewed after 2 weeks.

Outcomes

To evaluate the effectiveness of this procedure, a prospective randomized comparative study was performed where patients were randomized to undergo powered inferior turbinectomy on one side and submucous diathermy on the other. Nineteen patients were assessed by a preoperative and postoperative symptom score, endoscopic grading of turbinate hypertrophy, and acoustic rhinometry. The symptoms were scored individually for each side. This showed a significant improvement in symptoms of nasal patency on the powered turbinoplasty side in the immediate (first 3 weeks) postoperative period. The submucous diathermy

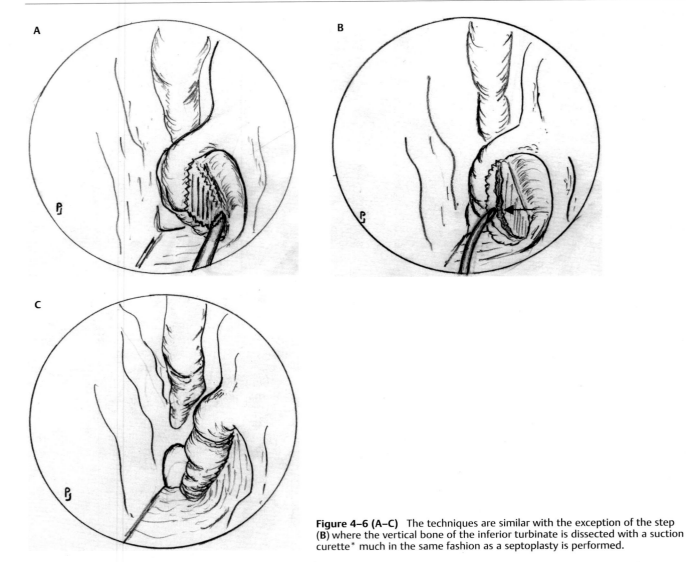

Figure 4–6 (A–C) The techniques are similar with the exception of the step (B) where the vertical bone of the inferior turbinate is dissected with a suction curette* much in the same fashion as a septoplasty is performed.

side continued to have nasal obstruction during this period. Objectively, there was also a statistically significant decrease in nasal crust formation at 3 weeks. After 3 weeks, objective nasal patency improved on the side that had undergone submucous diathermy, but the difference in symptomatic and objective nasal patency was maintained on the powered turbinoplasty side at 1, 3, and 6 months but was not present at 1 year. There was no difference in postoperative hemorrhage rates. Long-term follow-up was performed at 5 years and this showed that turbinate hypertrophy had recurred on the submucous diathermy side but not on the powered turbinoplasty side when the nasal cavity was assessed endoscopically and with acoustic rhinometry.

Figure 4–7 shows a typical view of an inferior turbinate in a patient who had undergone powered inferior turbinectomy.

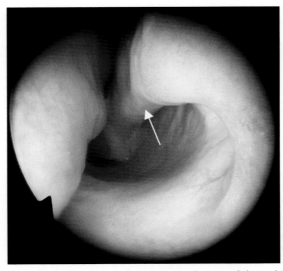

Figure 4–7 This picture demonstrates the size of the turbinate after 1 year (*white arrow*).

◆ ENDOSCOPIC SEPTOPLASTY

A significant percentage of patients have septal deviation that impedes adequate access to the middle meatus or to the axillary region of the middle turbinate. After the surgical principle that exposure is one of the keys to successful surgery, we recommend having a fairly low threshold in straightening such a deflection and thereby improving the access to the middle meatus and to the frontal recess. As the surgeon has the endoscopes all set up and ready to go, there seems little sense in using a headlight to perform an operation that is straightforward to perform with the endoscope. In addition, performing the surgery using the monitor allows all observers in the theater to view the surgery and has the significant advantage of allowing the surgeon to teach the operative steps to the junior resident. It is very difficult for the resident to follow the surgical steps if the surgeon performs the surgery using the headlight and speculum. The key to successful endoscopic septoplasty is instrumentation. A suction Freer elevator helps to keep the surgical field clear of blood, and it is extremely helpful to have an endoscope lens cleaner to remove any blood that may blur the end of the endoscope. If the septal deviation is to one side only, then it is advisable to perform the endoscopic sinus surgery (ESS) on the widely patent side and then perform the septoplasty with the incision on the side through which surgery had been performed. This decreases the likelihood of contaminating the endoscope as it is introduced through the nose.

Surgical Technique

The principle of endoscopic septoplasty is to preserve as much of the quadrilateral cartilage as possible. This is done by only elevating the mucosa off one side of the cartilage and leaving the other attached. In a large number of patients, the septum is too long and dislocates off the maxillary crest creating an anterior septal spur. As the cartilaginous septum is often too long, it bows and deviates aggravating the contralateral nasal obstruction. If there is a dislocation of the caudal end of the cartilaginous septum and the end of the septum protrudes into one of the nasal vestibules, this should be addressed with a hemi-transfixion incision rather than a Killian incision. If the deviation starts in the region of the lower border of the upper lateral cartilage, then a Killian incision is performed just beyond this landmark. The back of the scalpel is used to lift the presenting edge of the upper lateral cartilage. The vertical incision is started as high on the septum as possible, progressing to the floor of the nose and curving posteriorly as it reaches the floor of the nose, and a suction Freer elevator is used to elevate the mucosal flap in the subperichondrial plane (**Fig. 4–8**).

The flap is raised in a posterior direction before the dissection proceeds to the floor of the nose. Once the floor is reached, the flap is separated from the maxillary crest from posteriorly to anteriorly. If the cartilaginous septum is too long and is dislocated off the maxillary crest, a strip of cartilage needs to be removed from its lower insertion into the maxillary crest. The subperichondrial flap is brought down to the presenting edge of the spur, but the flap is not raised

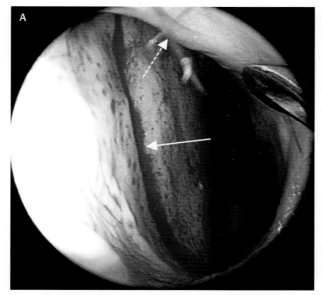

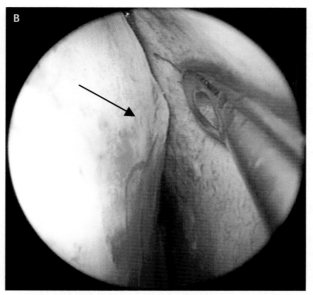

Figure 4–8 (**A**) A Killian incision (*white arrow*) has been performed just behind the leading edge of the upper lateral cartilage (*broken white arrow*). (**B**) The mucoperichondrial flap has been raised with a suction Freer elevator and the deviation at the junction of the cartilaginous and bony septum is seen (*black arrow*). Note the pearly white appearance of the cartilage indicating that the mucoperichondrium has been elevated in the correct plane.

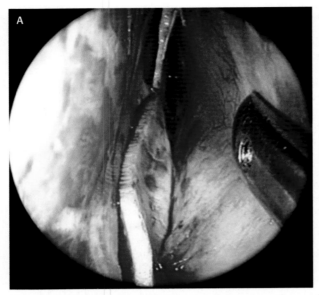

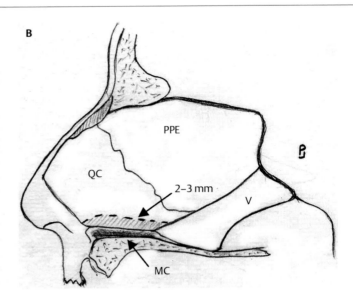

Figure 4–9 (**A**) The horizontal incision 2 to 3 mm above the maxillary crest has been made. This cartilage is gently elevated out of the groove of the maxillary crest starting anteriorly and moving posteriorly. (**B**) The quadrilateral cartilage (QC), perpendicular plate of the ethmoid (PPE), vomer (V), and maxillary crest (MC) are demonstrated. The 2 to 3 mm of cartilage to be excised above the maxillary crest are shaded.

over this deflection as it is likely to tear. Rather, using the sharp end of a regular Freer elevator, a horizontal incision is made above the spur through the cartilage from the bony cartilaginous junction ~2 to 3 mm above the maxillary crest up to the anterior Killian incision (**Fig. 4–9**).

The subperichondrial flap is raised on the opposite side of this inferior segment down onto the maxillary crest. This segment of cartilage is then elevated out of the maxillary crest starting anteriorly and working under the cartilage in the groove of the crest. In this manner, the mucosa over the anterior spur can often be preserved. If the maxillary crest is large or has a bony spur (**Fig. 4–10**), this can be trimmed back using a chisel. Usually, only the half of the crest that is protruding into the nasal cavity is removed because damage to the nerves that supply the incisor teeth is more common if the whole maxillary crest is removed.

To manage the posterior bony septum, the bony and cartilaginous junction is disarticulated up to the roof of the nose (**Fig. 4–10**). The suction Freer is used to develop the subperichondrial flap on the other side of the bony septum. Bony deviations are removed with special attention given to the bony septum directly under the nasal bones, which is often cancellous and quite thick. A great view of this is obtained with the endoscope, and deviated bone is resected as this bone will often obstruct the view of the insertion of the middle turbinate onto the lateral nasal wall—the so-called axilla of the middle turbinate.

No attempt is usually made to preserve bone in the posterior septum. The cartilaginous septum at this point has only had the lower 2 to 3 mm resected from it where it was dislocated from the maxillary crest. It still has the mucosal flap attached to one side and a subperichondrial flap raised on the opposite side. Superiorly, the cartilaginous septum is attached to the under surface of the upper lateral cartilages.

The cartilage has a free lower and posterior margin and if free of inherent bends or twists should hang relatively straight.

Management of the remaining quadrilateral cartilage depends upon there being any visible residual deviations within the cartilage. If there is a fracture line through the cartilage, this can be excised, and the remaining cartilage should then be straight. If, however, the cartilage has a bend or twist, the exposed surface is weakened with multiple incisions. The most difficult cartilaginous deviations are high anterior bends. These should be identified prior to surgery and the incision and flap elevation planned so that the concave surface of such a deviation is exposed during surgery. This allows multiple incisions and if necessary powered debridement with the microdebrider blade or septoplasty burr set on forward at a minimum of 6000 rpm.

If no tear of either mucosal flap has occurred, the scalpel is used to make a 2- to 3-cm horizontal incision on the floor of one of the mucosal flaps to ensure that no blood accumulates within the septum in the postoperative period.

After the ESS has been performed, a quilting suture is placed through the septum to hold the flaps together and to prevent hematoma formation. A 30 Vicryl on a cutting needle is used. A standard needle holder holds the needle with the shaft of the needle positioned between the jaws of the needle holder (**Fig. 4–11**). A knot is made at the end of the suture, and the needle is passed through the septum from one nasal cavity to the other.

Counterpressure is often required with the endoscope to allow the needle to pass from one nasal cavity to the other. The stitch is pulled through the septum until the knot reaches the mucosa in the other nasal cavity and prevents further passage of the suture. The suture is then placed some distance from its exit point through the septum into the other nasal cavity. This results in a quilting suture that keeps the

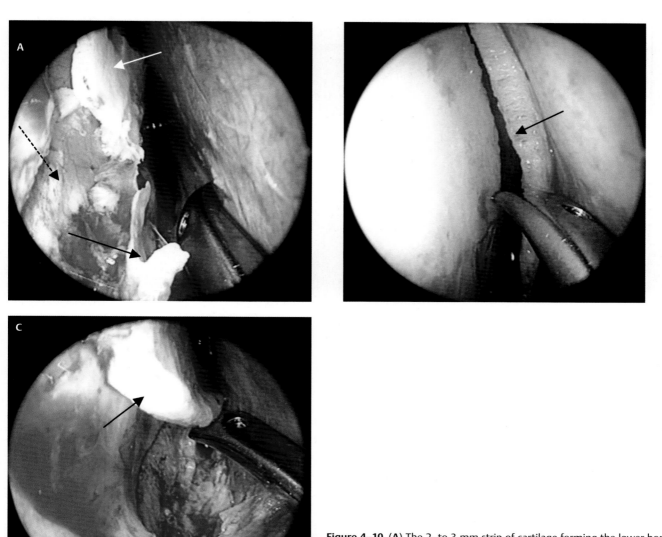

Figure 4–10 (**A**) The 2- to 3-mm strip of cartilage forming the lower border of the quadrilateral cartilage has been resected (*broken black arrow*). The maxillary crest is seen (*black arrow*) and the bony septum is indicated with a white arrow. (**B**) The cartilaginous septum has been dislocated from the posterior bony septum (*black arrow*). (**C**) The inferior bony septum has been resected and the thick upper bony septum remains (*black arrow*) and should be resected up to the roof of the nose.

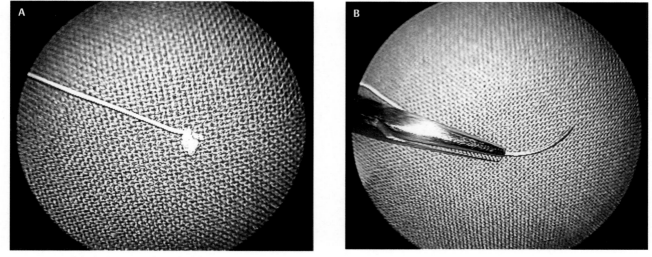

Figure 4–11 (**A**) The knot at one end of the suture is shown. (**B**) The shaft of the needle down the length of the needle-holding forceps is shown.

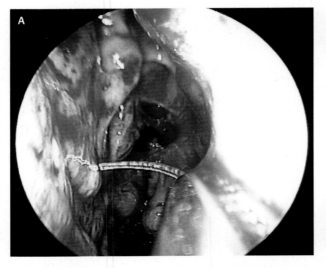

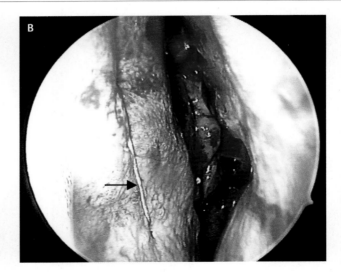

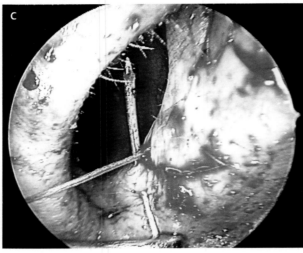

Figure 4–12 (**A**) The suture been passed through the septum from the left nasal cavity. (**B**) The quilting suture in the left septum is shown. (**C**) The suture catches a small bite of skin so it can be tied on itself in the right nasal vestibule.

two mucosal flaps of the septum apposed. The suture is used to appose the mucosal edges of the incision and is then tied on itself through the vestibular skin (**Fig. 4–12**).

References

1. Clement WA, White PS. Trends in turbinate surgery literature: a 35-year review. Clin Otolaryngol 2001;26:124–128
2. Lippert BM, Werner JA. Long-term results after laser turbinectomy. Lasers Surg Med 1998;22:126–134
3. Warwick-Brown NP, Marks NJ. Turbinate surgery: how effective is it? ORL J Otorhinolaryngol Relat Spec 1987;49:314–320
4. Gupta A, Mercurio E, Bielamowicz S. Endoscopic inferior turbinate reduction: an outcomes analysis. Laryngoscope 2001;111:1957–1959
5. Kawai M, Kim Y, Okuyama T, Yoshida M. Modified method of submucosal turbinectomy: mucosal flap method. Acta Otolaryngol Suppl 1994;511:228–232
6. Berenholz L, Kessler A, Sarfati S, Eviatar E, Segal S. Chronic sinusitis: a sequelea of inferior turbinectomy. Am J Rhinol 1998;12:257–261
7. Elwany S, Harrison R. Inferior turbinectomy: comparison of four techniques. J Laryngol Otol 1990;104:206–209
8. Moore GF, Freeman TJ, Ogren FP, Yonkers AJ. Extended follow-up of total inferior turbinate resection for relief of chronic nasal obstruction. Laryngoscope 1985;95:1095–1099

5

Uncinectomy and Middle Meatal Antrostomy Including Canine Fossa Puncture

Uncinectomy is the first step undertaken during endoscopic sinus surgery (ESS). If poorly performed, it may result in failure of the ESS procedure[1-3] and may result in orbital or lacrimal complications.[4,5] It is important that the anatomy of the uncinate and of the ethmoidal infundibulum is properly understood. The uncinate is a sickle-shaped bone extending from the frontal recess superiorly and attaching to the inferior turbinate inferiorly. If the uncinate is viewed in the parasagittal plane, the upward extension of the uncinate into the frontal recess cannot be seen. The middle and horizontal portions of the uncinate form a sickle-shaped bone attaching to the lacrimal bone and the ethmoidal process of the inferior turbinate and lying below the bulla ethmoidalis (**Fig. 5–1**).

The middle third of the uncinate arises from the lacrimal bone and lamina papyracea.[6] It projects posteriorly forming a gutter (the infundibulum) on its lateral aspect. It has a free edge that creates a space between this free edge and the bulla ethmoidalis.[6] This space is known as the hiatus semilunaris, as it is crescent shaped (**Fig. 5–1**). **Figure 5–2** illustrates the orbital attachment of the uncinate process, the infundibulum, and the hiatus semilunaris.

When viewed with an endoscope, only the medially projecting middle portion of the uncinate can be visualized (**Fig. 5–3**).

The superior portion of the uncinate that extends into the frontal recess will be considered in detail in Chapter 6. The attachment of the horizontal portion of the uncinate to the ethmoid process of the inferior turbinate is by a series of feet. This can clearly be seen in **Fig. 5–4** where the horizontal portion of the uncinate has been dissected free. Posteriorly, it may have a free end or it may attach to the palatine bone.

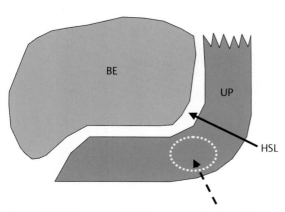

Figure 5–1 The parasagittal diagrammatic view of the uncinate process (UP) covering the natural ostium of the maxillary sinus (*broken black arrow*). The hiatus semilunaris (HSL) can be seen between the free edge of the uncinate process and the bulla ethmoidalis (BE).

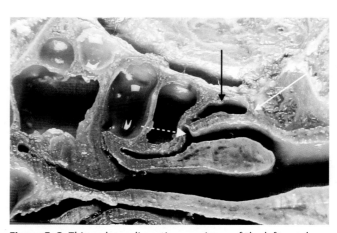

Figure 5–2 This cadaver dissection specimen of the left nasal cavity is cut in the axial plane with the anterior aspect of the specimen on the right. The white solid arrow indicates the uncinate attachment, the black arrow the infundibulum, and the broken white arrow the hiatus semilunaris (entrance to the infundibulum).

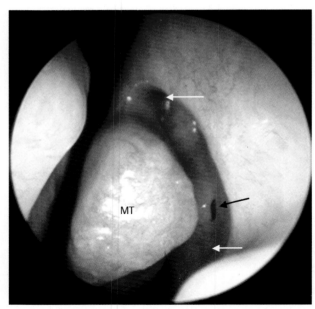

Figure 5–3 This photo is taken in the left nasal cavity. A concha bullosa (MT) and perforation of the uncinate (*black arrow*) are seen. The middle third of the uncinate lies between the two white arrows.

◆ UNCINECTOMY

The Swing-Door Technique

Removal of the Middle Part of the Uncinate

The swing-door technique[4] was devised in an attempt to achieve a complete removal of the midsection of the uncinate process and in so doing expose the natural ostium of the maxillary sinus. If there is doubt about the position of the free edge of the uncinate, a ball-tipped right-angled probe can be used to palpate its free edge confirming its position. The midpart of the uncinate is incised superiorly

and inferiorly. The superior incision is performed with a sickle knife just under the axilla of the middle turbinate (**Fig. 5–5**). The tip of the sickle knife cuts the soft bone of the uncinate from its posterior free edge until the tip of the knife can be felt to strike the hard bone of the frontal process of the maxilla. In this area, the uncinate attaches directly to the hard bone of the frontal process of the maxilla usually above the lacrimal bone. It is highly unlikely that this incision will penetrate the lacrimal sac or lamina papyracea and expose orbital fat.

The pediatric backbiter is passed into the middle meatus and opened. It is gently wriggled into the hiatus semilunaris so it engages the free edge of the uncinate process. It is easier to introduce the backbiter about midway up the middle portion of the uncinate before it is slid down the free edge until it comes to rest on the transition of the middle and horizontal parts of the uncinate. The uncinate is cut using sequential bites of the backbiter.[4] Usually (depending on the length of the uncinate and the size of the tooth of the backbiter), two to three bites are necessary (**Fig. 5–5**). If the backbiter can still palpate residual uncinate, then a final bite is made. The backbiter should be turned upward to an angle of 45 degrees before this final bite is made. This brings the tooth of the backbiter medial to the nasolacrimal duct and protects it from injury.

Next, a right-angled ball probe or curette is slid through the inferior incision behind the uncinate process fairly closely to the uncinate's insertion into the lateral nasal wall. The probe is pulled anteriorly and the uncinate is fractured at its insertion to the lateral nasal wall (**Fig. 5–6**).[4]

The posterior blade of a 45-degree upturned, through-cutting Blakesley forceps is placed through the inferior cut in the uncinate and the forceps pushed against the lateral nasal wall bringing the forceps hard up against the frontal process of the maxilla. The middle section of the uncinate is then removed flush with the lateral nasal wall (**Fig. 5–7**).

In most circumstances, the midportion of the uncinate can be removed in one piece. In **Fig. 5–8**, the superior, inferior, and anterior cuts as well as the free edge are labeled.

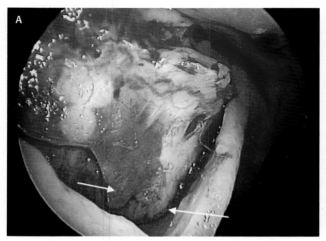

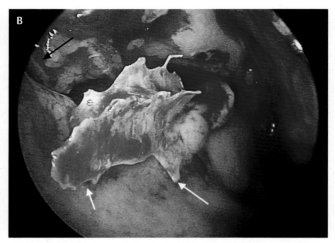

Figure 5–4 (A) The uncinate bone is displayed in situ with the medial mucosal flap dissected away from the bone. **(B)** The horizontal portion of the uncinate has been removed from between the two layers of mucosa. In both pictures, the feetlike attachments are indicated with white arrows. These feet attach to the ethmoidal process on the inferior turbinate.

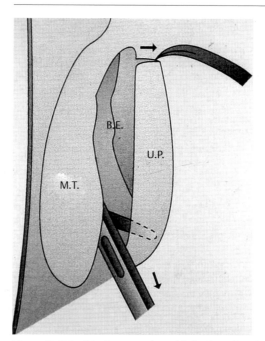

Figure 5–5 In this diagram, the sickle knife makes the upper cut directly under the axilla of the middle turbinate. A pediatric backbiter is introduced and the lower cut is made. BE, bulla ethmoidalis; UP, uncinate process; MT, middle turbinate. (From Wormald PJ, McDonogh M. The "swing-door" technique for uncinectomy in endoscopic sinus surgery. J Laryngol Otol 1998;112:547–551. Reprinted with permission.)

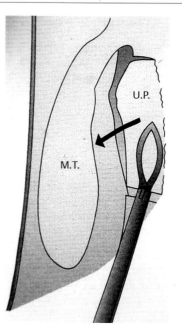

Figure 5–7 The 45-degree through-biting Blakesley is used to cut the uncinate flush with the lateral nasal wall. UP, uncinate process; MT, middle turbinate. (From Wormald PJ, McDonogh M. The "swing-door" technique for uncinectomy in endoscopic sinus surgery. J Laryngol Otol 1998;112:547–551. Reprinted with permission.)

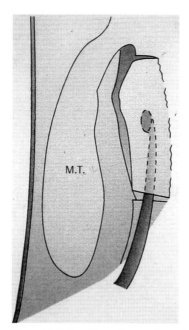

Figure 5–6 Insertion of a curette or ball probe behind the uncinate. The uncinate is fractured flush with the lateral nasal wall. MT, middle turbinate. (From Wormald PJ, McDonogh M. The "swing-door" technique for uncinectomy in endoscopic sinus surgery. J Laryngol Otol 1998;112:547–551. Reprinted with permission.)

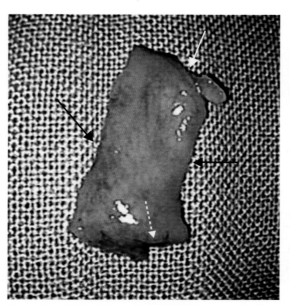

Figure 5–8 The middle section of the uncinate with superior (*white arrow*), inferior (*broken white arrow*), anterior cut edges (*black arrow*), and free edge (*broken black arrow*) labeled.

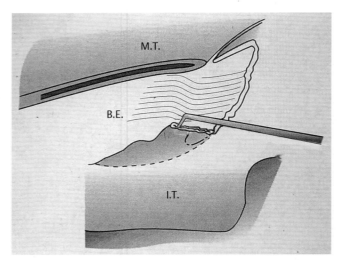

Figure 5–9 Diagram illustrating the double right-angled ball probe dissecting the bone of the horizontal portion of the uncinate process. BE, bull ethmoidalis; IT, inferior turbinate; MT, middle turbinate. (From Wormald PJ, McDonogh M. The "swing-door" technique for uncinectomy in endoscopic sinus surgery. J Laryngol Otol 1998;112:547–551. Reprinted with permission.)

Removal of the Horizontal Portion of the Uncinate

The 0-degree endoscope is changed for a 30-degree endoscope. This allows better visualization of the middle meatus and greater precision in the dissection. The next step is to dissect the horizontal portion of the uncinate bone out from between its two mucosal layers (**Fig. 5–9**).

The double right-angled ball probe is used to elevate the mucosa off the medial aspect of the uncinate. The bone is then fractured medially and the ball probe used to elevate the mucosa over the lateral aspect of the bone. Removal of this bone allows the mucosa covering the natural ostium to be delicately trimmed downward with the microdebrider exposing the natural maxillary ostium (**Fig. 5–10**). It also allows these

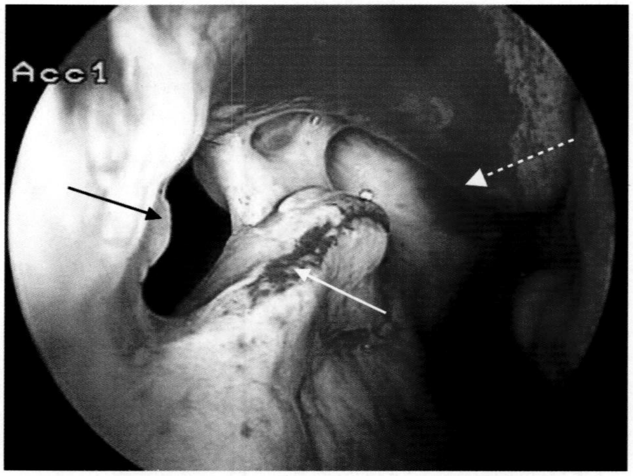

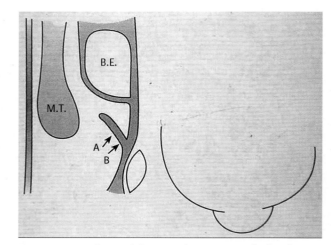

Figure 5–10 Intraoperative picture of the right maxillary ostium (*black arrow*) after removal of the horizontal portion of the uncinate with apposition of the mucosal edges (*white arrow*). The final common drainage pathway is indicated by the broken white arrow.

trimmed edges to lie directly apposed to each other without exposed bone separating these edges allowing these mucosal edges to heal by primary intention without scarring.

If there is any doubt as to the location of the natural ostium, the right-angled ball probe or right-angled olive tip suction can be placed directly behind the cut edge of the middle portion of the uncinate in the ethmoidal infundibulum. The probe or suction is slid down this natural gutter it must enter the natural ostium of the maxillary sinus. In this way, the natural ostium of the maxillary sinus should always be able to be located.

Results with the Swing-Door Technique

As part of the study comparing the swing-door[4] and traditional techniques of uncinectomy, we examined the results of 636 consecutive swing-door uncinectomies. There were no orbital penetrations with fat exposure, and all natural ostia of the maxillary sinuses were identified. However, there were four patients where the nasolacrimal duct was exposed and not opened and one patient in whom the nasolacrimal duct was opened. The important outcome was the ability of the surgeon to identify the natural ostium of the maxillary sinus in all 636 uncinectomies.

To compare the swing-door technique with the traditional technique of uncinectomy, a further 636 uncinectomies were performed using the traditional technique described below.[7] The traditional technique for uncinectomy starts with the identification of the uncinate's free edge. While the free edge is palpated, the surgeon attempts to gauge the site of the uncinate's insertion into the lateral wall of the nose. This decision is critical. If the surgeon starts too close to the uncinate insertion, the first incision may penetrate the lamina papyracea with a resultant prolapse of orbital fat. Surgeons tend to allow for such an error and leave a few millimeters of uncinate behind incising distal to its insertion (**Fig. 5–11**).

Figure 5–11 In this axial diagram, the surgeon will often have difficulty deciding exactly where the uncinate attaches to the lateral nasal wall and will usually make the incision into the uncinate as indicated by the "A" arrow as this gives a margin of safety when compared with the incision in the region of the "B" arrow, which may traverse the lamina papyracea and expose orbital fat. (From Wormald PJ, McDonogh M. The "swing-door" technique for uncinectomy in endoscopic sinus surgery. J Laryngol Otol 1998;112:547–551. Reprinted with permission.)

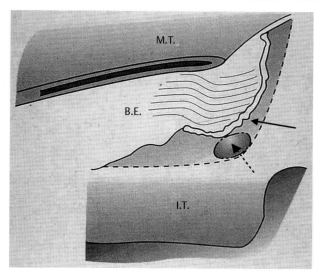

Figure 5–12 After the uncinectomy has been performed, 2 to 3 mm of residual uncinate remains (*solid black arrow*). This obscures visualization of the natural ostium (*broken black arrow*) and may not be located by the surgeon. This may result in a posterior fontanelle ostium being created. MT, middle turbinate; BE, bull ethmoidalis; IT, inferior turbinate. (From Wormald PJ, McDonogh M. The "swing-door" technique for uncinectomy in endoscopic sinus surgery. J Laryngol Otol 1998;112:547–551. Reprinted with permission.)

If too much uncinate remains, the ostium may remain hidden behind this residual uncinate. In this situation, the ostium should be sought behind the antero-inferior residual uncinate (**Fig. 5–12**).

Of 636 consecutives traditional uncinectomies, we were unable to locate the natural ostium of the maxillary sinus in 42. There were six cases of orbital fat exposure and no cases of nasolacrimal duct injury. In our hands, the swing-door technique was more reliable to identify the natural ostium of the maxillary sinus and was less likely to result in penetration of the orbit.

Complications of the Swing-Door Technique

The two areas at risk during uncinectomy are the orbit and the nasolacrimal duct.[4,5] To date, penetration of the orbit has not occurred with the superior horizontal incision of the middle part of the uncinate. This is due to the insertion of this part of the uncinate on the thick bone of the frontal process of the maxilla. The traditional technique of uncinectomy has a higher risk of orbital penetration. This is due to the knife penetrating the orbit during the anterior incision made into the uncinate at its insertion onto the lateral nasal wall.[4] This may result in the prolapse of orbital fat. Frequent palpation of the globe should be performed throughout the surgery. If inadvertent entry into the orbit or removal of the lamina papyracea has occurred, palpation of the globe will either cause a prolapse of orbital fat or cause the orbital periosteum to move. If orbital periosteum is exposed, care should be taken in this region during the rest of the surgery. If penetration of the orbit has occurred and orbital fat prolapse is seen, this should be left alone and not manipulated. The microdebrider should not be used in an

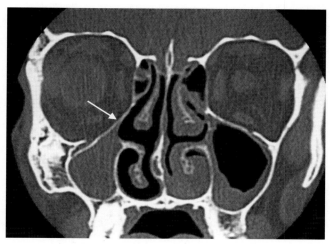

Figure 5–13 CT scan of a patient with a right atelectatic uncinate (*white arrow*). The uncinate is plastered against the lamina papyracea over a considerable length.

area where orbital fat has prolapsed as it can be sucked very rapidly into the blade with rapid removal of fat and damage to the medial rectus muscle. Damage to the nasolacrimal duct is less likely with the traditional technique than the swing-door technique as there is less use of the backbiter and therefore less risk to the nasolacrimal duct. If the nasolacrimal duct is opened, any small bony pieces are removed and the opening left as it is. Typically, no symptoms will result as the duct has not been obstructed. A crush injury of the duct has a worse prognosis as this may result in scar tissue formation within the duct with subsequent obstruction of the duct.

The surgeon should also be aware that collapse of the uncinate onto the lamina papyracea (so-called atelectatic uncinate) puts the orbit at greater risk of damage.[9] This occurs with complete opacification of the maxillary sinus with absorption of all gas within the sinus and resultant negative pressure sucking the uncinate laterally onto the lateral nasal wall. If this is long-standing, expansion of the orbit may occur with enophthalmos: the so-called silent sinus syndrome (**Fig. 5–13**). Anterior incisions into an atelectatic uncinate will result in a high incidence of orbital penetration and should not be used. The retrograde removal of the uncinate (swing-door technique) is preferred.

◆ PRESENCE OF A POSTERIOR FONTANELLE OR ACCESSORY OSTIUM

An accessory ostium is located within the posterior fontanelle of the maxillary sinus behind the natural ostium. Cadaveric studies have shown that 10% of the general population have an accessory ostium.[8] In addition, failure of the surgeon to locate the natural maxillary sinus ostium at surgery may result in the creation of a posterior fontanelle ostium. This is a common cause for ESS failure.[1–3] The presence of an accessory or posterior fontanelle ostium may result in the circular flow of mucus from the natural ostium of the maxillary sinus into the posterior fontanelle ostium with resultant recurrent chronic sinusitis symptoms (**Fig. 5–14**).

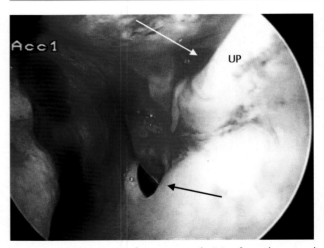

Figure 5–14 This picture shows mucus draining from the natural ostium (*white arrow*) behind the uncinate process (UP) into an accessory ostium (*black arrow*).

Patients who present with recurrent symptoms of sinusitis after ESS should have an endoscopic examination and, after appropriate medical treatment, a computed tomography (CT) scan. On clinical examination, the presence of a posterior fontanelle and circular flow of mucus should be sought. This can often be seen on endoscopy with a 30-degree endoscope. In addition, the CT scans of the patient should be closely scrutinized for presence of a natural ostium and a posterior fontanelle ostium or accessory ostium (**Fig. 5–15**).

If a posterior fontanelle ostium or accessory ostium is identified, this should be surgically joined to the natural ostium to prevent ongoing circular flow of mucus. This can be done by inserting a backbiter into the accessory ostium and coming forward to the natural ostium. After creating this tissue edge, the microdebrider is used to trim away excessive tissue.

◆ ENLARGING THE MAXILLARY OSTIUM

Currently, there is debate about whether enlarging the maxillary sinus ostium can be detrimental to the long-term health of the sinus.[10] The debate centers on the role of nitric oxide

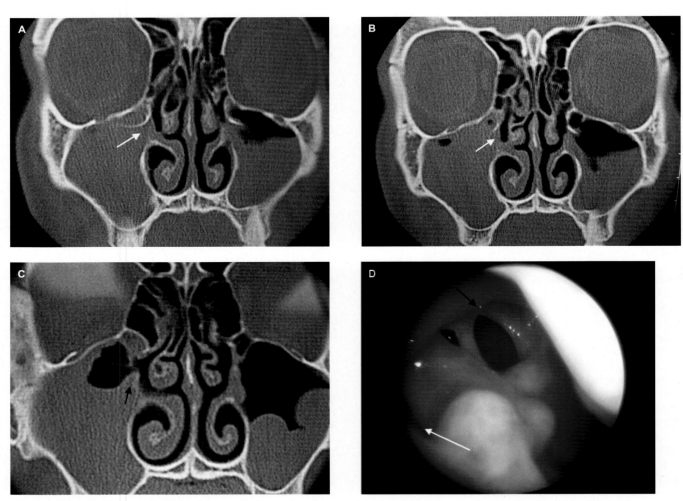

Figure 5–15 The endoscopic picture and corresponding series of sequential coronal CT scans reveal a partially obscured natural ostium (*white arrow* on photo and in CT scans [**A**] and [**B**]) and two accessory ostia (*black arrow* on photo and scan [**C**]).

(NO) in the sinuses.[10] NO is produced by nitric oxide synthase (NOS) in the mucosa of the sinuses.[11,12] There are three types of NOS with type II thought to be most important in the production of NO in the sinuses.[11–14] Type II is found in various cells in the nasal mucosa and is induced by bacterial inflammation.[14–17] NO is believed to play an important role in the local innate defense of the nasal sinus mucosa by stimulating ciliary motility and by inhibiting infection by bacteria, viruses, and fungi.[17] In the early stages of the development of ESS, many surgeons advocated enlargement of the maxillary ostium toward the posterior fontanelle.[18,19] This results in a very large maxillary ostium. Recently, there have been contrary opinions expressed where surgeons have argued that the proximity of the uncinate to the maxillary ostium results in a narrow transitional space that becomes easily obstructed and that removal of the uncinate alone is sufficient to restore the health of the maxillary sinuses.[20,21] Unfortunately, there are few data published to support either argument. Kennedy et al[18] described the natural size of the maxillary ostium to be 5×5 mm, which raises the possibility that significantly enlarging the ostium routinely may in some patients cause sufficient dilution of the sinus NO concentration to allow colonization of the sinus by bacteria with subsequent disease.

Our department recently published a study where we measured the size of the maxillary sinus ostium and correlated this with the concentration of NO found in both in the maxillary sinus and the nasal cavity.[10] There were 52 sinuses in the study with 22 sinuses having enlarged ostia and 30 sinuses having ostia less than 5×5 mm. This study showed that there was a significant decrease in NO concentration in sinuses and nasal cavities with large maxillary sinus ostia (greater than 5×5 mm). This does not mean that the study showed that a lower NO concentration predisposed patients to recurrent infections but only that a large maxillary ostium lowers the concentration of NO in the maxillary sinus and nasal cavity.[10] The association between large maxillary ostia and recurrent infections still needs to be formally studied. An example of a patient with recurrent maxillary sinus infection with a large maxillary antrostomy is presented in **Fig. 5–16**.

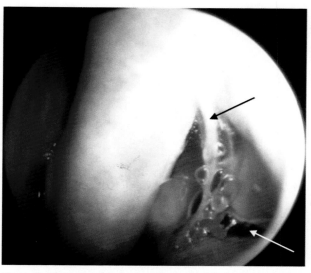

Figure 5–17 Mucus (*black arrow*) from the left frontal and ethmoid sinuses moving over the left small maxillary ostium (*white arrow*).

An additional consequence of removal of the posterior fontanelle during enlargement of the maxillary ostium may be dumping of secretions from the frontal sinuses and anterior ethmoids into the maxillary sinus. The natural drainage pathway of the frontal sinus and anterior ethmoids is above the natural ostium of the maxillary sinus along the base of the bulla ethmoidalis before crossing the posterior fontanelle and under the Eustachian tube to the nasopharynx. In **Fig. 5–17**, secretions can be seen coming from the frontal recess and anterior ethmoids across the natural ostium of the maxillary sinus.

Currently, the decision of whether the maxillary ostium is enlarged or not is dependent upon the degree of disease within the maxillary sinus. If the maxillary sinus has minimal disease with only mucosal thickening present on the CT scan (**Fig. 5–18**), then only the uncinate is removed.

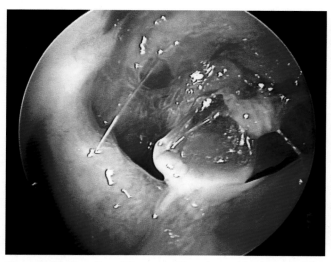

Figure 5–16 Secretions filling a maxillary sinus with a large middle meatal antrostomy on the left side.

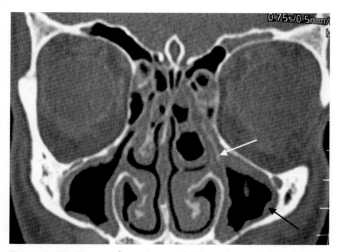

Figure 5–18 CT scan of a patient with bilateral mucosal thickening in the maxillary sinus (*black arrow*) with an obstructed ostio-meatal complex.

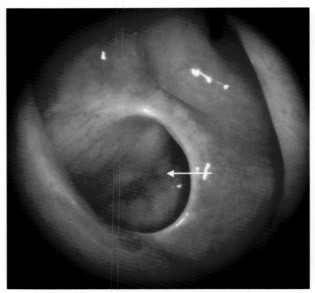

Figure 5–19 A patient with a large right maxillary antrostomy (*white arrow*) after having extensive sinus disease.

If the surgeon wishes to view the maxillary sinus, then a small enlargement of the maxillary ostium is performed. After removal of the horizontal bone of the uncinate, the mucosa is lowered onto the insertion of the inferior turbinate. In most cases, this is sufficient to view the majority of the maxillary sinus with a 70-degree telescope. If there is extensive polyp formation within the maxillary sinus or large amounts of thick and viscid secretions, particularly fungal mucin, then the maxillary ostium is opened into the posterior fontanelle and a large maxillary ostium created (**Fig. 5–19**). In patients with the Sampter triad and cystic fibrosis, a large maxillary antrostomy is usually created. This allows nasal douching to be effective in the maxillary sinus.

In **Fig. 5–20**, a polyp pedicled on the roof of the maxillary sinus is seen. Polyps that are based on the posterior roof and posterior wall of the maxillary sinus can usually be removed

through an enlarged maxillary ostium. If the majority of polyps or mucin remain after attempted removal through the large ostium, then a canine fossa trephine is performed as described below.

◆ THE SEVERELY DISEASED MAXILLARY SINUS

Grading

To date, when dealing with a severely diseased maxillary sinus, emphasis has been placed on the creation of the maxillary antrostomy and ensuring that natural ostium is incorporated into any antrostomy created.[3,4] Although establishment of a patent maxillary ostium is a vitally important part of the management of the severely diseased maxillary sinus, management of the sinus and its contents should not be ignored.[3] The diagnosis of the severely diseased maxillary sinus should be suspected if the maxillary sinus is completely opacified on the CT scan.[18] **Figure 5–21** shows examples of severely diseased maxillary sinuses.

However, the diagnosis can only be confirmed on endoscopy during surgery as the opacification may well be mucus, which is easily cleared through the natural maxillary ostium. The first step at surgery is to perform an uncinectomy and middle meatal antrostomy. A 70-degree endoscope is used to visualize the natural ostium and contents of the maxillary sinus. The extent of disease affecting the maxillary sinus should be graded according to **Table 5–1**.

Grades 1 and 2 are reversible with adequate clearance of mucus and aeration of the maxillary sinus, but grade 3 is irreversibly diseased (**Fig. 5–22**) and therefore the polyps and especially the thick eosinophilic mucus should be cleared before adequate re-epithelialization and eventually re-ciliation will occur.

If standard ESS techniques and instruments are used, the polyps and mucus from the posterior region of the maxillary sinus can be removed with angled microdebrider blades and curved forceps.[18] However, because of the two fulcrums that

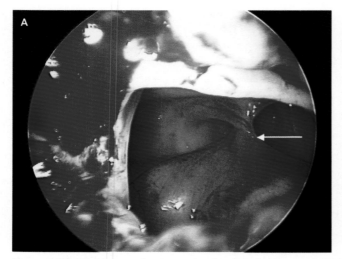
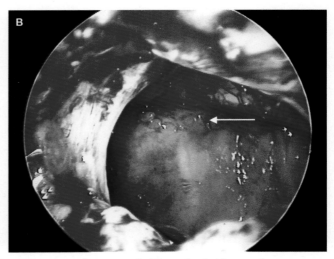

Figure 5–20 (**A**) A large polyp on a twisted pedicle (*white arrow*). (**B**) The maxillary sinus after removal of the polyp (*white arrow*).

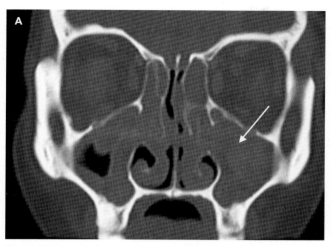

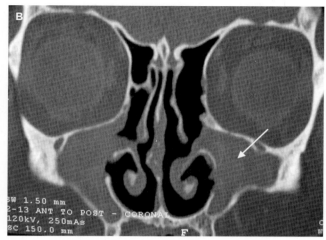

Figure 5–21 In both coronal CT scans (**A**) and (**B**), there is complete opacification of the left maxillary sinus with double densities indicative of fungal sinusitis. In (**B**), previous surgery had cleared the ethmoid cavity on the left and this remains disease free.

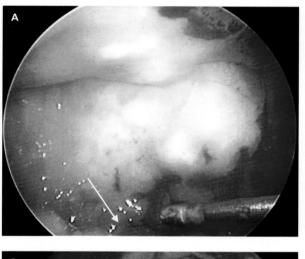

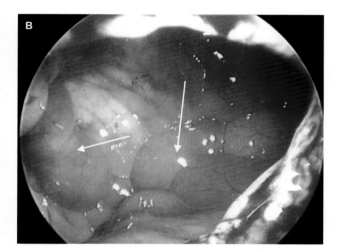

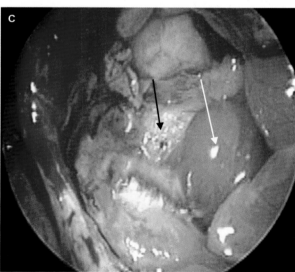

Figure 5–22 The following pictures of the left maxillary sinus were taken after a maxillary antrostomy has been performed and illustrate the grades of disease. (**A**) Grade 1: The mucosa is cobblestoned in the floor of the antrum (*white arrow*) with edema of the residual sinus mucosa. (**B**) Grade 2 (maxillary disease): The polyps are seen in the floor and posterior wall of the maxillary sinus (*white arrows*) and could be left and should reverse with medical treatment provided there is no eosinophilic mucin around the polyps. If mucin were present, a canine fossa trephine (CFT) should be performed. (**C**) The grade 3 maxillary sinus is completely filled with polyps (*white arrow*) and eosinophilic mucin (*black arrow*) and should be managed with a CFT.

Table 5–1 Grading and Management of the Diseased Maxillary Sinus

Grade	Endoscopic Findings	Suggested Surgery of Maxillary Ostium
1	Normal or slightly edematous mucosa (reversible disease)	Uncinectomy alone with visualization of the natural ostium
2	Edematous mucosa with small polyps (reversible disease) without significant eosinophilic mucus	Enlargement of the maxillary ostium to ~1 cm × 1 cm to allow suction clearance of maxillary, mucociliary clearance, and aeration
3	Extensive polyps and tenacious mucus (nonreversible disease)	CFP or CFT with complete clearance of polyps and mucus and creation of a large antrostomy

microdebrider blades and instruments have when passed through the maxillary antrostomy or inferior meatal antrostomy, polyps in the anterior, inferior, and medial regions cannot be reached. The anterior fulcrum is the nasal vestibule and the posterior fulcrum is the antrostomy or inferior meatal antrostomy site. If the blade or instrument is passed through the anterior wall of the maxillary sinus, it only has one fulcrum so a much greater degree of manipulation of the blade is possible (**Fig. 5–23**).

In current teaching, the maxillary sinus is managed by creating a large antrostomy and then removing whatever can be removed through the maxillary antrostomy. Polyps and thick tenacious mucus in the anterior region or floor of the nose require removal (**Fig. 5–22C**). In patients with severe and aggressive sinus disease such as allergic fungal sinusitis, nonallergic eosinophilic fungal disease (**Fig. 5–22C**), and nonallergic nonfungal eosinophilic disease, leaving eosinophilic mucin in the maxillary sinus may contribute to a rapid recurrence of disease.[18,19] Whether this is due to a continuing exposure to fungus in the eosinophilic mucin or due to ongoing inflammation from the toxic substances within the mucin such as major basic protein and other substances released by the eosinophils is unclear. In other patient groups such as Sampter triad and severe recurrent polyposis, it appears that if the maxillary sinus is left filled with polyps, these polyps do not resolve with only a maxillary antrostomy.

Removal of Polyps and Thick Mucin

We performed a study to establish whether clearing the polyps and mucus in a grade 3 maxillary sinus improved patient outcome.[18] All patients who had undergone ESS at the department over the prior 3 years were identified and their CT scans reviewed. If there was complete opacification of the maxillary sinus or sinuses, patients were included in the study. The researcher at that stage was not aware what surgical procedures had been performed or what the current status of the patient sinuses were. This was therefore an unselected patient cohort. The surgical notes were reviewed

and the patients were placed into two groups, depending upon whether the patient had undergone a large middle meatal antrostomy with clearance of all accessible polyps through the antrostomy or whether a canine fossa puncture/trephine (CFP/T) had been performed. If a trephine or puncture was performed, our standard practice is to place a microdebrider blade through this puncture/trephine site and perform a complete clearance of polyps under visualization of a 70-degree endoscope placed at the middle meatal antrostomy (**Fig. 5–24**).

The polyps and thick mucin were removed from the sinus under direct visualization with the 70-degree telescope. Care was taken not to strip the mucosa from the maxillary sinus. Only the polyp was taken while the base layer of mucosa underlying was preserved. This allowed rapid re-epithelialization after surgery and diminished crusting and secretion retention.

The patients in this study[18] underwent a magnetic resonance imaging (MRI) scan at a mean time since surgery of 19.9 months. On the MRI scan, the maxillary sinus was graded as normal, mucosal thickening less than 4 mm, mucosal thickening >4 mm but the sinus still aerated, or a completely opacified sinus (**Fig. 5–7**). This grading was confirmed on nasal endoscopy. In addition, the patients were asked to grade their sinus symptoms on a visual analogue scale and to complete the Chronic Sinusitis Survey (CSS) quality of life questionnaire. In the CFP group, the sinuses were normal in 62% of the patients compared with 12% in the patients that had undergone routine middle meatal antrostomy and as much maxillary sinus polyp resection as could be achieved through the natural ostium. The CSS symptom subscore and symptom score were statistically better in the CFP group indicating better symptom control in this group. If the overall disease burden was compared between the two groups using the Lund and Mackay score, it was found to be higher in the CFP group (Lund and Mackay = 10.3) compared with the group undergoing standard ESS techniques (Lund and Mackay = 8.6). In addition, all the other sinuses were treated in exactly the same manner with complete removal of all polyps and mucin from these sinuses and exposure of the natural ostium of the sinuses. This study confirmed the clinical perception that complete clearance of the severely diseased maxillary sinus plays a major role in the control of the disease and decreases the overall incidence and severity of recurrence of the disease.[18]

◆ CANINE FOSSA PUNCTURE

Technique

The old standard technique for CFP[20,21] was as follows[20]: The lip of the patient was elevated and the canine tooth identified (there are two front teeth either side of the midline before the canine tooth). The root of this tooth was traced with the finger under the lip until the canine fossa was palpated. One milliliter of 1:80 000 2% lignocaine and adrenalin was infiltrated in this region. A canine fossa trocar (Karl Storz, Germany) was placed in the fossa and directed posteriorly.

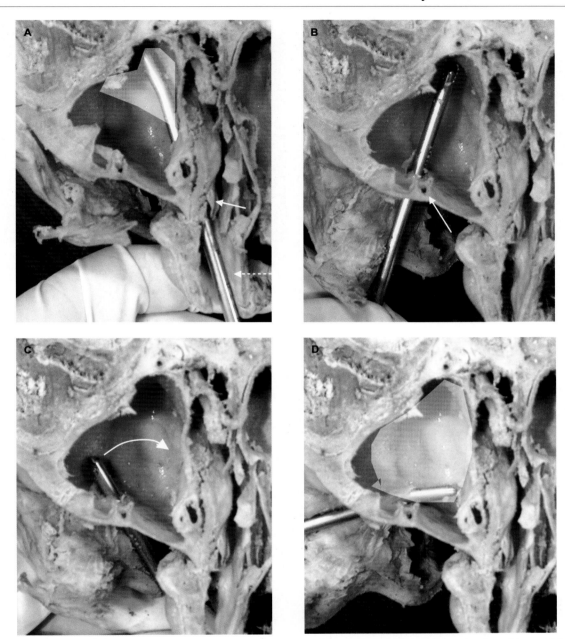

Figure 5–23 (A) The microdebrider blade has been passed through an inferior meatal antrostomy. Note the anterior fulcrum (nasal vestibule, *broken white arrow*) and the posterior fulcrum (inferior meatal antrostomy, *white arrow*). The region of the maxillary sinus that can be cleared through this access is shaded. This shaded region is smaller with a middle meatal antrostomy. The single fulcrum of the canine fossa puncture is indicated in (**B**), (**C**), and (**D**) illustrating how the entire maxillary sinus can be accessed as the blade only has a single fulcrum.

The trocar was introduced with a rotating forward motion. When the bone was too thick, a couple of firm taps with the palm of the hand was usually sufficient to drive the trocar through the bone. In some patients in whom the bone was thicker, however, the trocar needed to be tapped with a mallet. After the tip of the trocar was felt to fully penetrate the sinus, it was withdrawn and the microdebrider blade was introduced through the mucosal and bony hole into the maxillary sinus. The blade was kept closed during introduction to prevent soft tissues from been sucked into the debrider during passage into the maxillary sinus. Once the blade was in the maxillary sinus, the 70-degree telescope was introduced into the nasal cavity and the gate of the blade was opened. This helps remove most of the blood from within the sinus and allows the blade to be visualized within the sinus (**Fig. 5–24A**). This needs to be done before the blade is used to remove polyps. This visualization ensures that the blade is within the sinus and not in the orbit or soft tissues.

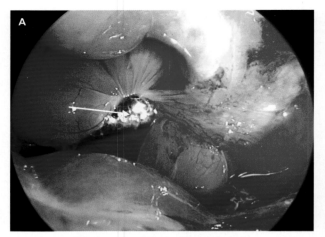

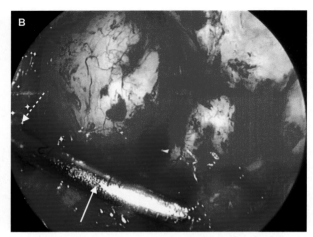

Figure 5–24 (A) The microdebrider blade has been passed through a CFT site in the anterior face of the maxillary sinus (*white arrow*). **(B)** The polyps have been removed from the sinus without stripping the basement membrane from the sinus (note no exposed bone). The debrider blade can be seen entering the sinus through the anterior wall (*broken white arrow*).

Complications

The incidence of complications with the old CFP technique performed at the same time as ESS was 75%.[20] A telephone survey revealed that the most common complications were cheek swelling, cheek pain, and facial pain. Most of these symptoms resolved within the first month after surgery. If the symptoms associated with the soft tissue dissection were removed, 28% of patients experienced a persistent significant complication of facial tingling, numbness, or continued pain. This incidence is similar to other studies where numbness of the upper lip and/or the upper teeth was seen in up to 38% of patients.[22] These persisting complications were thought to be a result of injury to branches of the infraorbital nerve. The infraorbital nerve divides before it exits the infraorbital foramen into the anterior superior alveolar nerve (ASAN) and the middle superior alveolar nerve (MSAN). These nerves traverse the anterior maxilla and supply sensation to the upper lip and teeth. Placement of the trocar through the anterior wall of the maxilla can injure these nerves and result in paresthesia and numbness of the upper lip and teeth. The risk of injury to this nerve increases if the trocar is placed too medially and cranially.[22] In most cases (91%), recovery from the paresthesia and numbness occurs within 12 months as the nerves either regrow or the area is reinnervated by nerves close by.[22] The area of numbness gradually shrinks then disappears.

The Neural Anatomy of the Anterior Maxilla

To determine the best way to avoid injury to these nerves, a cadaver-based study was undertaken in our department on 20 cadavers.[22] The soft tissue overlying the maxillae was removed and the underlying pattern of the ASAN and MSAN determined. The ASAN and the MSAN both run in the bone of the anterior face of the maxilla. The infraorbital nerve divides prior to exiting the infraorbital foramen (IOF) within the maxillary sinuses. The ASAN usually enters the anterior face of the maxilla just below the IOF and then traverses across the anterior face of the maxillary sinus. There were six patterns of branching of the ASAN and MSAN (types 1 to 6). The most common pattern was a single trunk of the ASAN (75%) with no branches (30%; type 1) (**Fig. 5–25A**) followed by multiple branches (25%; type 2) (**Fig. 5–25B**) and a single branch (20%; type 3). Type 4 was a double trunk with no branches (10%) (**Fig. 5–25C**), and type 5 was a double trunk with multiple branches (15%). The MSAN was present only as a single trunk with no branches (10%; type 6) and with multiple branches (13%; type 7) (**Fig. 5–25D**).

◆ NEW CANINE FOSSA PUNCTURE OR CANINE FOSSA TREPHINE[22,23]

Landmarks for Placing Trephine

To determine the region where neurologic injury would least likely occur, landmarks were determined on the cadavers as to the safest area to place the trephine.[23] The landmarks chosen were the intersection of the midpupillary line and a horizontal line drawn through the floor of the nose (**Fig. 5–26**). Canine fossa punctures were then performed on all 40 sides of the cadavers. In only 5 of the 40 punctures performed was there injury to one of the minor branches of the ASAN or MSAN confirming that these landmarks were the safest to perform a canine fossa puncture or trephine.

Rationale

One of the problems associated with canine fossa puncture is that the trocar is placed in a blinded manner. Although the soft tissue is dissected off the anterior face of the maxilla,

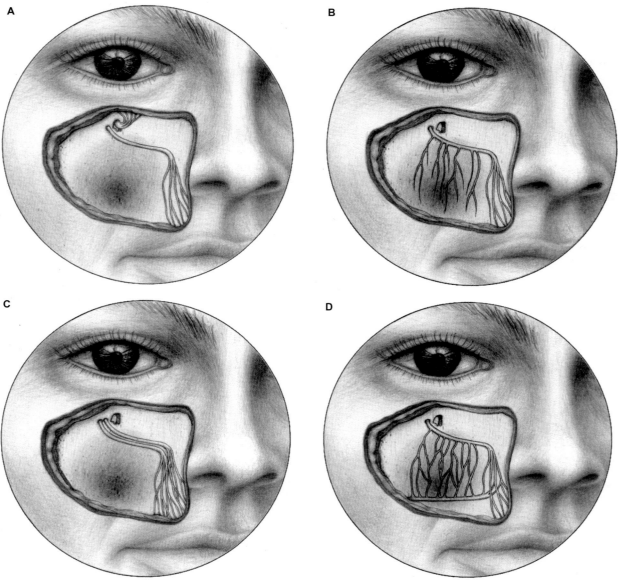

Figure 5–25 The most common nerve patterns are single trunk (75%) ([**A**] type 1 and [**B**] type 2). A double trunk is uncommon (10%) ([**C**] type 4). The MSAN is seen in 23% of patients and may have no branches (10%) or multiple branches (13%) ([**D**] type 7).

(From Robinson SR, Wormald PJ. Patterns of innervation of the anterior maxilla: a cadaver study with relevance to canine fossa puncture. Laryngoscope 2005;115(10):1785–1788. Reprinted with permission.)

the area through which the trocar is to be placed is not visualized and the ASAN or the MSAN could be damaged. In addition, placement of the trocar may cause fracture of the thin bone of the anterior wall of the maxilla around the puncture site. This is especially true if the trocar is not rotated with minimal pressure so that the edges of the trocar act as a drill as it penetrates the maxilla. If significant pressure is applied to the trocar, a fracture of the surrounding bone will often occur. This enlarges the area of trauma and in so doing increases the risk of possible associated neurologic injury. Also, the currently available canine fossa trocar (Karl Storz) is 4 mm in diameter. When a 4-mm debrider blade is placed through this opening, the fit is very snug, and when

the blade is manipulated within the maxillary sinus, this may cause fracture of the surrounding maxillary bone again increasing the potential risk of neurologic damage. To overcome these problems, an endoscope sheath* was developed with an extension to hold away the soft tissues (Medtronic ENT, Jacksonville, FL, USA).

Technique[23]

An ~6-mm incision is made in the gingivobuccal sulcus above and slightly lateral to the apex of the canine tooth. A suction Freer elevator is used to elevate the soft tissues off

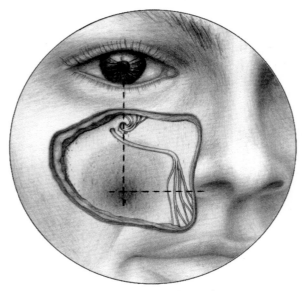

Figure 5–26 The landmarks for CFP/T are the intersection between a vertical line through the pupil and a horizontal line drawn through the floor of the nose. (From Robinson SR, Wormald PJ. Patterns of innervation of the anterior maxilla: a cadaver study with relevance to canine fossa puncture. Laryngoscope 2005;115(10):1785–1788. Reprinted with permission.)

the anterior face of the maxilla in a subperiosteal plane. Once this location is achieved, the endoscope soft tissue sheath blade* (Medtronic ENT) is placed into the incision and the soft tissues held away from the bone allowing the surgical plane to be endoscopically visualized (**Fig. 5–27**).

Dissection is continued in a superior and supero-lateral direction, exposing the canine fossa and the region lateral to the fossa where the midpupillary line and the line through the nasal floor intersect. If any nerve or branch of one of the

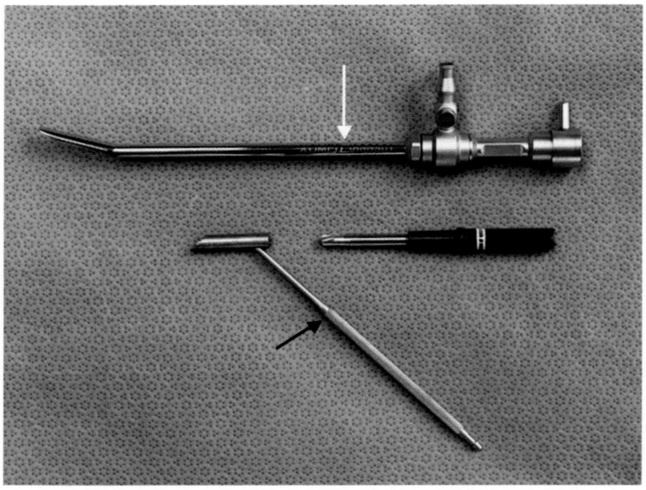

Figure 5–27 The maxillary trephination set* (Medtronic ENT) shows the endoscope sheath for holding the soft tissue away from the end of the endoscope (*white arrow*), the drill guide (*black arrow*), and the drill bit that fits into the end of the microdebrider.

nerves is seen (**Fig. 5–28**), further dissection is performed to create space so that the nerve can be avoided.

The canine fossa drill guide* (Medtronic ENT) is then placed on the anterior face of the maxilla at the intersection of the previously described lines. The canine fossa drill* (Medtronic ENT) is attached to the microdebrider handpiece and irrigation to the back of the drill guide. This allows irrigation of the burr during trephination. The drill should be used at 12,000 rpm for best results (lower revolutions may result in the burr sticking in the bone). A 5-mm-diameter hole is neatly drilled through the anterior face of the maxilla (**Fig. 5–28B**). A Frazier suction is used to remove any bone dust from the hole and surrounding soft tissues, and the 4-mm microdebrider blade is placed through the trephine into the maxillary sinus. Using a 70-degree endoscope placed transnasally at the maxillary antrostomy, the debrider blade can be opened and then visualized in the sinus. Activating the blade before it is visualized could result in damage if the blade had inadvertently been placed into the orbit or soft tissues (**Fig. 5–29**). The blade is then used to enlarge the maxillary sinus antrostomy. Any residual uncinate is removed, and the posterior fontanelle is removed up to the posterior wall of the maxillary sinus. Polypoid tissue and residual uncinate are removed from the anterior lip of the antrostomy. The widest possible view can now be obtained through the antrostomy, and the surgeon can remove the polyps and thick mucin from the maxillary sinus. Angled microdebrider blades are used for the lateral regions and anterior face of the maxillary sinus. The endoscope can also be placed through the trephine and the interior of the maxillary sinus inspected to ensure complete removal of polyps and mucin. Note that only the polypoid tissue and mucin are removed. The basement membrane of the maxillary sinus is retained. This allows speedy re-epithelialization in the postoperative period with re-ciliation and restoration of the maxillary sinus function (**Fig. 5–24**).

Clinical Study of Complications

To assess whether these new landmarks and technique reduced the incidence and severity of complications, a clinical study of 63 patients was performed.[23] Thirty-six patients had bilateral procedures resulting in 99 canine fossa punctures or trephines. Initial postoperative complication rate was reduced from 75% to 44% with only 3.3% of patients having a persisting neurologic complication after 6 months compared with 28.8% with the old CFP technique. In addition, the number of patients suffering from more than one side effect decreased from 70% to 31%. If the 99 sides were separated into patients who underwent canine fossa trephine ($n = 67$) as opposed to puncture ($n = 32$) with the new guidelines, a further reduction in complications is seen. In patients who had CFT and in whom the anterior face of the maxillary sinus was inspected for a visible ASAN or MSAN, the complication rate was 40%. This was significantly less than the 53% seen in patients who had a CFP and in whom the trocar was introduced in a blind manner. Also, the CFT patients recovered from their symptoms faster with an 83.3% full recovery in

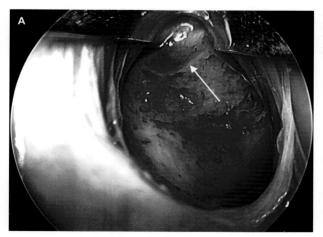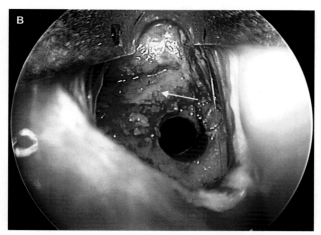

Figure 5–28 (**A**) The left ASAN (*white arrow*) is exposed and therefore (**B**) can be avoided during placement of the canine fossa trephine.

1 month compared with a 62.5% full recovery in CFP patients. Although both techniques used the described landmarks to place the trephine/puncture, it is thought that the additional visualization provided by the trephine technique allowed the ASAN and its branches to be seen and avoided.[23] In addition, the trephine technique creates a neat hole through which the debrider blade is passed, while the puncture technique potentially creates fracture lines in the anterior face of the maxilla that may disrupt the nerves running in the bone and cause injury to these nerves.

◆ POSTOPERATIVE CARE

Patients who have had either CFT or CFP are advised to rinse their mouths with saline after eating during the first few days, until the gingivobuccal incision seals. This incision is usually not stitched. All patients are advised to perform

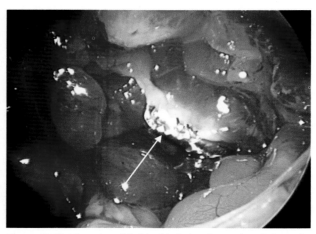

Figure 5–29 The microdebrider blade has been placed through a CFT access port and can be seen emerging from among the massive polyposis filling the left maxillary sinus.

saline douches starting the day after surgery and all patients receive 5 days of broad-spectrum antibiotics. Toilet of the nasal cavity and maxillary sinuses is performed at 2 weeks.

Conclusion

The severely diseased maxillary sinus should be dealt with in the same way as any other severely diseased sinus by removal of all polyps and mucus or pus. A large middle meatal antrostomy combined with canine fossa trephine or puncture using the landmarks described allows access to all regions of the maxillary sinus with the microdebrider blade. This in turn allows polyps and mucus to be removed with the retention of the basement membrane of the sinus and rapid postoperative healing with restoration of the function of the maxillary sinus.

Uncinectomy is the first and often the most important step of ESS.[1-4] If it is poorly performed, there is a significant likelihood that the ESS will fail.[1-4] Critical evaluation of the CT scan before uncinectomy is important so that an atelectatic uncinate can be identified before surgery is undertaken. In our hands, the swing-door technique of uncinectomy has few complications and a higher incidence of identification of the natural ostium.[4]

In revision ESS, the surgeon should specifically look for a posterior fontanelle ostium during both the clinical examination and the CT evaluation. It is critical that the natural ostium of the maxillary sinus is identified and if there is a posterior fontanelle or accessory ostium that the two ostia are joined to form a single ostium. The natural ostium should be enlarged posteriorly if there is evidence of significant disease within the maxillary sinus that needs to be addressed through the natural ostium.

A canine fossa puncture or trephine can be used to access anterior, medial, and inferior disease within the maxillary sinus. The patient should always be warned about the possibility of lip and teeth numbness after the surgery with a small risk of permanent numbness.

References

1. Owen R, Kuhn F. The maxillary sinus ostium: demystifying the middle meatal antrostomy. Am J Rhinol 1995;9:313–320

2. Richtsmeier WJ. Top 10 reasons for endoscopic maxillary sinus surgery failure. Laryngoscope 2001;111:1952–1956

3. Parsons DS, Stivers FE, Talbot AR. The missed ostium sequence and the surgical approach to revision functional endoscopic sinus surgery. Otolaryngol Clin North Am 1996;29:169–190

4. Wormald PJ, McDonogh M. The "swing-door" technique for uncinectomy in endoscopic sinus surgery. J Laryngol Otol 1998;112:547–551

5. Levine HL. Functional endoscopic sinus surgery: evaluation, surgery, and follow-up of 250 patients. Laryngoscope 1990;100:79–84

6. Yoon JH, Kim KS, Jung D. Fontanelle and uncinate process in the lateral wall of the human nasal cavity. Laryngoscope 2000;110:281–285

7. Stammberger H. Endoscopic endonasal surgery. Concepts in the treatment of recurring rhinosinusitis. Otolaryngol Head Neck Surg 1986;94:143–156

8. Jog M, McGarry GW. How frequent are accessory sinus ostia? J Laryngol Otol 2003;117:270–272

9. Joe JK, Ho SY, Yanagisawa E. Documentation of variations in sinonasal anatomy by intraoperative nasal endoscopy. Laryngoscope 2000;110:229–235

10. Kirihene RK, Rees G, Wormald PJ. The influence of the size of the maxillary sinus ostium on the nasal and sinus nitric oxide levels. Am J Rhinol 2002;16(5):261–264

11. Moncada S, Palmer RMJ, Higgs EA. Nitric oxide; physiology, pathophysiology, and pharmacology. Pharmacol Rev 1991;43:109–141

12. Nathan CF, Hibbs JB. Role of nitric oxide synthesis in macrophage antimicrobial activity. Curr Opin Immunol 1991;3:65–70

13. Bentz BG, Simmons RL, Haines GK, Radosevich JA, Förstermann U, Murad F. The yin and yang of nitric oxide: reflections on the physiology and pathophysiology of NO. Head Neck 2000;22:71–83

14. Nakane M, Schmidt HH, Pollock JS. Cloned human brain nitric oxide synthase is highly expressed in human skeletal muscle. FEBS Lett 1993;316:175–180

15. Arnal J-F, Flores P, Rami J. Nasal nitric oxide concentration in paranasal sinus inflammatory diseases. Eur Respir J 1999;13:307–312

16. Lundberg JO. Airborne nitric oxide: inflammatory marker and aerocrine messenger in man. Acta Physiol Scand Suppl 1996;633:1–27

17. Schlosser RJ, Spotnitz WD, Peters EJ. Elevated nitric oxide metabolite levels in chronic sinusitis. Otolaryngol Head Neck Surg 2000;123(4):357–362

18. Sathananthar S, Nagaonkar S, Paleri V, Le T, Robinson S, Wormald PJ. Canine fossa puncture and clearance of the maxillary sinus for the severely diseased maxillary sinus. Laryngoscope 2005;115(5):1026–1029

19. Desrosiers M. Refractory chronic sinusitis: pathophysiology and management of chronic rhinosinusitis persisting after endoscopic sinus surgery. Curr Allergy Asthma Rep 2004;4:200–207

20. Robinson SR, Baird R, Le T, Wormald PJ. The incidence of complications following canine fossa puncture performed during endoscopic sinus surgery. Am J Rhinol 2005;19(2):203–206

21. Bernal-Sprekelsen M, Kalweit H, Welkoborsky HJ. Discomforts after endoscopy of the maxillary sinus via canine fossa. Rhinology 1991;29:69–76

22. Robinson S, Wormald PJ. Patterns of innervation of the anterior maxilla: a cadaver study with relevance to canine fossa puncture. Laryngoscope 2005;115(10):1785–1788

23. Singhal D, Douglas R, Robinson S, Wormald PJ. The incidence of complications using a modified technique of canine fossa puncture. Am J Rhinol (submitted)

6

Anatomy of the Frontal Recess and Frontal Sinus with Three-Dimensional Reconstruction

In recent years, endoscopic sinus surgery (ESS) has become accepted as the treatment of choice for chronic sinusitis that is resistant to medical management.[1] As ESS has become more widely adopted, so the understanding of the complex and varied anatomy of the sinuses has improved.[2,3] However, the frontal recess and frontal sinus remain a challenge for surgeons. The anatomy is complex, varied, and can be confusing.[4,5] To better understand the anatomy of the paranasal sinuses, it is important to be aware of the embryology of the turbinates and sinuses. There are three to four embryologic lamellae or "ridges" that form from the lateral nasal wall and give rise to important structures in the nose. The first lamella forms the uncinate process, the second the middle turbinate, the third the superior turbinate, and the fourth (if present) the supreme turbinate (**Fig. 6–1**). The frontal, anterior ethmoid, and maxillary sinuses pneumatize from

the furrow between the uncinate and middle turbinate. The posterior ethmoids pneumatize from the furrow between the middle and superior turbinates and the sphenoid sinus from the furrow above the superior turbinate.

The key to safe surgery in the frontal recess is a clear understanding of the anatomy. This chapter explains how two-dimensional computed tomography (CT) scans in coronal, parasagittal, and axial planes can be used to create a three-dimensional (3-D) picture of the anatomy of the frontal recess. Such a 3-D picture allows the surgeon to plan a surgical approach to the frontal recess so that each cell in the frontal recess can be entered in a predetermined sequential manner and then removed. This allows the surgeon to be able to turn to the CT scan at any point during the dissection and identify the cell that is currently being dissected. This mental picture gives the surgeon greater confidence that the complex anatomy of the frontal recess and frontal sinus is fully understood and that removal of obstructing cells can be safely achieved. Insecurity during dissection in the frontal recess may result in either inadequate surgery with ESS failure or may increase the risk of injury to the skull base, orbit, and the anterior ethmoid artery.[4,6]

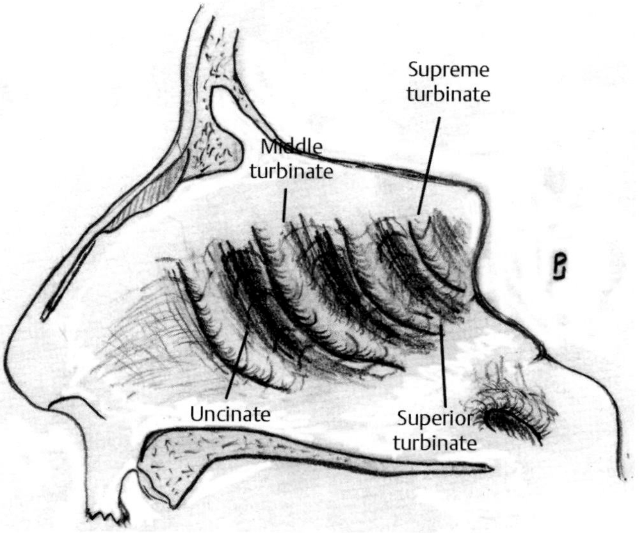

Figure 6–1 This drawing shows the four lateral lamellae and the corresponding structures into which they develop.

◆ BASIC ANATOMY OF THE FRONTAL RECESS AND FRONTAL SINUS

A common reason for ESS failure is inadequate removal of cells obstructing the outflow of the frontal sinus.[4,6] The location of the frontal recess creates anxiety for the surgeon as operating in this region places the lateral wall of the olfactory fossa (the thinnest part of the skull base), the anterior skull base (fovea ethmoidalis), the anterior ethmoidal artery, and the orbit at risk. The anterior wall of the frontal recess is formed by the thick bone of the frontal process of the maxilla, the so-called beak of the frontal process. The size of this beak will vary according to the degree of pneumatization of the agger nasi cell. If there is a large agger nasi cell, then the beak will be small. If, however, the agger nasi cell is absent or

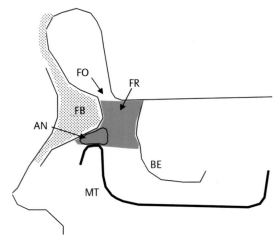

A

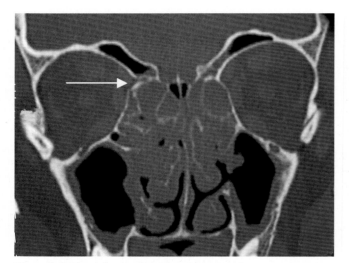

B

Figure 6–2 **(A)** This drawing illustrates the effect of a small, underpneumatized agger nasi cell (AN). The frontal beak (FB) is large and the AP diameter of the frontal ostium (FO) small. The frontal recess (FR) is shaded and extends from the beak to the bulla lamella (BE).

(B) This drawing illustrates the effect of a well-pneumatized agger nasi cell (AN) with a small frontal beak (FB) and large frontal ostium (FO). If the bulla lamella (BE) does not reach the skull base, a suprabullar recess (SBR) is formed. MT, middle turbinate.

underpneumatized, then the beak will extend significantly into the frontal recess and create a narrow frontal ostium as the beak approaches the forward projecting anterior skull base. Thus the anteroposterior distance from the skull base to the frontal beak is largely determined by the pneumatization of the agger nasi cell (**Fig. 6–2**).

The medial wall of the frontal recess is formed by the lateral wall of the olfactory fossa. The height of this wall is determined by the level of the cribriform plate. Keros[7] classified the depth of the olfactory fossa as a Keros type 1 (less than 3 mm), type 2 (3 to 7 mm), and a type 3 (>7 mm). Depending on the Keros type, a variable amount of the lateral wall of the olfactory fossa will be exposed during dissection in this region. The bone of the lateral wall of the olfactory fossa varies in thickness between 0.05 mm and 0.2 mm and provides little resistance to penetration.[8]

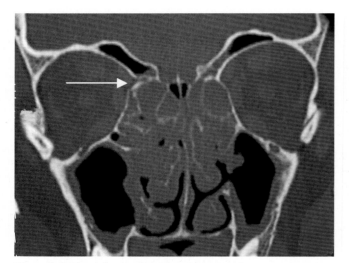

Figure 6–3 The right anterior ethmoidal artery is on a mesentery (*white arrow*). Note the pinching of the lamella papyracea as the artery exits the orbit.

The lateral wall of the frontal recess is formed by the lamina papyracea and the posterior wall by the upward continuation of the anterior face of the bulla ethmoidalis. On occasions, this anterior wall of the bulla ethmoidalis may not reach the skull base and a suprabullar recess is formed (**Fig. 6–2**). The frontal recess is then continuous with this recess.

The roof of the frontal recess is formed by the fovea ethmoidalis. This bone is relatively thick and normally provides significant resistance to penetration. In a study conducted in our department, we found that the right fovea ethmoidalis was higher than the left in 59% of patients.[9] It should also be noted that the roof (fovea ethmoidalis) may slope placing the medial aspect of the roof at a lower level than the lateral aspect. The anterior ethmoidal artery runs across the fovea ethmoidalis at a 45-degree angle from lateral to medial. In most instances, it can be found behind the upward continuation of the bulla ethmoidalis. When this is absent and a suprabullar recess is present, however, the anterior ethmoidal artery will be in the frontal recess. The anterior ethmoidal artery may lie in a mesentery suspended from the skull base in 14 to 43% of patients (in our study the incidence was 34%).[9] It is important that the CT scan is reviewed carefully before surgery to establish if the anterior ethmoidal artery is against the skull base or in a mesentery and if a suprabullar recess is present or not (**Fig. 6–3**).

If the anterior ethmoidal artery is cut during surgery (this is only likely if it is on a mesentery), it may retract into the orbit and cause bleeding within the orbital tissues. This creates an increase in the intraorbital volume with resultant proptosis. Increasing pressure stretches the optic nerve and may result in decreased arterial blood flow to the retina and subsequent loss of vision.

◆ THE UNCINATE PROCESS

The uncinate process has in the past been thought to be the key to the frontal recess.[8] This text adopts an alternate approach and suggests that the agger nasi cell is the key that unlocks the frontal recess.[10,11] The agger nasi cell is present in greater than 90% of patients.[12] As the agger nasi cell is the key, it is important to understand the interaction between the uncinate and the agger nasi cell. The interaction between the upward continuation of the uncinate and the agger nasi cell is often poorly understood. The attachment of the root of the uncinate into either the lamina papyracea, skull base, or middle turbinate has been well described (**Fig. 6–4**),[5,8,13] but how this upward continuation of the uncinate interacts with the agger nasi cell and anterior ethmoidal cells in the frontal recess is sometimes poorly understood.

Attachment of the Uncinate to the Lamina Papyracea

In most cases, the uncinate/medial wall of the agger nasi cell implants on the lamina papyracea. In a large proportion of these patients, this upward extension will give off a leaflet of bone to the bulla lamella forming a plate of bone that divides the frontal recess vertically from posterior to anterior[14,15] as it extends from the bulla ethmoidalis to the medial wall of the agger nasi cell and onto the frontal beak. In this situation, the frontal sinus will drain medial to this plate (**Fig. 6–5**).

If the relationship of a single large agger nasi cell (AN) to the frontal sinus ostium (FS) is considered, it is better understood

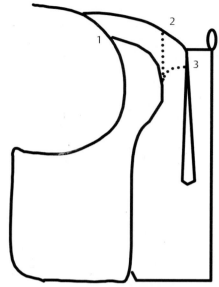

Figure 6–4 The classic description of the insertions of the uncinate process. *1,* insertion into the lamina papyracea; *2,* insertion into the skull base; *3,* insertion into middle turbinate. (From Wormald PJ. The agger nasi cell: the key to understanding the anatomy of the frontal recess. Otolaryngol Head Neck Surg 2003:129:497–507. Reprinted with permission.)

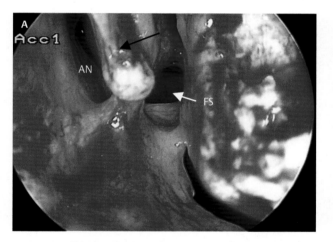

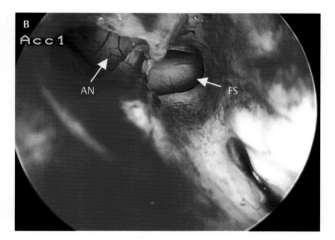

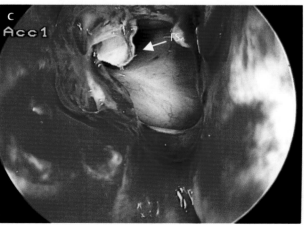

Figure 6–5 Intraoperative pictures in the right frontal recess illustrating (**A**) the upward continuation of the uncinate (*black arrow*) forming the medial wall of the agger nasi cell (AN); (**B**) the further removal of the medial wall/uncinate superiorly revealing the roof of the agger nasi cell (AN) and frontal ostium (FS); and (**C**) in which a small residual part of the roof of the agger nasi cell remains. The frontal sinus ostium (FS) can be seen.

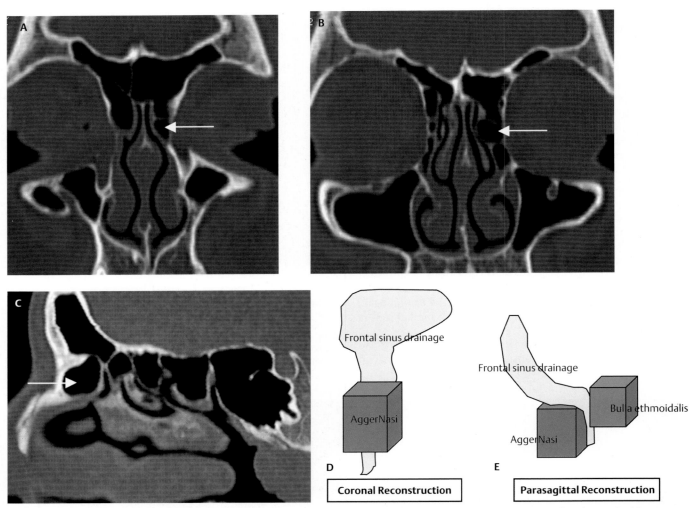

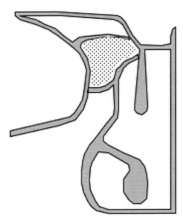

Figure 6–6 (A–E) Coronal and parasagittal CT scans illustrating a single agger cell (*white arrow*) on the left side. Note that the 3-D building block reconstructions have been done in the AP (coronal) and parasagittal planes.

by viewing the coronal and parasagittal scans. This example shows the simplest anatomic configuration of the frontal recess. The next important step is to decide where the frontal sinus drains in relation to these cells.[16–18] This concept is illustrated in **Fig. 6–6**.

Attachment of the Uncinate to the Middle Turbinate

The second anatomic variation to consider is that of a larger agger nasi cell. A large cell may push the upward continuation of the uncinate medially so that it attaches to the middle turbinate (**Fig. 6–7**).

This configuration alters the drainage of the frontal sinus as the agger nasi cell pushes the frontal drainage pathway posteriorly. Therefore, the surgeon can no longer access the frontal recess medial to the uncinate. Access is obtained by passing the curette along the frontal sinus drainage pathway behind the posterior wall of the agger nasi cell and fracturing the posterior wall and roof of the agger nasi cell forward to fully expose the frontal ostium.

Figure 6–7 A diagram illustrating how a single large agger nasi cell pushes the insertion of the uncinate onto the middle turbinate. (From Wormald PJ. The agger nasi cell: the key to understanding the anatomy of the frontal recess. Otolaryngol Head Neck Surg 2003;129:497–507. Reprinted with permission.)

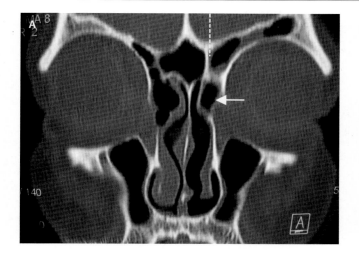

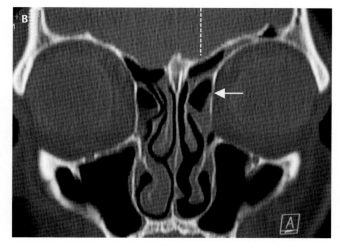

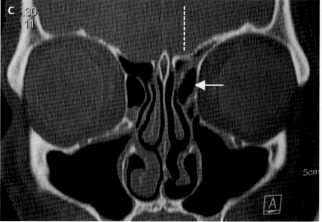

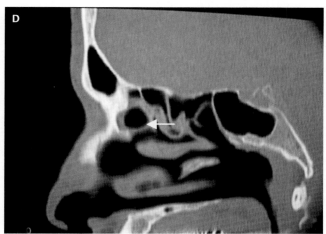

Figure 6–8 (A–C) In these CT scans, the agger nasi cell is indicated by the *white arrow*, and the *broken line* indicates the position of the parasagittal CT scan. (**D**) The uncinate can be seen to be pushed

medially by the agger nasi cell, touching the middle turbinate before turning more posteriorly to form the posterior wall and roof of the agger nasi cell and implanting on the lamina papyracea.

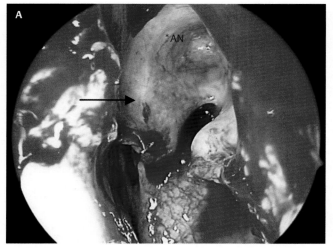

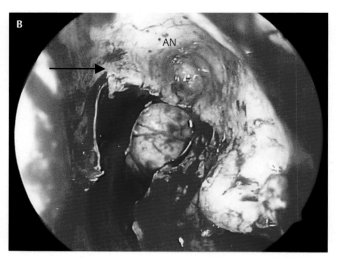

Figure 6–9 (A, B) These left-sided operative pictures are taken of the patient in the CT scans of **Fig. 6–8**. The *black arrow* indicates the uncinate process that forms the medial wall of the agger nasi

cell and attaches to the middle turbinate before progressing superiorly to form the roof of the agger cell and implanting on the lamina papyracea.

The following series of CT scans and operative dissection pictures illustrates the upward continuation of the uncinate that forms the medial wall of the agger nasi cell and has been pushed by this cell to insert on the middle turbinate before progressing superiorly, forming the roof of the agger nasi and then implanting on the lamina papyracea (**Fig. 6–8 and Fig. 6–9**).

Attachment of the Uncinate to the Skull Base

The third scenario involves the further upward continuation of the uncinate onto the skull base. In a small percentage of patients, the uncinate may have no relationship with the agger nasi cell. Usually in this configuration, the uncinate will progress superiorly to implant on the skull base. The following series of CT scans and anatomic dissections illustrates this variation (**Fig. 6–10**).

The uncinate can be seen passing medial to the agger nasi cell and implanting at the junction of the middle turbinate and skull base. The broken line indicates the position of the parasagittal scan. Alternatively, the uncinate process may form the medial wall of a fronto-ethmoidal cell that is sitting above the agger nasi cell. This fronto-ethmoidal cell may push the upward continuation of the uncinate superiorly to attach onto the skull base (**Fig. 6–11**). The variations associated with the fronto-ethmoidal cells will be considered below with the discussion on the classification of the frontal ethmoidal cells. The following cadaver dissection and CT scan illustrate a cell on the right side pushing the insertion of the uncinate onto the skull base.

The Agger Nasi Cell[10]

There are a large number of possible variations in the anatomy of the frontal recess. To gain a functional understanding of the anatomy of the frontal recess, the simplest configurations should be understood first before more complex variations are tackled. The simplest anatomic configuration is

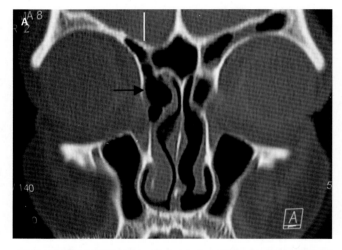

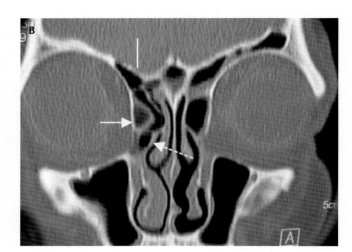

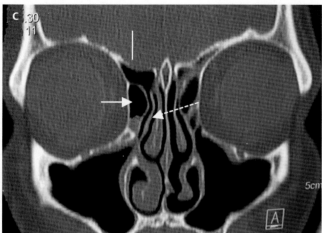

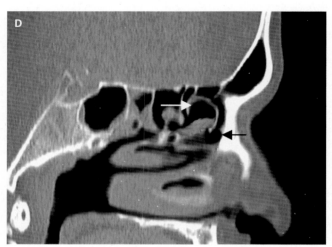

Figure 6–10 (A–D) On the right side of this coronal CT scan, the *white arrow* indicates the agger nasi cell. (**A, D**) The *black arrow* indicates the space anterior to the agger nasi cell. (**A–C**) The *solid white vertical line* indicates the position of the parasagittal CT scan (**D**). (**B, C**) The *broken white arrow* indicates the uncinate process separate from the agger nasi cell.

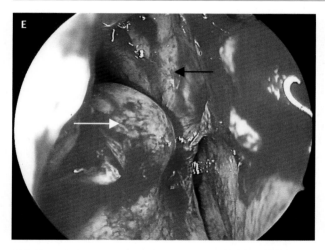

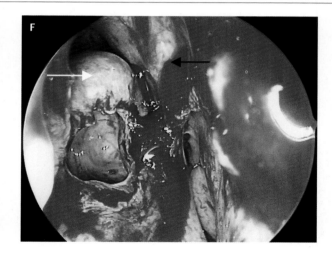

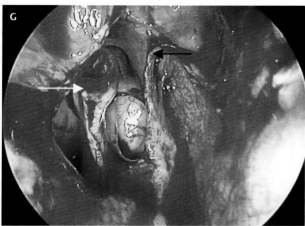

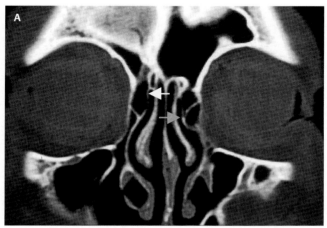

Figure 6–10 (*Continued*) These are the right-sided operative pictures of the patient in the CT scan of **Fig. 6–10. Fig. 6–10E** corresponds with the CT scan in **Fig. 6–10A** and shows the agger nasi cell intact (*white arrow*) and the *black arrow* indicates the uncinate process as it progresses upward to implant on the junction of the middle turbinate and the skull base. Part (**F**) shows the anterior face of the agger nasi cell opened with the uncinate process (*black arrow*) seen to be separate from the agger nasi cell. Part (**G**) shows the uncinate (*black arrow*) implanting onto the skull base. The *white arrow* indicates the remaining roof of the agger nasi cell.

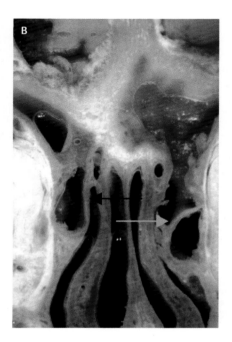

Figure 6–11 (A, B) The CT scan is taken of the cadaver dissection specimen pictured beside it. On the right, the uncinate process (*white arrow*) is pushed up toward the skull base and onto the middle turbinate by a small cell sitting above and medial to the agger nasi cell. On the left, the upward continuation of the uncinate can be seen forming the roof of the agger nasi cell (*gray arrow*). Note the frontal sinus draining directly above the agger nasi cell.

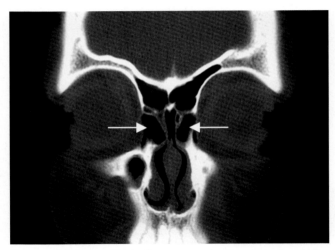

Figure 6–12 CT scan illustrating agger nasi cells anterior to middle turbinate insertion (*white arrows*).

Computed Tomography Scans of the Agger Nasi Cell

Transition from Frontal Sinus to Frontal Recess on the Coronal Computed Tomography Scans

The surgeon reviewing a patient's CT scans before surgery needs to understand how the anterior coronal CT scan through the agger nasi cell relates to the frontal beak and frontal sinus and how to be able to tell on coronal sequential CT scans when the transition from frontal sinus to frontal recess occurs. **Figure 6–6** is a diagrammatic illustration of how a coronal CT scan through the anterior half of the agger nasi cell and through the frontal sinus can be identified on a coronal CT scan.

If line *1* is drawn in the coronal plane, the frontal beak can be seen as continuous ridge of bone with the frontal sinus above it (diagonally shaded area in **Fig. 6–13 and Fig. 6–14**). This line (line *1*) is anterior to the uncinate and one can still see the continuous ridge of bone of the beak (floor of the frontal sinus). This makes it simple to differentiate the frontal sinus (above the beak) from the frontal recess. Line *2* in **Fig. 6–14** shows a coronal cut through the uncinate process behind the beak. This illustrates the transition from the frontal sinus to the frontal recess with loss of the continuity of bone (illustrated as the "frontal beak" in **Fig. 6–13**) and by the presence of the uncinate. This coronal cut illustrates the posterior part of the agger nasi cell's relationship to the superior extension of the uncinate process. This part of the uncinate forms the medial and posterior medial wall of the agger nasi cell and represents the relationship between the anterior agger nasi cell (shaded with dots) and the frontal beak and the floor of the frontal sinus (diagonally shaded area).

The diagonally shaded area in **Figs. 6–13 and 6–14** is the frontal sinus above the frontal beak. The frontal beak forms the floor of the frontal sinus. Frontal ethmoidal cells

the single agger nasi cell without frontal ethmoidal cells. The agger nasi cell is the most anterior ethmoidal cell and is present in 93% of people.[12] The agger nasi cell forms a bulge on the lateral nasal wall anterior to the middle turbinate. If coronal sequential CT scans are evaluated in an anterior to posterior direction, the agger nasi cell can be seen before the middle turbinate comes into view (**Fig. 6–12**).[5,12]

Note that the uncinate has a relationship only with the posterior half of the agger nasi cell and not with the anterior half, which is why the uncinate cannot be seen on the coronal CT scans taken through the anterior half of the agger nasi cell as seen in **Fig. 6–12**. This relationship can be viewed in **Fig. 6–13 and Fig. 6–14**.

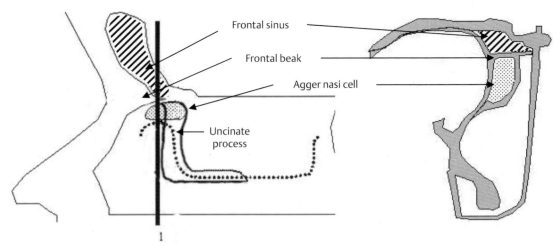

Figure 6–13 A diagrammatic illustration of a parasagittal view of the agger nasi cell with line *1* representing a coronal cut through the anterior aspect of the agger nasi cell anterior to the middle turbinate. The diagonally striped, shaded area represents the area of the

frontal sinus above the frontal beak (*black arrow*). (From Wormald PJ. The agger nasi cell: the key to understanding the anatomy of the frontal recess. Otolaryngol Head Neck Surg 2003;129:497–507. Reprinted with permission.)

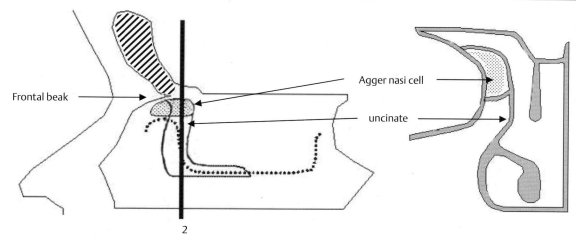

Figure 6–14 A diagram of the parasagittal view with line *2* representing a more posterior coronal cut through the posterior aspect of the agger nasi cell. (From Wormald PJ. The agger nasi cell: the key to understanding the anatomy of the frontal recess. Otolaryngol Head Neck Surg 2003;129:497–507. Reprinted with permission.)

pushing into this shaded area are classified as Kuhn type 3 cells (**Table 6–1**).[14] From these diagrams, it can be seen that most of the agger nasi cell is anterior to the uncinate but the posterior half of the agger nasi cell has an intimate relationship with the upward extension of the uncinate process (**Fig. 6–15**).[10]

Transition from Frontal Sinus to Frontal Recess on the Axial Scans

The surgeon should also be able to differentiate on the axial scans when transition occurs from the frontal sinus to the frontal recess. The frontal sinus scans should be viewed from the top down (cranial to caudal). The frontal sinus is relatively easy to identify; as it narrows toward the frontal ostia, it forms a square (**Fig. 6–16**). At this level, the posterior wall of the two frontal sinuses forms a straight line (**Fig. 6–16**). As the skull base turns posteriorly, these squares elongate posteriorly but still maintain a roughly rectangular shape. This is the transition stage from frontal sinus to frontal recess (**Fig. 6–16D**). As the posterior ends of these boxes become pointed, so the scans reach the frontal recess (**Fig. 6–16E**). **Figures 6–16A, B** show the square formation of the frontal sinuses. The transition region is between **Fig. 6–16D and 6–16E**. Note

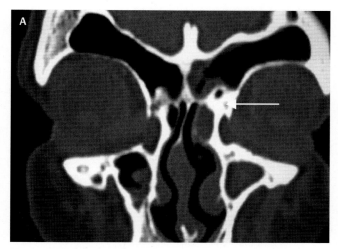

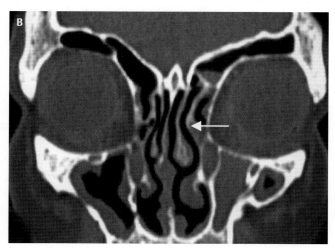

Figure 6–15 (**A**) Coronal CT scan anterior to uncinate with the floor of the frontal sinus (frontal beak) illustrated by *white arrow* on the left. (**B**) Coronal CT scan through the uncinate process (*white arrow*) with the uncinate forming medial wall and roof of agger nasi cell on the left.

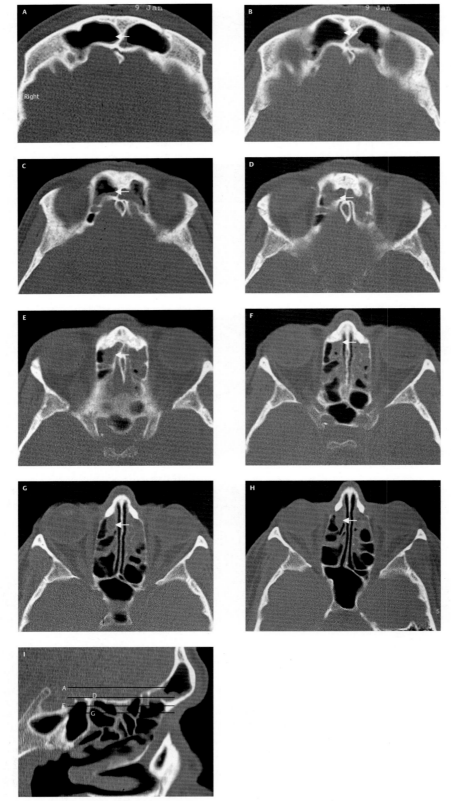

Figure 6–16 (A–H) Sequential axial CT scans of the approximate levels of cuts are demonstrated in (**I**), the parasagittal CT scan. The transition from frontal sinus to frontal recess is between axial CT scans (**D**) and (**E**). (**E**) Note the development of the nasion with thick bony beak visible. *White arrows* demonstrate the drainage pathway of the frontal sinus on the right side.

Table 6–1 Kuhn Classification of Frontal Recess and Frontal Sinus Cells

Cell	Description
Agger nasi cell	
Supraorbital ethmoid cells	
Frontal cells	
Type 1	Single frontal recess cell above agger nasi cell
Type 2	Tier of cells in frontal recess above agger nasi cell
Type 3	Single massive cell pneumatizing cephalad into frontal sinus
Type 4	Isolated cell in the frontal sinus
Frontal bulla cells	
Suprabullar cells	
Interfrontal sinus septal cell	

Source: Data from Kuhn FA. Chronic frontal sinusitis: the endoscopic frontal recess approach. Operative techniques. Otolaryngol Head Neck Surg 1996;7:222–229.

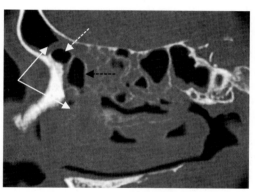

Figure 6–17 In this CT scan, the region between the divergent *solid white arrows* is the frontal process of the maxilla. In this example, we have a large agger nasi cell (*broken black arrow*) and a T3 frontal ethmoidal cell (*broken white arrow*).

how the bone of the anterior wall changes at each of these levels. In **Figs. 6–16A, B**, the bone of the anterior wall of the frontal sinus is even and relatively flat and not very thick. The anterior wall bone becomes much thicker as the upper region of the frontal beak is reached (**Fig. 6–16C**). In **Figs. 6–16D, E**, the anterior wall is curved indicating that the nasion has been reached. In **Fig. 6–16D**, the nasion is fully developed and the frontal beak bone is thick. Also note how the posterior wall has become pointed as the axial cut goes into the frontal recess toward the anterior ethmoidal arteries. This artery is seen in its canal in **Fig. 6–16D** on the right side.

Classification of Anatomic Variants of Frontal Recess and Frontal Sinus

A single agger nasi cell in the frontal recess is only one of the many anatomic variations. In 1995, Fred Kuhn classified the cells seen in the frontal recess and frontal sinus as presented in **Table 6–1**.[14] This classification still forms the basis of our current classification although we have made significant modifications (**Table 6–2**). One of the important modifications is defining more precisely the types of cells that occur in the frontal recess and frontal sinus. The first cells to be considered are the frontal ethmoidal cells. For a cell to be called a frontal ethmoidal cell, it needs to satisfy two criteria: first it must be an anterior ethmoidal cell, and second it should be in close proximity to the frontal process of the maxilla. The frontal process of the maxilla is the bone forming the anterior wall of the frontal recess (**Fig. 6–17**).

Table 6–2 Modified Classification of Frontal Recess and Frontal Sinus Cells*

Cell	Description
Agger nasi cell	*Cell that is either anterior to the origin of the middle turbinate or sits directly above the most anterior insertion of the middle turbinate into the lateral nasal wall*
Frontal ethmoidal cells	*An anterior ethmoidal cell that needs to be in close proximity (touching) to the frontal process of the maxilla*
Type 1	Single frontal ethmoidal cell above agger nasi cell
Type 2	Tier of frontal ethmoidal cells above agger nasi cell
Type 3	Frontal ethmoidal cell that pneumatizes cephalad into the frontal sinus through the frontal ostium but not extending beyond 50% of the vertical height of that frontal sinus on the CT scan that is evaluated (is usually found in the lateral region of the frontal ostium)
Type 4	*A frontal ethmoidal cell that extends more than 50% of the vertical height of the frontal sinus in the scan in which it is evaluated. Originally termed an isolated cell in the frontal sinus, but in our experience isolated cells in the frontal sinus are extremely rare and seldom clinically important.*
Frontal bulla cells	This is a cell that originates in the suprabullar region but pneumatizes along the skull base into the frontal sinus along the posterior wall of the frontal sinus.
Suprabullar cells	These are suprabullar cells (*cells above the bulla ethmoidalis*) that do not enter the frontal sinus.
Intersinus septal cell (also termed "interfrontal sinus septal cell" in Kuhn classification)	This cell is associated with the frontal sinus septum and compromises the frontal ostium by occupying part of the frontal ostium. *It is always medially based and opens into the frontal recess.*

*The modifications from the original Kuhn classification are in italics.

Source: Data from Kuhn FA. Chronic frontal sinusitis: the endoscopic frontal recess approach. Operative techniques. Otolaryngol Head Neck Surg 1996;7:222–229.

This bone goes on to form the frontal beak. The frontal ethmoidal cells are further divided depending on how many there are and how far these cells extend into the frontal sinus through the frontal ostium.[16] Kuhn classified frontal ethmoidal cells into types 1 to 4.[14] However, we have modified this classification by clearly defining a frontal ethmoidal cell and by redefining the type 3 and 4 cells (**Table 6–2**).

◆ THE BUILDING BLOCK CONCEPT FOR RECONSTRUCTION OF THE ANATOMY OF THE FRONTAL RECESS

Arranging Building Blocks for Cells

To reconstruct in three dimensions the cells in the frontal recess, building blocks are arranged, one block for each cell.[10,18] This is done as an aid to the dissection of the frontal recess. When operating in this area, the surgeon needs to know exactly which cell is being dissected and in what sequence each sequential cell will be opened so that the frontal recess can be safely and competently cleared. To build a mental picture of the cells in the frontal recess, the coronal CT scans are viewed first. The first cell seen on the coronal CT scan that is anterior to and directly above the insertion of the middle turbinate is, in most cases, the agger nasi cell (**Fig. 6–18**).[10,18] This cell should now be identified on the parasagittal CT scan. Make sure that you use all the information available to you to confirm that the cell seen on the coronal scan is indeed the cell that you have identified on the parasagittal scan. Ask yourself if the cell has air or whether it is partially or completely opacified. Check on both the coronal and parasagittal scans that the cell that you have identified has the expected amount of opacification. A building block is now placed for this cell (**Fig. 6–18**).

The cell directly adjacent (above) to the agger cell is now identified (**Fig. 6–19**). This cell is followed in each coronal

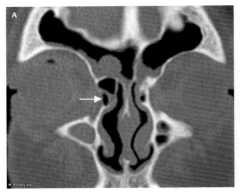

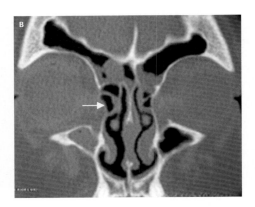

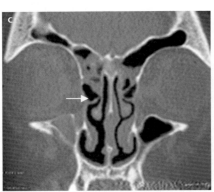

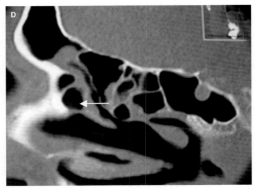

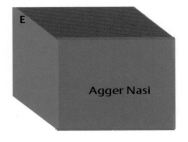

Figure 6–18 **(A)** In this CT scan, the first cell just above the origin of the middle turbinate is marked with a *white arrow*. Follow this cell posteriorly into **(B)** and **(C)** (*white arrows*) then identify this cell in **(D)**, the parasagittal CT scan (*white arrow*). Place a building block for this cell in your 3-D reconstruction. **(E)**

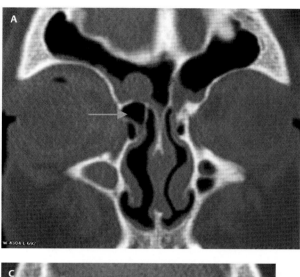

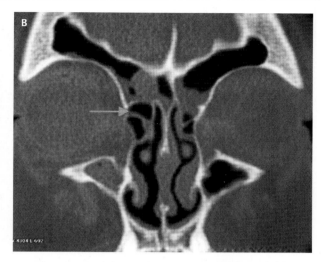

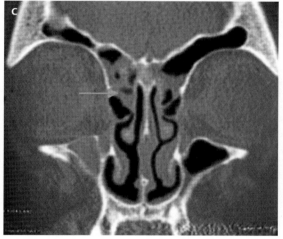

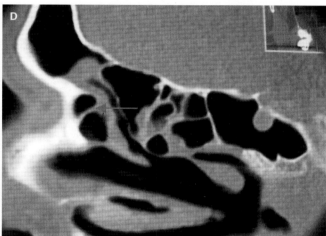

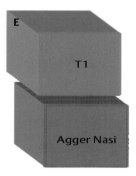

Figure 6–19 (A–E) The cell directly above the agger nasi cell is identified in (**A**, *gray arrow*), the first coronal CT scan and followed in the subsequent coronal scans. This cell (T1) is then identified in (**E**), the parasagittal scan, and a building block placed for it directly above the agger nasi cell.

sequential scan and is again identified on the parasagittal scan by again using all the information available. A building block is placed to represent this T1 cell. There are no other cells associated with the second cell in this example, but if there were, they would be identified in the same manner, and a building block would be placed for each additional cell.

In most patients, a suprabullar cell is present. This cell can be difficult to identify on the coronal scan if the septation between it and the frontal drainage pathway is not

actively sought. This cell lies against the skull base so the skull base forms its roof (**Fig. 6–20**). It is often confused with the frontal sinus drainage pathway especially if it projects forward toward the frontal ostium. A building block should be placed for this cell and another for the bulla ethmoidalis, which lies directly below this cell (**Fig. 6–20**). This sequential identification of each cell first on the coronal scan and then on the parasagittal scan allows the surgeon to begin to build up a 3-D picture of the anatomy of the frontal recess.

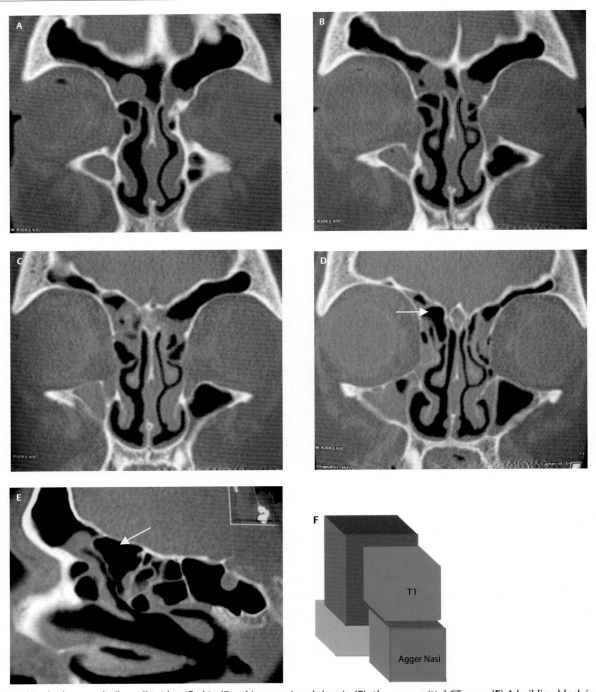

Figure 6–20 (A–F) The suprabullar cell is identified in (**D**, *white arrow*) and then in (**E**), the parasagittal CT scan. (**F**) A building block is placed to represent this cell. A building block is also placed for the small bulla ethmoidalis cell below the suprabullar cell.

Identifying Drainage Pathways, a Critical Concept in Frontal Recess Dissection[16–18]

However, it is not just the cellular construction and the relationship of cells with one another that is important but also the drainage pathway of the frontal sinus around these cells.[16–18] It is critical to identify the drainage pathway of the frontal sinus on the CT scan and then to mentally place

this pathway in the 3-D reconstruction of the anatomy of the frontal recess. The axial CT scans of the frontal sinus and frontal recess are the most helpful in evaluating the drainage pathway. Sequential axial scans are viewed starting in the frontal sinus and progressively following the frontal sinus drainage pathway into the frontal recess. An example of this is presented in **Fig. 6–21**. The black arrows indicate the frontal sinus on the axial CT scans. As the axial

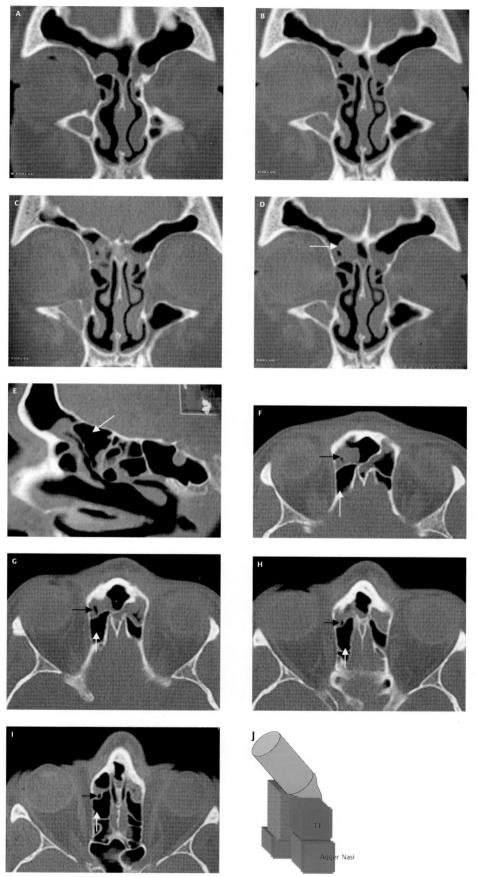

Figure 6–21 (A–J) The axial CT scans (**F–I**) are added to the coronal and parasagittal scans. The *black arrows* in (**F**) to (**I**) indicate the frontal sinus and its drainage pathway. Note how this pathway gets compressed between the T1 cell and the suprabullar cell in (**I**). The suprabullar cell is indicated with a *white arrow* in CT scans (**F**) to (**I**). This posterior and lateral drainage pathway has been added to the 3-D reconstruction in this figure.

scans are followed inferiorly, the T1 cell in the frontal recess comes into view (axial scan **I** in **Fig. 6–21**). Note the change in shape of the frontal sinus during the transition from the frontal sinus to the frontal recess and the thickening of the bone in the region of the nasion where the frontal beak is formed.

During this transition, the anterior wall (beak) also becomes more bowed in the region of the nasion (**Figs. 6–21H, I**). This is the region of the frontal ostium. In this example, the drainage pathway is pushed posteriorly between the suprabullar cell and the T1 cell. During the dissection of the frontal recess, instruments (probes or curettes) are passed along this pathway and the identified cells fractured to clear the pathway.[16] Usually, the pathway is medial or posterior to the cell(s) and the cell(s) can be fractured laterally or anteriorly quite safely. However, when the pathway is anterior, care needs to be taken when fracturing the cell wall posteriorly against the skull base. When the drainage pathway is lateral, the cell wall should be removed by a very gentle fracture if the bone is thin or by placing the instrument as far posterior to the cell wall as possible and fracturing the cell wall anteriorly. For removing residual bony fragments, a through-cutting giraffe forceps can be used. Instruments should not be passed through the roof of a cell as occasionally the surgeon may be confident that he or she is in a cell with space between the roof of the cell and the skull base, but if mistaken and he or she is in the space above the cell, pushing the instrument through the "roof" of the cell will result in the instrument entering into anterior cranial fossa. If instruments are passed along pathways, and this can be done very gently without undue force or pressure, cell walls can be fractured safely clearing the drainage pathway of the frontal sinus without endangering the anterior cranial fossa or the orbit.[16–18]

◆ ANATOMICAL VARIATIONS OF THE FRONTAL RECESS AND FRONTAL SINUS

The Type 1 Cellular Configuration

A T1 configuration is one frontal ethmoidal cell above the agger nasi cell (**Fig. 6–22**). This configuration of a single cell associated with the agger nasi cell is common but also may induce significant variability into the frontal recess. The 3-D conceptualization of this arrangement is two building blocks sitting one on top of the other. The lower building block is the agger nasi cell, and the upper block represents the T1 cell.

The Type 2 Cellular Configuration

A type 2 (T2) configuration consists of two or more frontal ethmoidal cells in association with the agger nasi cell (**Fig. 6–23**). These cells are most commonly seen directly above the agger nasi cell and push the implantation of the uncinate higher on the lamina papyracea.

The CT scan (**Fig. 6–23**) illustrates the T2 configuration on the right side with cell *1* representing the agger nasi cell and cells *2* and *3* the frontal ethmoidal cells above it. Review of the parasagittal scan (not shown here) would confirm the position and placement of these cells. Note that the type 2 frontal ethmoidal cells do not reach above the frontal beak and therefore do not migrate into the floor of the frontal sinus, and removal of these cells does not involve the frontal ostium.[17] If **Fig. 6–6** is reviewed, the diagonally shaded area represents the inferior (floor) part of the frontal sinus.

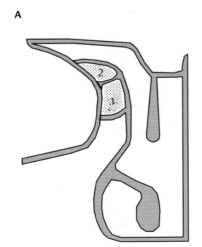

A

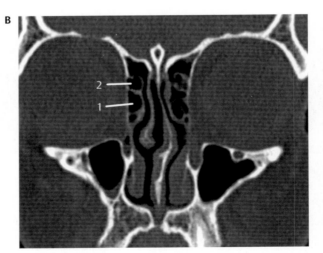

B

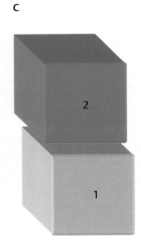

C

Figure 6–22 (A–C) The cell numbered *1* is the agger nasi cell and the cell numbered *2* is the T1 cell. ([A] From Wormald PJ. The agger nasi cell: the key to understanding the anatomy of the frontal recess. Otolaryngol Head Neck Surg 2003;129:497–507. Reprinted with permission.)

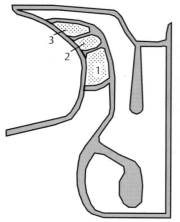
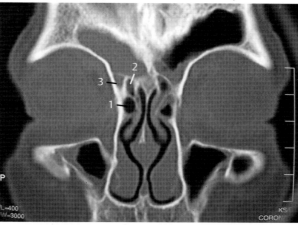
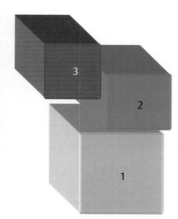

A–C

Figure 6–23 (A–C) The cell numbered *1* is the agger nasi cell, and the cells numbered *2* and *3* are T2 cells. ([A] From Wormald PJ. The agger nasi cell: the key to understanding the anatomy of the frontal recess. Otolaryngol Head Neck Surg 2003;129:497–507. Reprinted with permission.)

Type 3 Cellular Configuration[17]

Further pneumatization of these frontal ethmoidal cells into the floor (inferior part) of the frontal sinus above the frontal beak (into the diagonally shaded area in **Fig. 6–6**) is classified as type 3 (T3) configuration (**Fig. 6–24**). If the section where the frontal sinus becomes the frontal recess is reviewed (**Figs. 6–13 and 6–14**), the transition from the frontal sinus to the frontal recess occurs when the continuous bony line that forms the floor of the frontal sinus disappears. For the cell to be pushing into the floor of the frontal sinus, the cell needs to be visualized above this bony line in the floor of the frontal sinus. T3 cells are usually found in the lateral aspect of the frontal sinus ostium and push the drainage pathway medially and narrow (obstruct) the drainage pathway of the frontal sinus (white arrow, **Fig. 6–24**). The bony beak can be visualized forming the floor of the frontal sinus on the left side of **Fig. 6–24A** (broken white arrow).

The parasagittal scan (**Fig. 6–24B**) shows air in the roof of the T3 cell. In addition, on the parasagittal scan, a cell can be seen above the bulla (suprabullar cell) that almost touches the K3 cell as it pneumatizes forward. This creates a narrowing of the frontal outflow track.

Type 4 Cellular Configuration

The original definition of a T4 cell was an isolated cell within the frontal sinus.[14] This is a very rare occurrence. Most cells appearing as isolated frontal sinus cells are frontal bulla cells that have pneumatized along the skull base into the frontal sinus and protrude from the posterior wall of the frontal sinus into the sinus. A T4 cell is a frontal ethmoidal

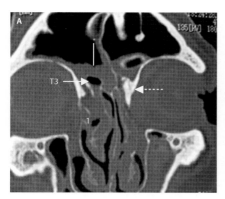
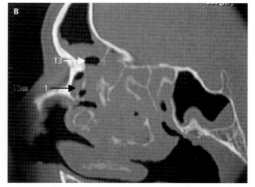
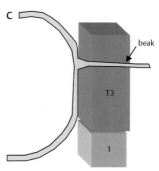

Figure 6–24 (A–C) CT scans of a frontal ethmoidal cell (T3) on the right side pushing into the floor of the frontal sinus. The 3-D reconstruction illustrates this point. The parasagittal scan is taken along the *white line* marked with an asterisk (*). The frontal beak (floor of the frontal sinus) is the bony continuity marked by the *white broken arrow* in the coronal scan (**A**) and by the "beak" in the 3-D reconstruction. The agger nasi cell is numbered *1*.

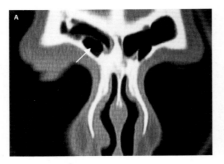
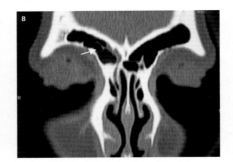
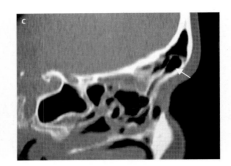

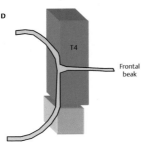

Figure 6–25 In coronal CT scans (**A**) and (**B**), the T4 cell in the right frontal sinus is indicated with a *white arrow*. In parasagittal CT scan (**C**), the T4 cell can be seen pneumatizing from the frontal ethmoidal cell directly above the agger nasi cell. Part (**D**) is a 3-D reconstruction of the cells.

cell that pneumatizes through the frontal ostium and extends further than 50% of the vertical height of the frontal sinus (**Fig. 6–25**).

Clinical Difference between a Type 3 and a Type 4 Cell[17]

If we assume that with very few exceptions all apparent isolated frontal sinus cells originate in the frontal recess or from the bulla ethmoidalis/suprabullar cell, then what is the value in discriminating between T3 and T4 cells? In a recent article,[17] we suggested that it is worthwhile to discriminate between very extensive pneumatization of a frontal ethmoidal or bulla frontalis cell and a cell that pushes only part way into the frontal sinus.[17] Most T3 cells that push into the floor

of the frontal sinus can be removed from below through the frontal ostium. Cells that pneumatize extensively into the frontal sinus may require additional access (combined approach, endoscopic modified Lothrop or osteoplastic flap)[14,17] for removal to be achieved. On review of the patients included in that study,[17] we suggested it would be clinically relevant to create an artificial demarcation between T3 and T4 cells based on the height that the cell extends into the frontal sinus. If the cell extends further than 50% of the height of the frontal sinus on the coronal scans, then the cell is a T4 cell (by our definition) rather than a T3 cell (**Fig. 6–26**). Such a T4 cell would usually not be able to be removed from below unless the frontal ostium was particularly large in its anteroposterior dimension. Further discussion on the selection and techniques used to remove T3 and T4 cells (and frontal bulla cells) is to be found in Chapter 7.

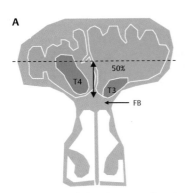
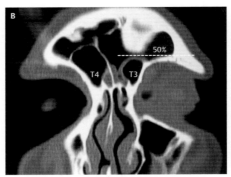
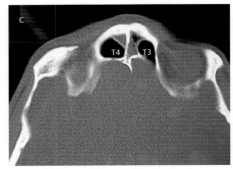

Figure 6–26 (**A**) A drawing of a T3 and T4 cell illustrating that the T3 is less than 50% of the height of the frontal sinus on the coronal scan and that the T4 is greater than 50% of the frontal sinus. FB, frontal beak. In coronal CT scan (**B**), the T4 and T3 cells are illustrated. The axial CT scan (**C**) illustrates how these cells have migrated up the lateral walls of the frontal ostia into the frontal sinuses pushing the drainage pathways medially. (From Wormald PJ, Chan SZX. Surgical techniques for the removal of frontal recess cells obstructing the frontal ostium. Am J Rhinol 1(4):221–226. Reprinted with permission.)

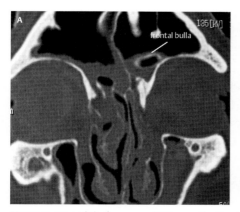
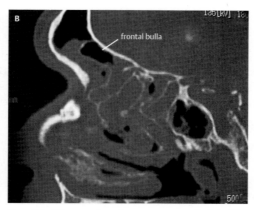
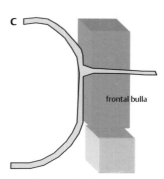

Figure 6–27 In (**A**), the coronal CT scan, the frontal bulla cell (*white arrow*) again appears as an isolated frontal sinus cell, but when (**B**) the parasagittal scan is reviewed, it can be clearly seen pneumatizing from the suprabullar region (*white arrow*).

The posterior wall of the frontal sinus slopes and the definition of a T4 cell (>50% of the height of the frontal sinus on the coronal CT scan under review) is used for the more anterior coronal CT scans as opposed to the CT scans performed in the region of the transition from the frontal sinus to the frontal recess.

Frontal Bulla Cells

Frontal bulla cells are cells that take origin in the suprabullar region and are therefore technically suprabullar cells. They become frontal bulla cells when they migrate through the frontal ostium into the frontal sinus. The skull base always forms the roof of these cells, and they are seen on the parasagittal to hug the skull base as they migrate into the frontal sinus (**Fig. 6–27**). On the axial CT, they can be clearly seen on the posterior wall of the frontal sinus. If these cells protrude

off the skull base in an anterior manner, they will often appear as an isolated cell in the frontal sinus (**Fig. 6–27A**). The clinical importance of these cells is that they push the drainage pathway of the frontal sinus anteriorly, and to be removed, the curette or probe needs to be passed anterior to their wall and the cell wall carefully fractured in a posterior direction.

Intersinus Septal Cells

Intersinus septal cells (ISSCs) are associated with the intersinus septum of the frontal sinus. This cell pneumatizes from the frontal recess through the frontal ostium and its medial wall is the intersinus septum of the frontal sinus. This cell may vary in size, but it always pushes the frontal sinus drainage pathway laterally. If this cell is large, it may significantly compromise the drainage of the frontal sinus (**Fig. 6–28**),

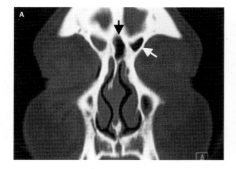
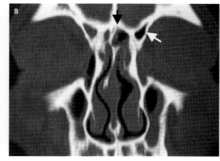
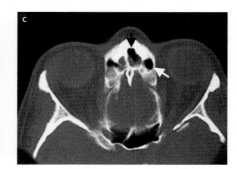
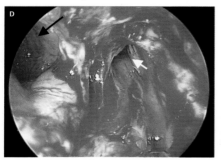

Figure 6–28 In (**A, B**), the coronal CT scans and (**C**) the axial CT scan, the *black arrow* indicates the intersinus septal cell opening into the left frontal sinus and pushing the drainage pathway of the frontal sinus laterally (*white arrow*). (**D**) The picture taken during surgery shows the large opening into the intersinus septal cell (*black arrow*) and the small lateral ostium of the frontal sinus (*white arrow*).

61

and if the lateral wall of the cell is thick, it may not be possible to fracture this wall, and removal with normal handheld instruments may not be possible. In these patients, we do not advocate drilling this septum as the drill always creates significant mucosal trauma often leading to a scarred or stenosed frontal ostium as healing takes place.

◆ IDENTIFYING THE FRONTAL SINUS DRAINAGE PATHWAYS IN THE DIFFERENT ANATOMIC VARIATIONS

Cellular Configurations and Associated Drainage Pathways

In the preceding pages, the various cellular configurations have been detailed. Although it is vital to determine the number of cells in the frontal recess and their relationship to the frontal ostium, it is equally important to understand how these cells interact with the drainage pathway of the frontal sinus.[16–18] One of the most difficult tasks is to determine with each cellular variation where the particular drainage pathway is. In the following examples, the cellular configuration is first established and then for each configuration the drainage pathway is determined. Once the drainage pathway has been identified, the surgeon can work out where to slide the frontal sinus probe or curette so that the cells can each be removed sequentially, clearing the drainage pathway and exposing the frontal sinus ostium.

Type 1/Type 2 Variations

◆ **Configuration with a Posterior Drainage Pathway** To construct the 3-D picture, the first step is to identify the

agger nasi cell on the coronal CT scan and to identify this cell in the parasagittal CT scan (**Fig. 6–29**). The next cell seen in the coronal scans sits directly above this agger nasi cell, and the T1 cell is numbered 2. This cell is also identified on the parasagittal CT. Building blocks are placed for both these cells. The bulla ethmoidalis cell is noted on the parasagittal CT and a building block placed for this cell as well.

The next step is to work out how the frontal sinus drains around these cells. This is a crucial step, as it will determine where the surgeon places instruments during the surgical dissection. Typically, the surgeon will be faced with several potential drainage pathways once the agger nasi cell has been removed. When looking into the frontal recess, he or she needs to know if the pathway is posterior/medial/lateral or anterior as this will determine where the probe or curette is placed. Once this instrument is slid up the pathway, the obstructing cells can be fractured and removed with safety. Failure to correctly identify the frontal drainage pathway on the CT scan will cause indecision and may result in the probe being placed in the incorrect position and potentially, if force is used, may breach the skull base. In this example, the T1/T2 cell occupies the entire anterior region of the frontal recess and pushes the drainage pathway posteriorly. This can be clearly seen in the axial CT scans in the accompanying **Fig. 6–30**. Drawings of the axial scans from the frontal sinus into the frontal recess are presented in conjunction with the axial CT scans to help identify the drainage pathway and follow it from the frontal sinus into the frontal recess.

The first two steps were to construct a 3-D picture and to place the drainage pathway in this 3-D picture. The combined 3-D reconstruction is presented in **Fig. 6–31**.

If the surgeon had created a 3-D mental picture of the anatomy before the surgery, he or she would have visualized that after the agger nasi cell had been removed, the T1 cell

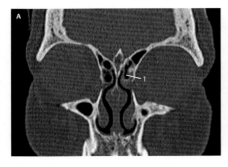
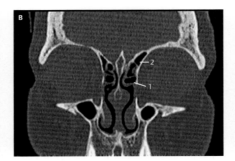
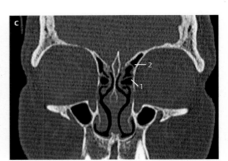
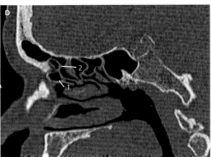
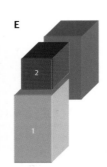

Figure 6–29 The agger nasi cell (*1*) and T1 cell (*2*) are first identified on (**A–C**) the coronal scans and then on (**D**) the parasagittal CT. (**E**) A building block is placed for each of these cells. The bulla ethmoidalis cell is seen on the parasagittal scan and a block placed for this cell.

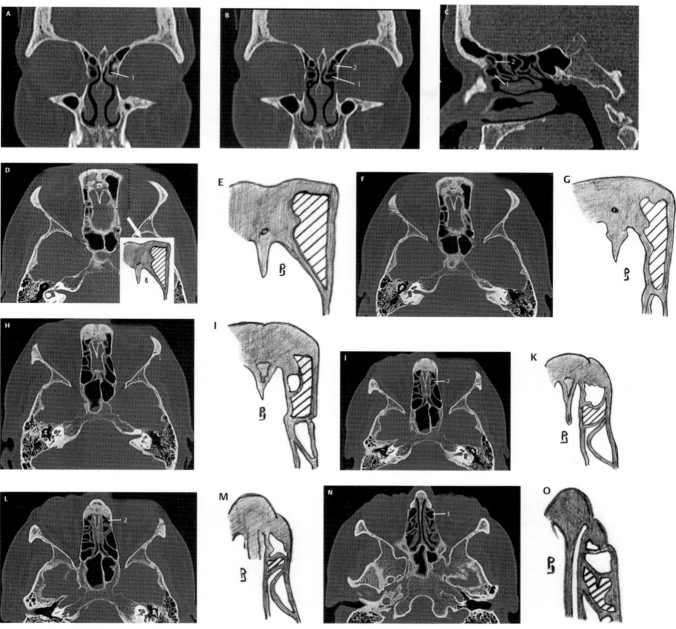

Figure 6–30 (A, B) The coronal CT scans, (**C**) the parasagittal CT scan, and (**D, F, H, J, L, N**) axial CT scans are presented. The frontal sinus drainage pathway on each of the axial CT scans is illustrated on (**E, G, I, K, M, O**) the accompanying drawings (*shaded area*), and this pathway can be followed from the frontal sinus into the frontal recess around the cells in the frontal recess.

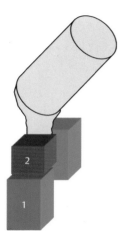

Figure 6–31 Cell *1* is the agger nasi cell and cell *2* is the T1 cell. Note the frontal sinus drainage pathway is posterior to the T1 cell (*2*) and anterior to the bulla ethmoidalis.

would be visible in the medial region of the frontal recess and the frontal sinus drainage pathway would be visible posterior to this cell.

◆ **Type 1/Type 2 Configuration with a Medial Drainage Pathway** This is one of the more common configurations where the T1/T2 cell sits directly above the agger nasi cell

and pushes the drainage pathway of the frontal sinus in a medial direction. This is caused by the upward continuation of the uncinate process forming the medial wall of not only the agger nasi cell but also of the T1/T2 cell before finally implanting on the lamina papyracea. In this example, the T1 cell is seen first and is identified on the parasagittal CT scan (**Fig. 6–32**). The agger nasi cell is small and is seen in

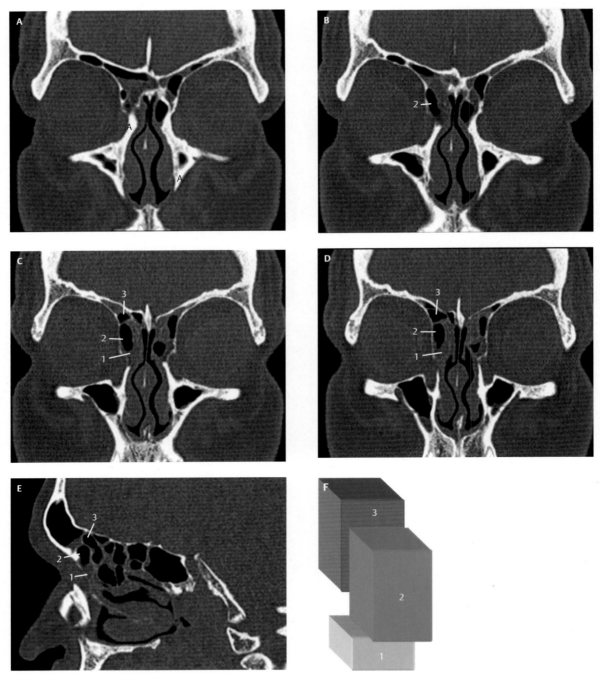

Figure 6–32 On the right side on (**A–D**), the coronal CT scans, the T1 cell (*2*) and agger nasi cell (*1*) are identified. These cells are then identified on (**E**) the parasagittal CT scan. The suprabullar cell (*3*) is

seen in (**C**) the coronal CT scans and in (**E**) the parasagittal CT scan. (**F**) A 3-D image is created with the building blocks.

the coronal CT scan (**Fig. 6–32C**) just as the insertion of the middle turbinate comes into view. The agger nasi cell (numbered *1*) should also be identified on the parasagittal scan. On the coronal CT scan, a cell appears on the skull base (numbered *3*). This is a suprabullar cell and is clearly seen on the parasagittal CT scan (**Fig. 6–32E**). To create the 3-D image, a building block is placed for each one of these cells.

The next step is to identify the drainage pathway in this example. The series of axial CT scans are used and the frontal sinus identified. The frontal sinus is followed inferiorly into the frontal recess. Note how the first cell seen on the axial scans is the suprabullar cell (numbered *3*) and that the drainage pathway is initially anterior to this cell before it becomes medial to both this cell and the T1 cell (**Fig. 6–33**).

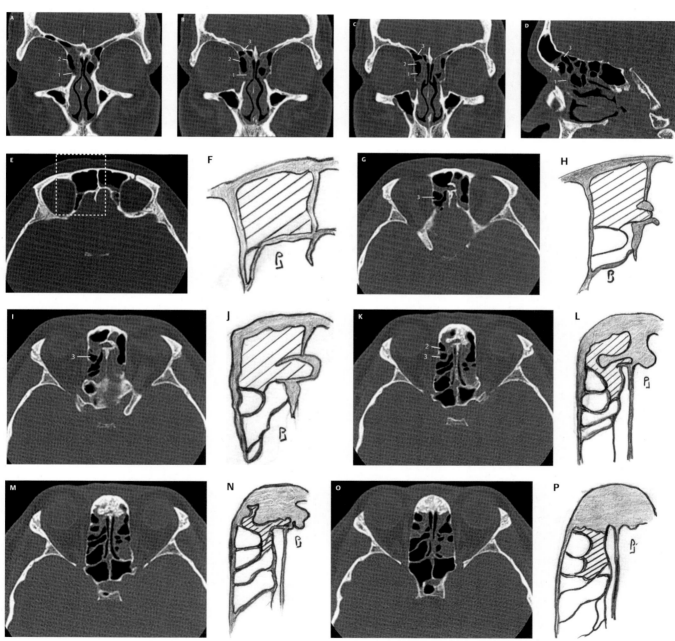

Figure 6–33 (A–D) The axial CT scans (**E, G, I, K, M, O**) are added so that the frontal sinus drainage pathway can be followed from the frontal sinus into the frontal recess. Note how the pathway passes initially anteriorly to the suprabullar cell (*3*) before passing medial to both the suprabullar cell and the T1 cell (*2*).

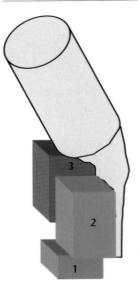

Figure 6–34 The 3-D picture of the cells in the frontal recess (*1*, agger nasi cell; *2*, T1 cell; *3*, suprabullar cell) complete with the frontal sinus drainage pathway.

To complete the 3-D image, the frontal sinus drainage pathway is drawn into the building block 3-D picture (**Fig. 6–34**). This allows the surgeon to have a complete understanding of the anatomy of this frontal recess and to have a surgical plan to place the probe or curette and remove the frontal recess cells thereby clearing the frontal ostium.

◆ **Type 1/Type 2 with an Anterior Drainage Pathway** If the T1/T2 cell expands so that it touches the suprabullar cell and the frontal process of the maxilla in the lateral region, it will push the drainage pathway of the frontal sinus antermedially (**Fig. 6–35**). This T1/T2 configuration is illustrated by the following example on the left side. The first cell identified in scan (B) is the agger nasi cell numbered *1*. Directly above this cell is the frontal ethmoidal T1 numbered *2*. A building block is placed for each of these cells. In the parasagittal scan (E), the suprabullar cell numbered *3* and bulla ethmoidalis numbered *4* can be seen. Building blocks are also placed for these cells.

It is important to be able to pick the drainage pathway of the frontal sinus around these cells. In this patient, the frontal sinus drains antermedial to the T1 cell as the T1 cell is attached to the anterior skull base and laterally to the frontal process of the maxilla (**Fig. 6–36**). Again, if we follow the drainage

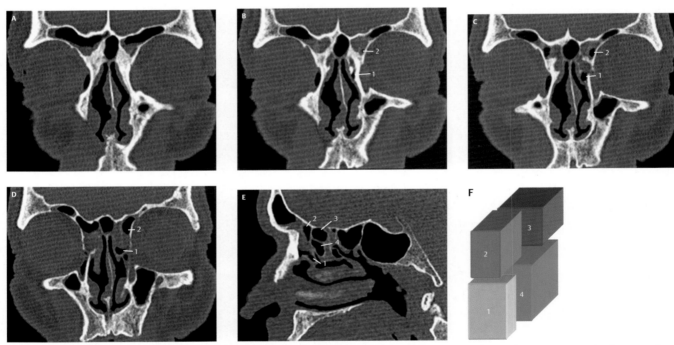

Figure 6–35 (A–D) The coronal CT scans are viewed and each sequential cell identified and followed from anterior to posterior. **(F)** A building block is placed for each cell. Additional cells can be seen in **(E)** the parasagittal scan that are not seen in the coronal scans as the coronal scans do not go far enough posteriorly. Building blocks are also placed for these cells.

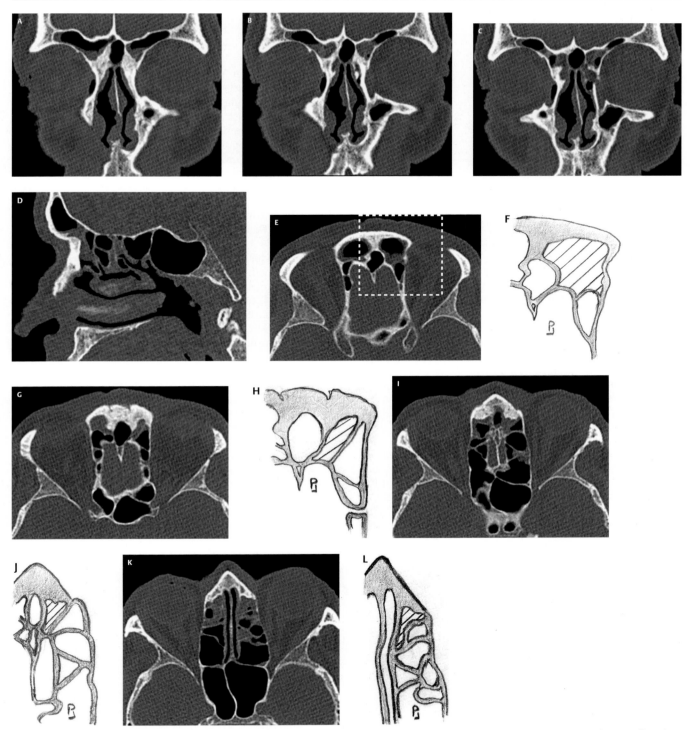

Figure 6–36 (A–L) The following series of CT scans includes (**E–L**) the axial scans with associated drawings to illustrate how the T1 cell pushes the frontal sinus drainage pathway antermedially.

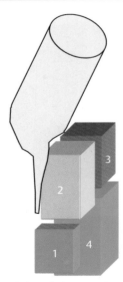

Figure 6–37 This frontal sinus drainage pathway is placed in the 3-D picture. The T1 cell (*2*) pushes the pathway antermedially.

pathway of the frontal sinus from the frontal sinus inferiorly into the frontal recess on the axial CT scans, the relationship between the pathway and the T1 cell is clearly seen.

If we now add this drainage pathway to the 3-D picture, a clear understanding of the relationship of these frontal recess cells and the drainage pathway should be established (**Fig. 6–37**).

To add a clinical perspective, the following intraoperative pictures of this example are shown (**Figs. 6–38A, B**). The surgeon should be able to visualize the configuration of the frontal recess cells and drainage pathway and should be able to

picture this in his or her mind before surgery is commenced. When the surgeon looks up into the frontal recess, the T1/T2 cell should be seen anteriorly with the drainage pathway antermedially.

Once the agger nasi cell is removed and the T1 cell identified, the surgeon should know where to look for the frontal sinus drainage pathway. In this patient, if attempts were made to push probes posterior to the cell, injury and penetration of the skull base would be possible. If the pathway is recognized, however, a small probe can be slid up between the T1 cell and the medial wall of the olfactory fossa and the cell fractured laterally thereby clearing the frontal recess. Review the Chapter 6 tutorials and video on the accompanying DVD to see how this configuration was dissected and how it compares to your mental 3-D reconstruction of the anatomy.

◆ **Type 1/Type 2 with a Lateral Drainage Pathway** If a T1/T2 cell abuts the insertion of the middle turbinate as it inserts to the skull base, the frontal sinus drainage pathway may be pushed laterally. This is relatively uncommon but is important to recognize when it occurs. It is more common for a medially based cell to be situated much higher and for it to be in contact with the frontal sinus septum and is termed an *intersinus septal cell* (ISSC; see below). Recognition of a T1/T2 cell situated medially in the frontal recess will allow the frontal sinus drainage pathway to be sought laterally and allow this cell to be safely removed and the frontal ostium to be fully exposed. The following example shows the medially placed T1 cell with the lateral drainage pathway (**Fig. 6–39**).

Now that the 3-D reconstruction of the cells has been made, the drainage pathway of the frontal sinus into the frontal recess is established. This is done by following the frontal sinus inferiorly into the frontal recess. Note in

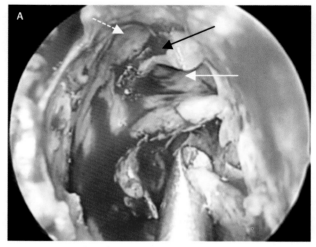

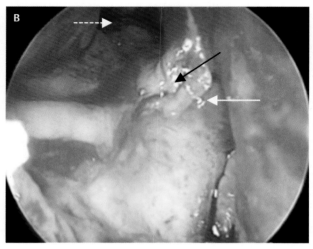

Figure 6–38 In (**A**), the frontal sinus drainage pathway is indicated with a *broken white arrow*. The anterior wall of the T1 cell is indicated with a *solid black arrow* and the cell itself indicated with a *solid white arrow*. The suction curette indicates the suprabullar

cell. Part (**A**) is prior to removal of the anterior wall of the cell, and in (**B**), after the wall has been removed, the frontal ostium is seen (*broken white line*) with the insertion of the T1 cell indicated by the *solid black line* and the cell by the *solid white line*.

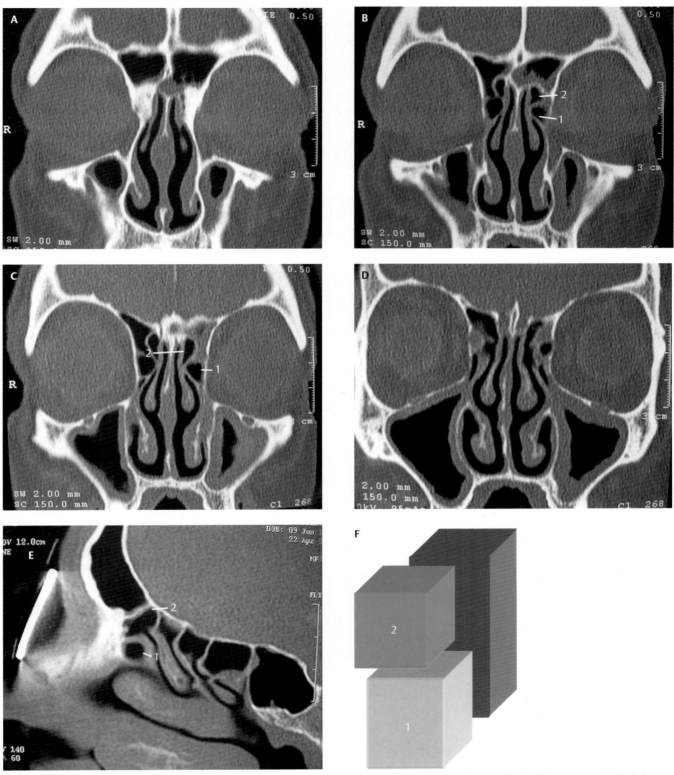

Figure 6–39 The agger nasi cell (*1*) and the T1 cell (*2*) are identified on (**A–D**) the coronal CT scans and on (**E**) the parasagittal CT scan. (**F**) A building block is placed for each of these cells. A large bulla ethmoidalis extending to the skull base is seen behind these cells on (**E**) the parasagittal CT scan and (**F**) a building block is also placed for this cell.

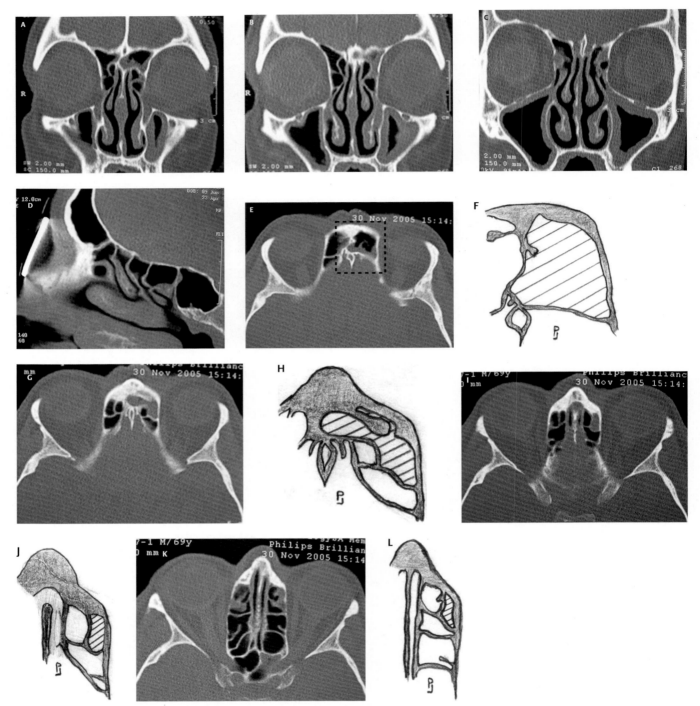

Figure 6–40 (A–L) When **(E–L)** the axial CT scans and accompanying diagrams are reviewed, note how the frontal sinus drainage pathway is first pushed anteriorly **(G)** then laterally **(I, K)**.

Fig. 6–40 the shaded region progressing from the frontal sinus lateral to the T1 cell and then medial to the agger nasi cell.

Although the axial CT scans are the primary scans we use to follow the frontal sinus drainage pathway, it is also important to view the coronal CT scans as well. In this example, the frontal drainage pathway can be clearly seen in the coronal CT scans as well as the axials but what can also be seen from the coronal scans is how the frontal sinus drainage pathway swings below the T1 cells to move over the roof of the agger nasi cell to continue medial to this cell into the nasal cavity. This pathway can now be placed with

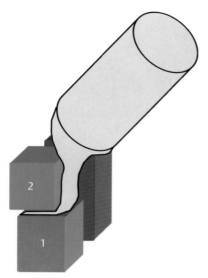

Figure 6–41 When both the coronal CT scans and axial CT scans are viewed together, note how the drainage frontal sinus pathway drains initially lateral to the T1 cell before swinging medial to the agger nasi cell.

the building blocks to form the 3-D picture providing the surgeon with a clear understanding of the left frontal recess (**Fig. 6–41**).

If the surgeon had a clear 3-D picture of the anatomy, then he or she would be able to visualize the T1 cell in the medial region of the frontal recess and the frontal sinus drainage pathway draining lateral to it. To aid the surgeon's conceptualization of this situation prior to any surgery being performed, the following clinical intraoperative pictures are provided (**Fig. 6–42**). Make sure that this is how you visualized the frontal recess after looking at the scans, and if not, redo the scans until the clinical pictures are what you would expect to see.

Type 3/Type 4 and Intersinus Septal Cell Variations

◆ **Type 3/Type 4 with a Medial Drainage Pathway** In most cases, a T3 cell will enter the frontal ostium laterally pushing the frontal sinus drainage pathway medially (**Fig. 6–43**). In this example, on the right side the T3 cell occupies most of the frontal ostium as it pushes through the ostium into the floor of the frontal sinus. The steps for creating a 3-D image remain to identify each cell seen in each sequential coronal CT scan on the parasagittal scan. In this case, the T3 cell is the first one identified, followed by a small agger nasi cell and a small medial cell. The suprabullar cell also pushes forward onto the back wall of the T3 cell (**Fig. 6–43**).

The next step is to identify the drainage pathway of the frontal sinus. This is best appreciated in the axial CT scans and drawings. Note how the frontal drainage pathway is narrowed progressively as the T3 cell occupies more and more space and squeezes the frontal drainage pathway medially. The small medial cell (numbered 3) again pushes this pathway more antermedially by occupying some of the medial drainage space (**Fig. 6–44**).

Once the frontal sinus drainage pathway around the cells has been established, this can be drawn on the 3-D image giving the surgeon a clear understanding of the anatomy of the frontal recess and allowing a surgical plan to be developed for the frontal recess dissection (**Fig. 6–45**).

In some patients with very large T3 cells, only the medial wall that occupies the frontal ostium may need to be removed, and the roof of the cell may be left if this no longer obstructs the frontal sinus drainage pathway. This is usually only done if there is technical difficulty in reaching the roof or dome of the cell or if the roof is too thick to fracture easily with a probe or a curette. A T4 cell is a cell that usually enters the frontal sinus along the lateral wall of the frontal ostium pushing the drainage pathway medially. However, in the coronal plane it can be

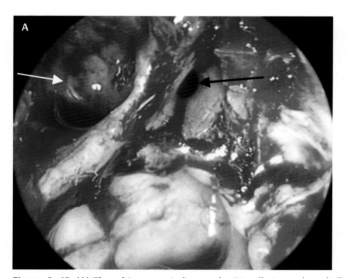

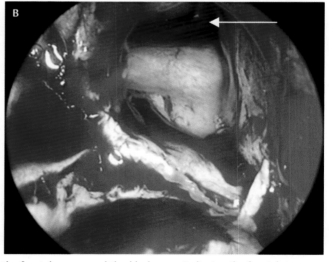

Figure 6–42 (**A**) The *white arrow* indicates the T1 cell situated medially in the frontal recess, and the *black arrow* indicates the frontal sinus drainage pathway. (**B**) The *white arrow* indicates the frontal ostium after the T1 cell has been removed.

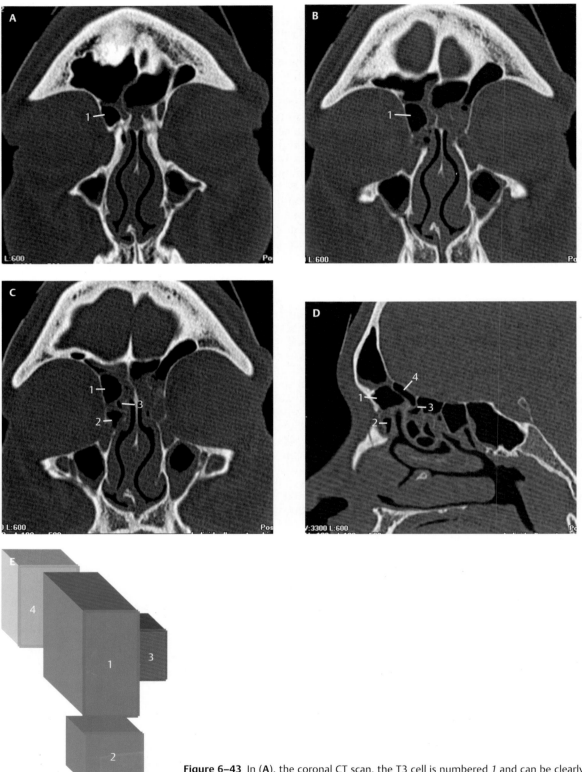

Figure 6–43 In (**A**), the coronal CT scan, the T3 cell is numbered *1* and can be clearly seen on (**E**) the parasagittal scan. Note the small medial cell numbered *3* in (**C**) the CT scans.

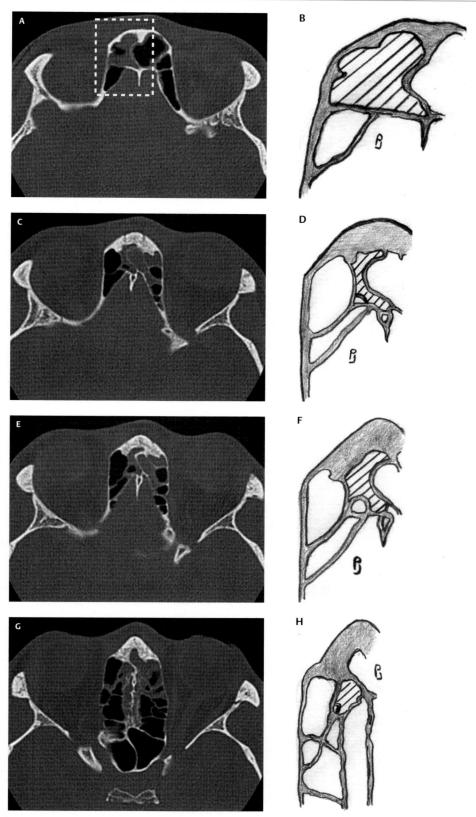

Figure 6–44 (A, C, E, G) The coronal, parasagittal, and axial CT scans are presented with (**B, D, F, H**) drawings of the medial frontal sinus drainage pathway (*shaded area*) on the right side of the patient. (**A, C**) Note in these axial CT scans the small medial ethmoidal cell pushing into the drainage pathway from behind. This cell was numbered *3* in the previous figure.

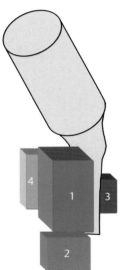

Figure 6–45 The frontal sinus drainage pathway is medial to the T3 cell (*1*) and lateral to the cell numbered *3*.

seen that the cell extends more than 50% of the vertical height of the frontal sinus on the scan. The decision as to whether it would be possible to remove this is based on the anterior-posterior dimension of the frontal ostium best evaluated on the parasagittal scan. In this case, the frontal ostium is widely patent and the T4 cell was able to be removed from below. If this is not believed to be the case, then a modified Lothrop is performed for access and

in all cases this provides more than adequate access to be able to remove T4 cells.

◆ **Type 3/Type 4 with a Posterior Drainage Pathway** This situation occurs when a frontal ethmoidal cell pneumatizes through the frontal ostium and occupies the entire anterior region of the frontal ostium pushing the frontal sinus drainage pathway posteriorly. In some instances, this pathway can be very narrow and there may be significant risk when trying to manipulate a probe or curette through this narrow space due to the proximity of the skull base. In most patients, this portion of the skull base (fovea ethmoidalis) is quite thick and there should be resistance to penetration. This should be checked on the CT scan prior to the probe being placed. In the following example, the T3 cell almost reaches 50% of the vertical height of the frontal sinus on the coronal scan, and therefore it is marginal if this cell should be termed a T3 or a T4 cell (**Fig. 6–46**). In addition, this patient has undergone prior surgery, and the agger nasi cell and bulla ethmoidalis have been removed.

Once the 3-D picture has been created, the drainage pathway of the frontal sinus around these cells needs to be established. In **Fig. 6–47**, the T3 cell can be seen occupying most of the frontal ostium and pushing the drainage pathway of the frontal sinus posteriorly but anterior to the residual suprabullar cell.

If the frontal sinus drainage pathway is now added to the 3-D picture, its posterior course can be clearly seen and understood (**Fig. 6–48**).

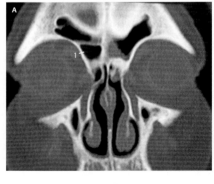
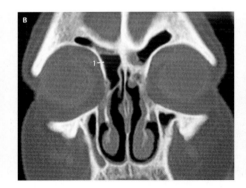
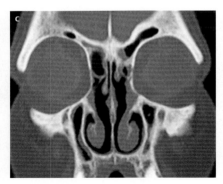

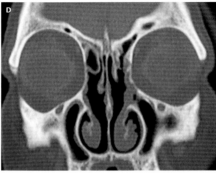
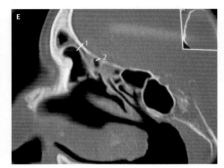
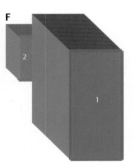

Figure 6–46 (A–D) In these coronal CT scans, the large T3 cell (*1*) occupies almost the entire frontal recess. (**E**) In the parasagittal CT scans, a small residual suprabullar cell (*2*) is seen just posterior to the T1 cell on the skull base. A building block is placed for each of these cells to create the 3-D picture.

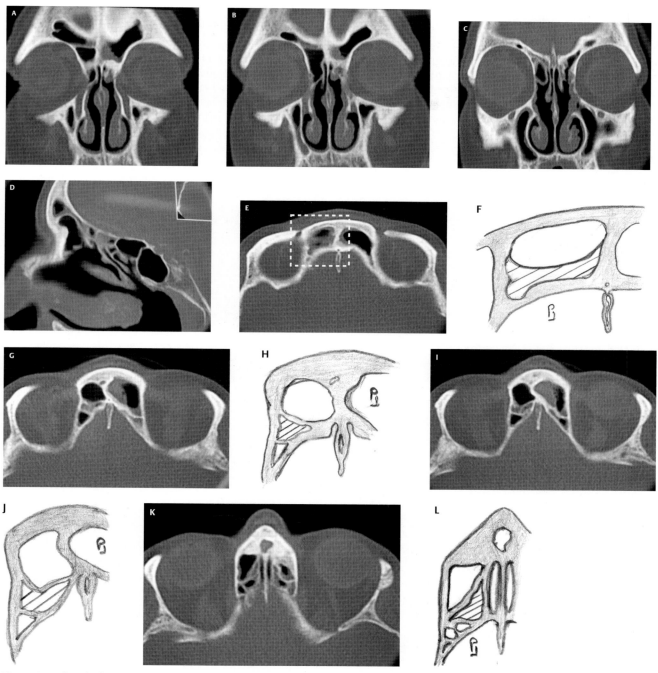

Figure 6–47 (E, G) These axial CT scans and (**F, H**) the accompanying drawings illustrate the frontal sinus drainage pathway (*shaded area*). Note how compressed this pathway becomes and how closely associated it is with the posterior wall of the frontal sinus and fovea ethmoidalis. Fortunately in the patient, this region of the skull base has thick bone and the risk of skull base penetration while placing the probe or curette should be low. If the surgeon remains concerned, a frontal mini-trephine can be placed, as discussed in Chapter 7.

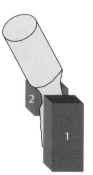

Figure 6–48 The frontal sinus drainage pathway can be seen behind the T3 cell and anterior to the residual suprabullar cell.

◆ **Type 3/Type 4 and Intersinus Septal Cell with an Anterior Drainage Pathway** If the T3/T4 cell is large and fills the frontal ostium, it will push the drainage pathway either medially, posteriorly, or anteriorly. The direction it pushes the drainage pathway is primarily dependent upon where the cell is based (anteriorly, laterally, or posteriorly) and

what other cells are present in the frontal ostium/recess. If for example an ISSC is present, this will further narrow the frontal sinus drainage pathway and this cell will tend to push the pathway laterally. In such a case, the pathway will be squeezed between these two cells. An example of this anatomic variation is presented in **Fig. 6–49**. In **Fig. 6–49B**,

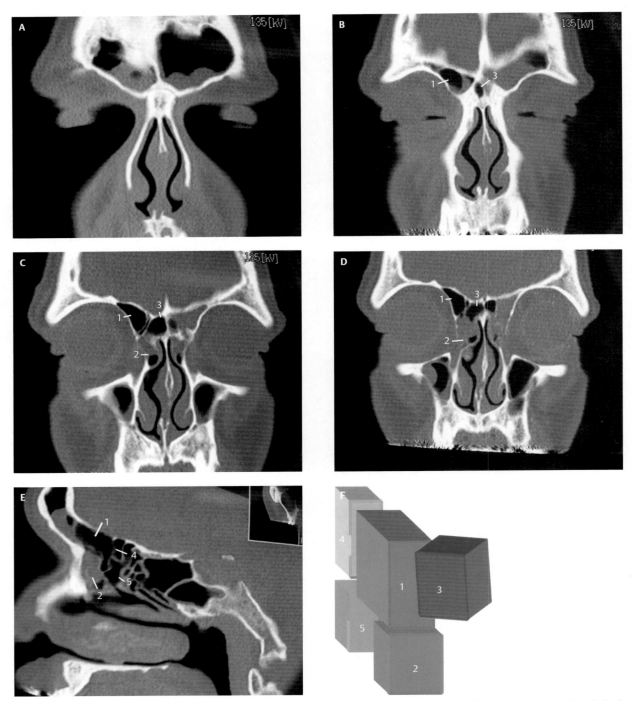

Figure 6–49 **(A)** In this CT scan, no cells are seen. **(B)** In this scan, the T3 cell is seen as the beginning of the ISSC (numbered *3*). **(C)** The agger nasi cell (numbered *2*) is first seen on this scan.

(E) In this scan, the suprabullar cell (numbered *4*) and the bulla ethmoidalis (numbered *5*) are also seen. **(F)** A building block is placed for each numbered cell.

the T3 cell is numbered *1* and the ISSC is numbered *3*. The T3 cell extends further through the frontal ostium than the ISSC and initially pushes the drainage pathway anteriorly. As the drainage pathway continues inferiorly, the ISSC is encountered, which squeezes the pathway between itself and the T3 cell. If a building block is placed for each of these cells seen and for the bulla ethmoidalis (cell number *5*) and suprabullar cell (cell number *4*), a 3-D picture of this complex cellular configuration is established.

To work out the frontal sinus drainage pathway, the axial scans are viewed from cranial to caudal. As the frontal sinus is followed into the frontal recess, its pathway is initially pushed anteriorly by the T3 cell, then as the pathway reaches the ISSC, it is squeezed between the T3 cell and the ISSC (**Fig. 6–50**).

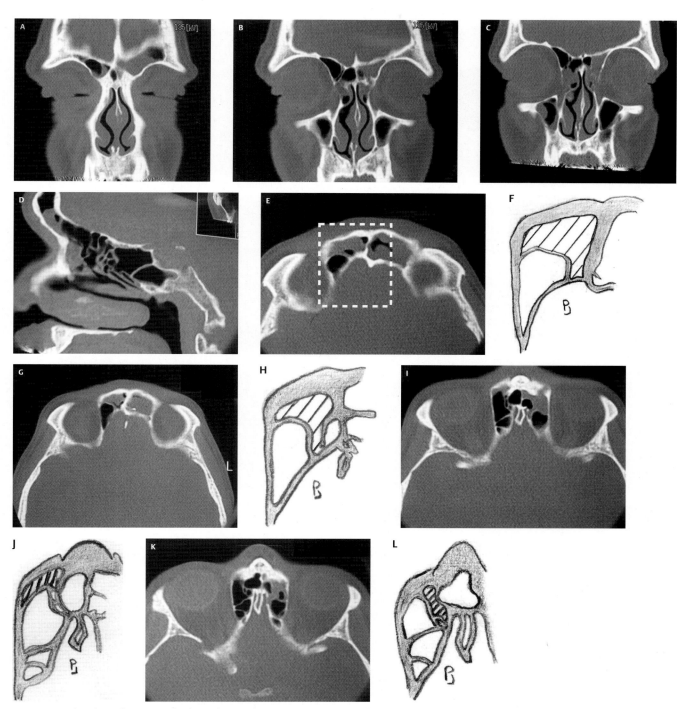

Figure 6–50 (A–L) To determine the frontal sinus drainage pathway, the frontal sinus is followed from within the frontal sinus (axial CT scan [**E**]) into the frontal recess (**G**) and (**H**). Note how the drainage pathway is first squeezed anteriorly and the ISSC is seen (in scans [**F**] to [**H**]), between the ISSC and the T3 cell.

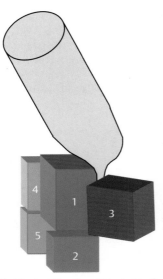

Figure 6–51 Block *1* is the T3 cell and block *3* is the ISSC. Note how the drainage pathway is squeezed between these cells.

If the 3-D image is reviewed, the frontal sinus drainage pathway can be placed among these cells. This allows the surgeon to decide exactly where the probe or curette should be placed so that it can be slid up the drainage pathway and the cells that are obstructing the frontal ostium can be removed (**Fig. 6–51**).

To further illustrate this complex anatomic arrangement of cells, the following intraoperative photograph shows the ISSC and T3 cell (**Fig. 6–52A**); the curette (**Fig. 6–52B**) illustrates where the drainage pathway would be sought after the CT scans had been thoroughly evaluated and the 3-D reconstruction performed and drainage pathway determined. **Figure 6–52C** is the frontal ostium once these cells have been removed.

Frontal Bulla Cell with Anterior Drainage Pathway

This cell has been commonly confused with the type 4 cell of the original Kuhn classification in which a type 4 cell was defined as an isolated cell within the frontal sinus. In **Fig. 6–53**,

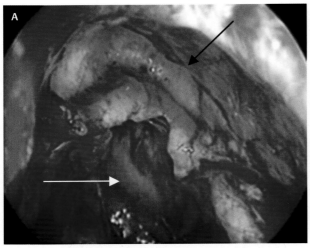

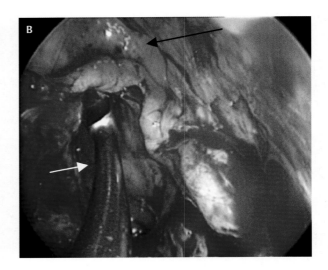

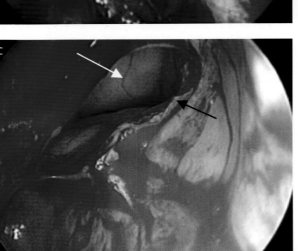

Figure 6–52 (A) This operative photograph shows the ISSC extending from the intersinus septum (region of the *black arrow*) laterally and the T3 cell (*white arrow*). Note that the roof of the T3 cell is higher than that of the ISSC as could be seen in the CT scans. **(B)** The curette is placed into the drainage pathway and slid into the frontal sinus allowing both the ISSC and the T3 cell walls to be fractured and removed from the frontal ostium. **(C)** The frontal ostium after removal of the ISSC and T3 cell walls. The *white arrow* indicates the frontal sinus and the *black arrow* the edge of the ISSC wall where it attaches to the intersinus septum.

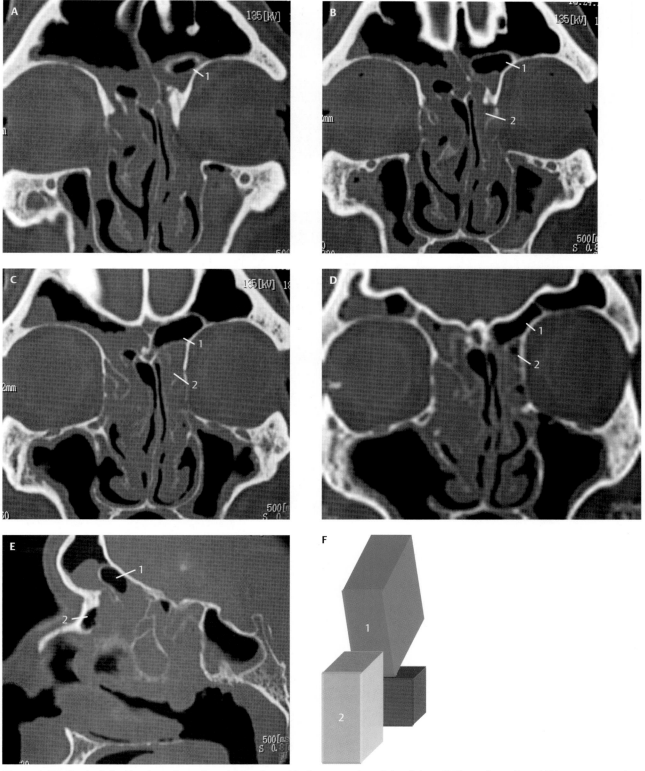

Figure 6–53 On the left side, the cell numbered *1* is a frontal bulla cell. (**A–D**) This can be followed in the coronal sequential CT scans into the suprabullar space. (**E**) The parasagittal CT scan illustrates the origin of the cell. The cell numbered *2* is an agger nasi cell. (**F**) A building block is placed for each cell seen to complete the 3-D conceptualization of the anatomy in this region.

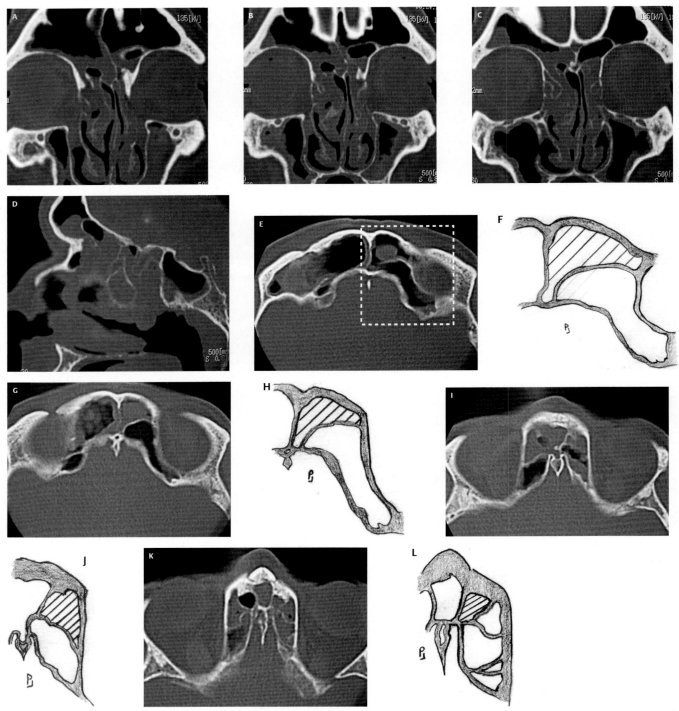

Figure 6–54 (A–L) In the axial CT scans (**E–H**), note how on the left the suprabullar cell attaches to the posterior wall of the frontal sinus (skull base) as it creeps along the skull base into the frontal sinus. It pushes

the frontal sinus drainage pathway anteriorly. This can be seen on the axial CT scan drawings where this pathway is shaded allowing this drainage pathway to be clearly followed on the scans.

the cell numbered *1* appears to be an isolated cell in the frontal sinus. When this cell is followed posteriorly and viewed on the parasagittal scan, however, it is quite clear that this is a frontal bulla cell that originates in the suprabullar space and pneumatizes forward along the skull base into the frontal sinus.

In **Fig. 6–54**, the frontal sinus drainage pathway can be followed from the frontal sinus into the frontal recess. Note how the sinus drains anterior to the frontal bulla cell and then medial to the agger nasi cell.

If the 3-D picture is reviewed and the frontal sinus drainage pathway is placed, a true 3-D image of both the

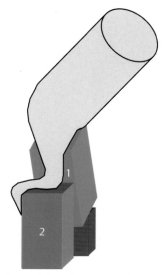

Figure 6–55 The frontal sinus drainage pathway is initially pushed anteriorly to the bulla frontalis cell (numbered *1*) before moving medial to the agger nasi cell (numbered *2*).

anatomy and the pathway is formed. This allows planning of each step of the surgical resection of the frontal bulla cell (**Fig. 6–55**).

◆ CONCLUSION

The anatomy and common variations that occur in the frontal recess are poorly understood by a large number of endoscopic sinus surgeons. The agger nasi cell is proposed as the key to the understanding of this complex area. Fine-cut coronal and parasagittal reconstructed CT scans aid the identification of each individual cell and allow the surgeon to formulate a clear and precise surgical plan. Axial scans are useful for the identification of the frontal sinus drainage pathway. Before surgery is performed in the frontal recess, the surgeon needs to fully review all the CT scans in the three planes and assume that he or she is in a surgical simulator. The surgeon should be able to mentally create an image of the cellular structure in the frontal recess and then be able to place the frontal sinus drainage pathway in this 3-D picture. The surgeon should then go through the surgical steps to be performed. For example: create an axillary flap, raise the flap, remove the anterior wall of the agger

nasi cell, place the curette medial or behind the agger nasi cell, and remove this cell (medial wall and roof). Identify the residual cells and the frontal sinus drainage pathway around these cells. Place the suction curette along the frontal sinus drainage pathway without force and fracture the cell and remove the cell(s) exposing the frontal ostium. Such a surgical plan formulated from a thorough understanding of the anatomy allows a confident dissection of a complex and difficult area.

References

1. Kaliner MA, Osguthorpe JD, Fireman P, et al. Sinusitis: bench to bedside. Current findings, future directions. J Allergy Clin Immunol Suppl 1997;99:S829–S847

2. Davis WE, Templer J, Parsons DS. Anatomy of the paranasal sinuses. Otolaryngol Clin North Am 1996;29(1):57–74

3. Schaefer SD, Manning S, Close LG. Endoscopic paranasal sinus surgery: indications and considerations. Laryngoscope 1989;99:1–5

4. Kennedy DW, Senior BA. Endoscopic sinus surgery - a review. Otolaryngol Clin North Am 1997;30:313–330

5. Stammberger H, Kennedy D. Paranasal sinuses: anatomic terminology and nomenclature. Ann Otol Rhinol Laryngol Suppl 1995;167:7–16

6. Thawley SE, Deddens AE. Transfrontal endoscopic management of frontal recess disease. Am J Rhinol 1995;9(6):307–311

7. Keros P. Über die praktische Bedeutung der Niveauunterschiede de Lamina cribrosa des Ethmoids. Laryngol Rhinol Otol (Stuttg) 1965;41:808–813

8. Special endoscopic anatomy. In: Stammberger H, Hawke M, eds. Functional Endoscopic Sinus Surgery - The Messerklinger Technique. Philadelphia, PA: B.C. Decker Publishers; 1991;61–90

9. Floreani SR, Nair SB, Switajewski MC, Wormald PJ. Intranasal endoscopic ligation of the anterior ethmoidal artery – a cadaver study. Laryngoscope 2006;116:1263–1267

10. Wormald PJ. The agger nasi cell: the key to understanding the anatomy of the frontal recess. Otolaryngol Head Neck Surg 2003;129:497–507

11. Kew J, Rees G, Close D, Sdralis T, Sebben R, Wormald PJ. Multiplanar reconstructed CT images improves depiction and understanding of the anatomy of the frontal sinus and recess. Am J Rhinol 2002;16(2):119–123

12. Bolger WE, Butzin CA, Parsons DS. Paranasal sinus bony anatomic variations and mucosal abnormalities: CT analysis for endoscopic sinus surgery. Laryngoscope 1991;101:56–64

13. Wake M, Takeno S, Hawke M. The uncinate process: a histological and morphological study. Laryngoscope 1994;104:364–369

14. Kuhn FA. Chronic frontal sinusitis: the endoscopic frontal recess approach. Operative techniques. Otolaryngol Head Neck Surg 1996;7:222–229

15. Kim KS, Kim HU, Chung IH, Lee JG, Park IY, Yoon LH. Surgical anatomy of the nasofrontal duct: anatomical and computed tomographic analysis. Laryngoscope 2001;111:603–608

16. Wormald PJ. The axillary flap approach to the frontal recess. Laryngoscope 2002;112(3):494–499

17. Wormald PJ, Chan SZX. Surgical techniques for the removal of frontal recess cells obstructing the frontal ostium. Am J Rhinol 2003;17(4):221–226

18. Wormald PJ. Surgery of the frontal recess and frontal sinus. Rhinology 2005;43(2):83–85

19. Jacobs JB. 100 years of frontal sinus surgery. Laryngoscope 1997;107:1–36

7

Surgical Approach to the Frontal Sinus and Frontal Recess

The frontal recess has always been considered to be the most difficult area to dissect.[1-4] This is largely due to its location behind the beak of the frontal bone.[5] There are three major philosophies regarding the management of disease of the frontal recess and sinus. The minimal invasive sinus technique, or MIST, advocates management of the maxillary sinus and associated transitional spaces (hiatus semilunaris and ethmoidal infundibulum) without performing surgery in the frontal recess.[6-8] This philosophy states that treatment of the maxillary sinus and associated transitional spaces will result in clearance of the frontal recess and sinus disease. There are few published papers supporting this theory, and all publications come from the same group of investigators.[6-8] Until there is substantial evidence that this approach works for a broad spectrum of frontal sinus and frontal recess disease, we do not advocate this approach. The second philosophy is that the frontal recess and frontal sinus should only be operated upon if there are symptoms that can be directly ascribed to the frontal sinus such as frontal headache and pain. Whereas we agree that surgery on a diseased frontal sinus or recess that is symptomatic is appropriate, we disagree that this is the only indication for surgery in this region. Patients who present with nasal obstruction, postnasal drip, purulent rhinorrhea, or anosmia or who have radiologic disease in the frontal sinus or recess need to have this region surgically addressed. These patients have their diseased maxillary sinuses, ethmoid and sphenoid sinuses addressed, and it makes no sense that just because they do not have localized frontal pain or tenderness, the frontal sinus should not be addressed as well. It has been well recognized that retained or residual cells in the frontal recess/sinus is one of the most common causes of endoscopic sinus surgery (ESS) failure.[1,2]

In this chapter, we present our graduated approach to surgery of the frontal recess and sinus. In the easy frontal recess and sinus, simple maneuvers in terms of endoscopy and surgical access (axillary flap) are advocated and are in most cases sufficient to allow clearance of the frontal recess

and frontal ostium. In the difficult frontal recess or sinus, the additional technique of frontal sinus mini-trephination is presented. These difficult patients may also benefit from the surgeon having computer-aided surgical navigation available.

The mainstay of our surgical technique is the axillary flap technique. This technique has similarities to the frontal sinus rescue procedure described by Kuhn et al[9] in that mucosal flaps are raised during the surgery on the frontal ostium. However, the major difference is that the frontal sinus rescue procedure is designed for the management of patients who have failed previous standard ESS and have a stenosed frontal ostium. The axillary flap technique is designed for all patients undergoing frontal recess or sinus procedure including previously operated patients. The central concept of the axillary flap procedure is removal of the anterior wall of the agger nasi cell. This is not new and was described by May and Schaitkin[10] as part of their naso-frontal approach (NFA 1) to the frontal sinus. Schaefer and Close[11] have advocated a similar approach with removal of the bone above the insertion of the middle turbinate. The major difference between these approaches and the axillary flap approach is the elevation of a mucosal flap that can be replaced at the end of the procedure to cover the raw exposed bone that is seen after removal of the anterior wall of the agger nasi cell. This prevents granulation tissue from forming over the exposed bone with subsequent scarring and cicatrization of this area. Such scarring can pull the upper extension of the middle turbinate laterally and close off the anterior aspect of the frontal recess. This may in turn lead to blockage of the frontal outflow tract and result in recurrent frontal sinusitis.

May and Schaitkin advocated enlarging the frontal ostium in their NFA II and III approaches.[10] This is unnecessary and not advocated in the vast majority of patients as the removal of residual cells within the frontal recess with the exposure of the frontal ostium is usually sufficient to achieve resolution of frontal sinusitis. It is our philosophy that where patients have cells in the frontal recess or frontal ostium that obstruct the outflow of the frontal sinus, these should be removed without enlarging the frontal ostium. Even very small frontal ostia can function well if their outflow pathway is not obstructed and the patients should be given the opportunity to see if the natural size of their frontal ostium is sufficient. In some patients, especially those with severe mucosal disease, this ostium may become edematous and obstruct, and if this causes symptoms, then enlargement of the ostium is indicated. However, this occurs in the minority of cases and it is not possible to predict which patients with a particular frontal ostium size will obstruct and become symptomatic. In most patients, the only way to enlarge a frontal ostium is with a drill. Drilling in the frontal ostium without creation of the largest possible ostium is likely to result in an intense fibrous reaction from the exposed raw bone and in most cases will increase the likelihood of postoperative scarring and stenosis. As can be seen in Chapter 9, enlargement of the frontal ostium is usually done with a modified Lothrop procedure and very rarely with a Draf type 2 (unilateral enlargement of the frontal ostium) procedure due to the increased incidence of fibrosis and stenosis seen with unilateral drilling on the frontal ostium.[12] This is especially true for patients who have severe mucosal disease and in whom the inflammatory process continues in the postoperative period.[13]

◆ INDICATIONS FOR FRONTAL RECESS AND FRONTAL SINUS SURGERY

Our philosophy is that a patient who has undergone appropriate medical therapy (including systemic steroids) and is then found to have mucosal thickening in the frontal recess or sinus should have all cells cleared from the frontal recess and the frontal ostium exposed (**Fig. 7–1**).[13–16] In patients without significant disease of the frontal recess, only the diseased sinuses are addressed, and the frontal recess is left untouched. Partial surgery of the frontal recess is never indicated. If only the roof of the agger nasi cell is removed or one of the frontal ethmoidal cells is removed, scarring is likely to result. The cells in the frontal recess are usually in close approximation, and partial clearance of cells will very likely result in adhesions forming between these closely approximated surfaces with obstruction of the drainage pathway of the frontal sinus. Our philosophy is an all-or-nothing approach. The frontal recess is either left entirely alone or all the cells are removed from the recess with visualization of the frontal ostium.

◆ PREOPERATIVE PATIENT EVALUATION

Understanding the Anatomy and Planning the Surgery

In a patient who is to undergo frontal recess and sinus surgery, the computed tomography (CT) scans need to be carefully assessed and the three-dimensional (3-D) reconstruction of the anatomy performed (see Chapter 6). Once the surgeon has a clear understanding of the anatomy, a surgical plan should be formulated. An example of such a plan is presented in **Fig. 7–2**. In this patient, after uncinectomy and middle meatal antrostomy, an axillary flap is performed to expose the anterior face of the agger nasi cell. This is removed with the Hajek Koeffler punch (Storz) and the agger nasi cell visualized. The malleable frontal sinus curette* (Medtronic ENT) is placed posteromedially to the agger nasi posterior wall and roof and the cell removed by fracturing it forward. The resultant debris is removed with a microdebrider. The residual roof of the agger nasi cell is cleared and the T3 cell visualized. After careful assessment

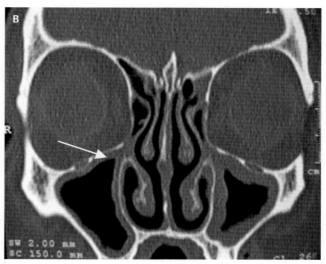

Figure 7–1 In coronal CT scan (**A**), note the mucosal thickening in the left frontal sinus (*white arrow*) and recess with a normal right frontal sinus and recess. In coronal CT scan (**B**), note the mucosal thickening of the right maxillary sinus (*white arrow*). In this patient, the left frontal recess would be cleared of cells and the frontal ostium identified while on the right side no surgery would be performed in the frontal recess. Both maxillary sinuses would be surgically addressed.

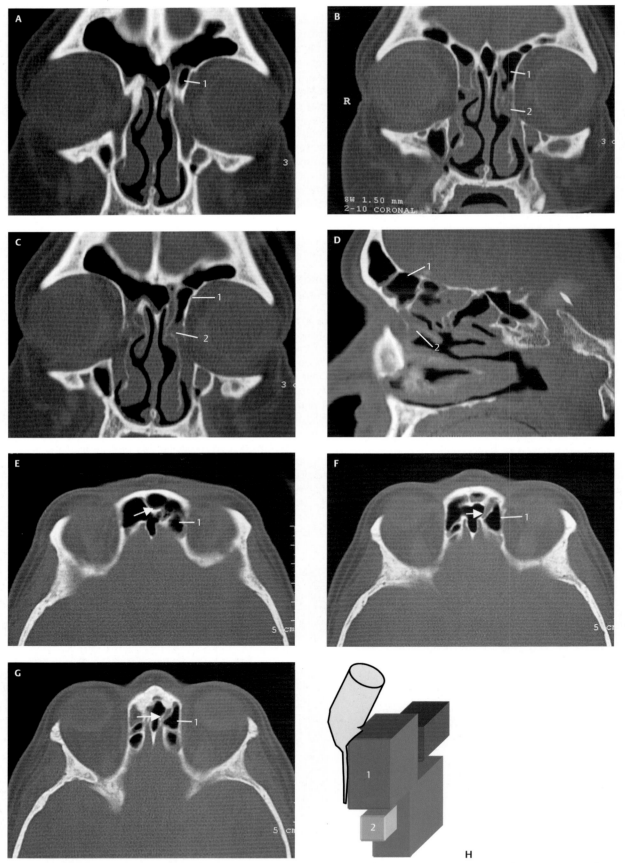

Figure 7–2 (A–H) The T3 cell is numbered *1* in (**A–C**) the coronal CT scans and (**D**) the parasagittal CT scan and the agger nasi cell is numbered *2*. In (**E–G**), the axial CT Scans, the T3 cell is numbered *1* with the frontal sinus drainage pathway medial to this cell (*white arrow*).

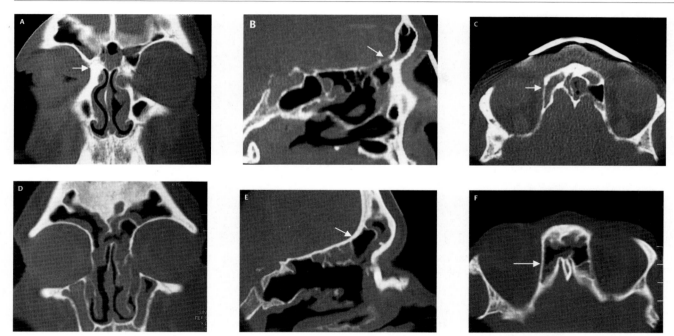

Figure 7–3 (A–F) The patient in CT scans (**A–C**) has a very narrow AP diameter. In (**A**), the clue to the narrow AP diameter is the thick bone (*white arrow*) on either side of the frontal ostia, which is not present in the equivalent coronal CT scan of the patient with a wide AP diameter as seen in (**D**). In the parasagittal CT scans (**B, E**), the difference between (**B**) with a narrow AP and (**E**) with a wide AP is apparent (*white arrow*). On the axial CT scans (**C, F**), the difference in the AP diameter is again apparent (*white arrow*).

of the axial scans, we know that the frontal sinus drains medially around this cell and the suction curette is slid along this drainage pathway into the frontal sinus and the cell fractured laterally and removed. An angled microdebrider blade is used to clear debris, and small residual bony fragments are cleared with giraffe forceps and the malleable frontal sinus hooked probe* (Medtronic ENT). The frontal ostium is visualized but all mucosa around the frontal ostium is preserved.

Factors Affecting the Degree of Difficulty of the Surgery

Surgeons should recognize potentially difficult frontal recesses by studying the CT scans at the time the patient is listed for surgery.[13–16] Recognition of potential difficulties can aid the surgeon when discussing the likelihood of success of the procedure and the probable need for further surgery such as enlargement of a very narrow frontal ostium. In addition, the likelihood of possible ancillary procedures such as a mini-trephination of the frontal sinuses can be assessed and discussed with the patient. The need for computer-aided surgical navigation is assessed at the same time. The surgeon should assess the degree of difficulty of the surgery, and if the case is too difficult for the surgeon's level of expertise, the patient should be referred to a specialist rhinologist. The following features should be sought on the CT scan.

Narrow versus Wide Anteroposterior Diameter of the Frontal Ostium

Patients who have a wide anteroposterior (AP) diameter will usually have a technically easier operation and will in most cases have a better prognosis for maintenance of health of the sinuses after surgery. This reflects the postoperative size of the frontal ostium that can be achieved without drilling on the ostium. **Figure 7–3** illustrates a patient with a narrow AP diameter compared with a patient with a wide AP diameter. Note the space available to operate in the wide-diameter patient.

Single Agger Nasi Cell or Simple T1/T2 Configuration

Single agger nasi cell is the simplest configuration in the frontal recess, and after removal of this cell, the frontal ostium can be identified (**Fig. 7–4**). A simple cell configuration of one or two associated frontal ethmoidal cells is also relatively easy to deal with in the frontal recess.

Frontal Ethmoidal Type 3 and 4 Cells Obstructing the Frontal Sinus Ostium

Even after an axillary flap approach, these cells can be difficult to access, and surgery often requires an angled endoscope thereby increasing the difficulty of the surgery. In addition, a

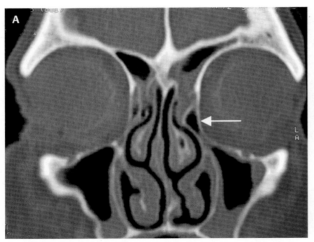
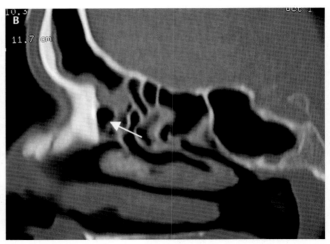

Figure 7–4 In coronal CT scan (**A**), the left frontal recess has a single agger nasi cell (*white arrow*). This can be clearly seen on the parasagittal CT scan (**B**) (*white arrow*). This is the simplest configuration seen in the frontal recess.

high T3 or T4 cell can be confused with the frontal sinus, and the CT scans should be reviewed to ensure that the drainage pathway of the frontal sinus is identified and instrumented. These cells need to be removed to allow adequate ventilation and drainage of the frontal sinus. An example of this is given in **Fig. 7–5**.

Small Frontal Sinus with Poorly Pneumatized Agger Nasi Cells and Small Frontal Ostium

This can be problematic if the frontal sinus is completely opacified and the surgeon wishes to ensure the pus or inspissated mucus is cleared from the sinus. Failure to clear thick mucus or pus from the frontal sinus may allow the inflammatory process to continue in the postoperative period in the region of the frontal ostium. This delays the healing proc-

ess and can increase the risk of scarring and adhesions in the frontal region. An example of a small frontal sinus ostium is presented in **Fig. 7–6**.

New Bone Formation in the Region of the Frontal Ostium

New bone formation in the region of the frontal ostium and recess often indicates osteitis of the surrounding bone. If the new bone obstructs the frontal ostium, removal will often leave vascular and inflamed exposed bone that will usually produce significant fibrosis and scar tissue. Re-stenosis and obstruction of the frontal ostium will often result. An example of the CT scan appearance of new bone formation is shown in **Fig. 7–7**. Cultures of removed bone should be performed and patients then be started on appropriate antibiotics. Consideration should also be given to suppressing the

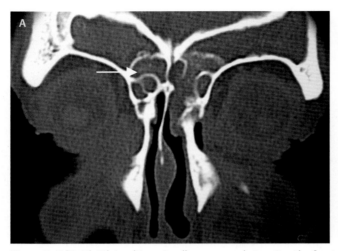
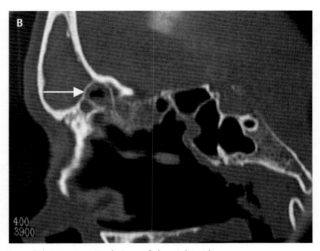

Figure 7–5 (A, B) Bilateral type 3 cells are seen obstructing the frontal ostium. (**B**) A parasagittal view of the right side.

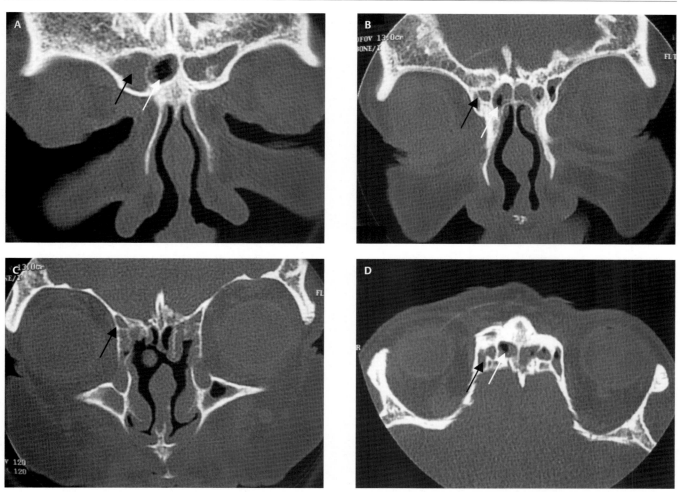

Figure 7–6 (A–D) This patient has a combination of an intersinus septal cell (*white arrow*) and a small frontal sinus on the right (*black arrow*) and on the left. The small drainage pathway of the frontal sinus on the right is marked with a black arrow in scans (**B–D**).

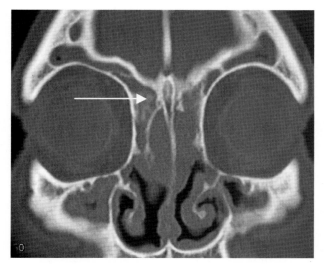

Figure 7–7 New bone formation is seen in the right frontal recess (*white arrow*).

inflammatory response during the healing period. This can be done by giving a 3-week course of oral steroids. Alternatively or in combination with the oral steroids, the mini-trephine cannulas can be left in place for 3 to 4 days postoperatively and the frontal sinuses irrigated with prednisolone drops after saline douching. This serves two purposes as it keeps the frontal ostium clear of blood clot, which can contribute to fibrosis and scarring, and the prednisolone diminishes the inflammatory response in the immediate postoperative period.

Previous Surgery with Scarring of the Frontal Recess

Previous surgery, especially amputation of the middle turbinate with lateralization of the remnant, with associated scar tissue formation can make exposure of the frontal ostium difficult. Diagnosis is made both on the CT scan appearance and on endoscopy. The CT scan can show residual cells and new bone formation and the endoscopy can confirm the

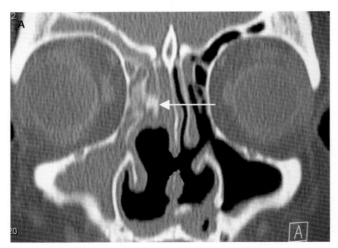

Figure 7–8 (A, B) The amputated right middle turbinate is marked with a *white solid arrow* in both the CT scan and on the endoscopic view. The uncinate remains and abuts the retained anterior ethmoid cells obstructing the drainage of the frontal sinus. Significant scarring is seen between the lateralized residual middle turbinate and lateral nasal wall (uncinate) on the endoscopic view.

presence of scar tissue in the frontal recess. An example is shown in **Fig. 7–8**.

Extensive Disease in the Frontal Recess

Some patients may have extensive and severe disease in the frontal recess (**Fig. 7–9**). In this example, the patient has allergic fungal sinusitis with expansion of the frontal recess and double densities visible on soft tissue settings (*white arrow*). The frontal recesses in this patient were filled with highly vascular polyps and inspissated fungal material. Not only were the normal anatomic landmarks distorted in this patient but also there was extensive bleeding in the frontal recess as the polyps were removed. As previously stated, such vascularity can significantly increase the degree of difficulty for the surgeon during removal of the polyps and cells and during identification of the frontal ostium.

Resected Middle Turbinates and Patients with Few or No Operative Landmarks

Patients who have previously had resection of their middle turbinates can be difficult to manage as the absence of the middle turbinate has removed the most important operative landmark (**Fig. 7–10**).

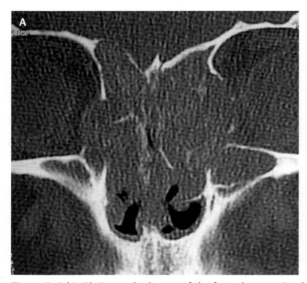

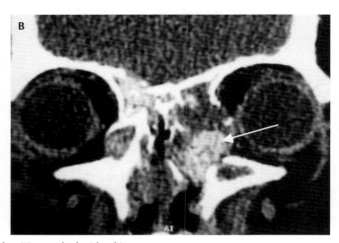

Figure 7–9 (A, B) Expansile disease of the frontal recess. Double densities marked with *white arrow*.

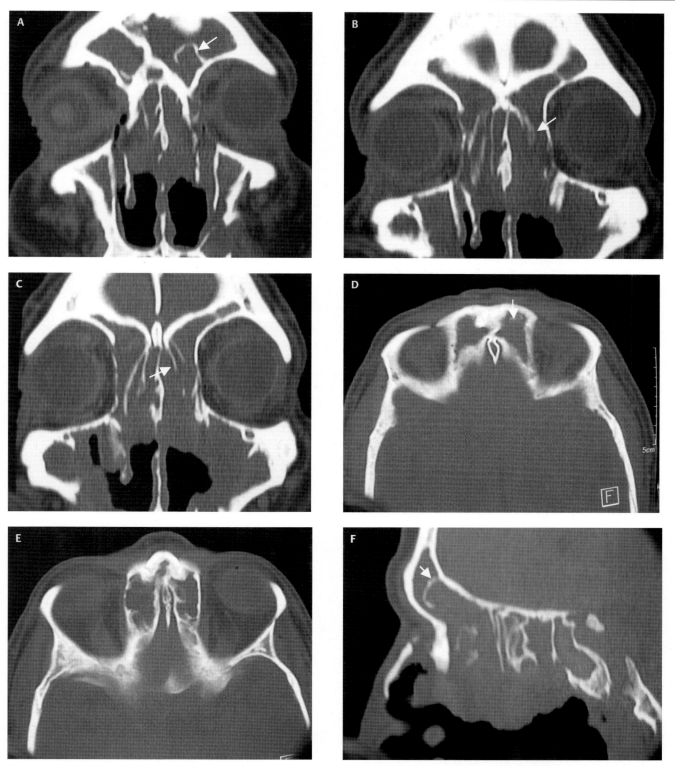

Figure 7–10 (A–F) In scan (**A**), the *white arrow* indicates a residual T4 cell in the frontal sinus. In scans (**B, C**), the *white arrow* indicates the previously resected middle turbinate. Note the absence of the inferior turbinate on the left side from previous surgery. In scans (**D**) and (**F**), the *white arrow* indicates the anterior wall of the T4 cell. Note extensive polyps visible on all scans.

◆ SURGICAL TECHNIQUE

If there are polyps present, identification of the residual middle turbinate can be difficult (**Fig. 7–11**). The first step is to identify the maxillary ostium and to clear the maxillary sinus of polyps using the maxillary trephination procedure if necessary (see Chapter 5). This will allow positive identification of the lamina papyracea, an important landmark in the further dissection of the frontal recess. The next step is to gently debride the polyps to reveal the underlying bony structures: the septum, olfactory recess, residual middle turbinate, and posterior bony choanae. If the anatomy is still unclear, the polyps in the region of the posterior bony choanae and the anterior face of the sphenoid should be removed. As the polyps are cleared, the residual superior turbinate may come into view. If this has also been previously resected, then the polyps should be cleared from the skull base. The fovea ethmoidalis and olfactory fossa are normally in the same horizontal plane in this posterior region of the ethmoids, and gentle removal of polyps (without bone removal) should safely expose the skull base and residual superior turbinate. The previously identified lamina papyracea is an important additional landmark.

The next step is to identify the ostium of the sphenoid sinus (the method is described in Chapter 8) and enlarge the natural ostium of the sphenoid. This will allow the skull base to be positively identified and the dissection can then be brought along the skull base anteriorly. The surgeon needs to check the CT scan to identify the position of the anterior ethmoid artery and whether it is suspended within a mesentery or not. Using the lamina papyracea as the lateral landmark, the skull base as the superior landmark, and the beak of the frontal maxillary process as the anterior landmark, the frontal recess can be identified. In most patients, a small stump of residual middle turbinate can be seen, and an axillary flap is performed and the axilla opened with a Hajek

Koeffler punch. Now that all the landmarks for the frontal recess are established, the clearance of the frontal recess can continue according to the 3-D reconstruction of the anatomy of that recess with localization of the frontal sinus drainage pathway and stepwise removal of each remaining cell in the frontal recess.

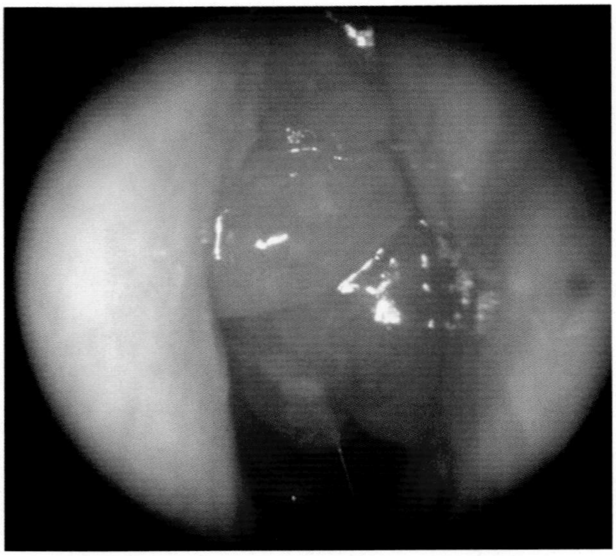

The following techniques are used for frontal recess and frontal sinus dissection:

1. Endoscopy
2. The axillary flap technique
3. Mini-trephination of the frontal sinus
4. Computer-aided surgery (CAS), or image-guided surgery

The combination of endoscopy utilizing the least-angled endoscope with the axillary flap technique is used for all frontal recess and sinus dissections. Frontal sinus mini-trephination and CAS are used in the more difficult frontal recess dissections.

Endoscopy

The classic description of the technique for dissection in the frontal recess and frontal sinus involves the use of 30-degree, 45-degree, and 70-degree endoscopes.[2–4] It is also recognized that the more angulated the endoscope, the greater the degree of difficulty of the dissection because of surgeon disorientation and the manipulation of angled instruments. A recent paper[17] described increasing unwanted trauma within the nose and sinuses from the passage of angulated instruments during dissection.[17] **Figure 7–12** shows the

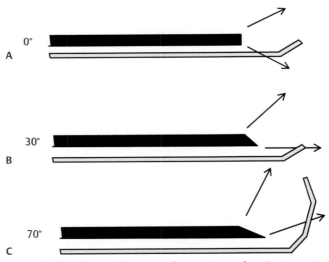

Figure 7–12 When a 0-degree endoscope is used, an instrument passed beneath the scope will be in the center of the field of view as demonstrated in (**A**). If a 30-degree endoscope is used and a similar instrument is passed beneath the scope, the instrument tip is on the extreme periphery of the field of view. If the tip of the instrument is brought into the center of the field of view, the endoscope is pushed upward by the instrument and the area of dissection may no longer be visible. If a 45-degree or 70-degree endoscope is used, the instrument needs to be sufficiently angulated to be able to be placed in the center of the field of view as demonstrated in (**C**).

Figure 7–11 Massive nasal polyps with no identifying landmarks visible.

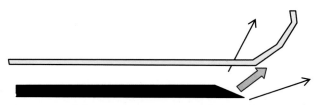

Figure 7–13 If the instrument is positioned above the scope, the undersurface of the instrument is visualized (*black arrow*) and the working tip is not seen. This can be potentially dangerous if the working tip of the instrument is in a potentially vulnerable region of the frontal recess.

increasing angulation of instruments required to keep the tip of the instrument in the center of the field of dissection with increasing angulation of the endoscope.

As illustrated in Chapter 1, the vast majority of surgery is conducted with the endoscope placed above the instrument. If the endoscope is placed below the instrument, the working tip of the instrument cannot be visualized (**Fig. 7–13**).

The degree of difficulty is further increased if the surgical field is bloody. It can take longer for an angled endoscope (30 degree or 70 degree) and a curved instrument to be positioned in the frontal recess before surgical dissection can take place. If bleeding in the surgical field is profuse, the surgical field may be covered in blood before the dissection begins. This situation may lead to frustration for the surgeon at the slow progress of surgery, and the surgeon may be tempted to proceed with dissection despite poor visibility. This can potentially lead to inadvertent injury to the skull base, lamina papyracea, or anterior ethmoidal artery. As with any surgical procedure, the wider the exposure, the easier the operation becomes. Most surgeons can recall a situation when they needed the aid of a senior colleague during a procedure, and that the first thing that the senior surgeon did was to widen the incisions to improve the surgical access. The axillary flap technique was designed to try to overcome some of the problems mentioned above by optimizing access

to the frontal recess and allowing a large part of the dissection in the frontal sinus to be performed with a 0-degree telescope (**Fig. 7–14**).[13–16]

The Axillary Flap Technique

The first step in the axillary flap approach is to make an incision ~8 mm above the axilla of the middle turbinate and to bring this forward by ~8 mm.[15] The incision is turned vertically down to the level of the axilla. It is then carried back under the axilla onto the root of the middle turbinate (**Fig. 7–15**). A no. 15 scalpel blade on a no. 7 BP scalpel blade holder is used to make these incisions.

The full-thickness mucosal flap is then raised with a suction Freer elevator. It is important to ensure that the tip of the suction Freer is on bone when the flap is being raised and that the flap extends behind the root of the middle turbinate (**Fig. 7–16**). The flap is connected at its inferior edge to tissue under the axilla of the middle turbinate. This needs to be separated from the flap with a sickle knife or scalpel (see videos on the accompanying DVD) before the flap is tucked between the middle turbinate and the septum. Failure to expose the vertical bone of the middle turbinate just below where it attaches to the lateral nasal wall will often result in this bridge of tissue remaining. If this bridge of tissue is pulled on by an instrument or suction, then the flap will be pulled from between the turbinate and septum into the frontal recess. Here it may either be inadvertently removed by a microdebrider or instrument or irritate the surgeon by requiring it to be tucked away regularly before surgery can proceed. By exposing the vertical upper bony part of the middle turbinate, the surgeon ensures that the bridge of tissue is divided, and once the flap is tucked between the middle turbinate and septum, it should not be seen again until it is retrieved at the end of surgery to cover the raw bone of the newly created axilla.

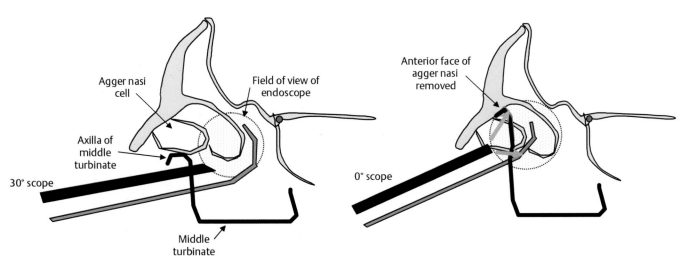

A

B

Figure 7–14 **(A)** This drawing illustrates the need to use an angled endoscope to view the frontal recess with the axilla intact (the visual field is the shaded circle). After opening the anterior wall of

the agger nasi cell **(B)**, a 0-degree endoscope can be used to view and operate in the frontal recess without having to use angled endoscopes and instruments.

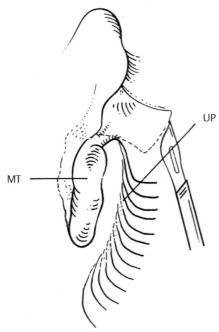

Figure 7–15 The middle turbinate (MT) and uncinate process (UP) are marked in the left nasal cavity. The scalpel blade outlines the incisions for the axillary flap above the insertion of the middle turbinate on the left lateral nasal wall. (From Wormald PJ. The axillary flap approach of the frontal recess. Laryngoscope 2002;112:494–499. Reprinted with permission.)

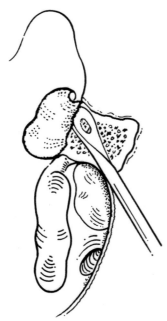

Figure 7–16 Suction Freer elevates the axillary flap. Identification of the root of the middle turbinate is necessary before the flap is tucked between the turbinate and septum. (From Wormald PJ. The axillary flap approach of the frontal recess. Laryngoscope 2002;112:494–499. Reprinted with permission.)

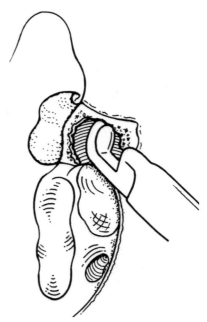

Figure 7–17 The Hajek Koeffler punch removes the anterior face of the agger nasi cell. (From Wormald PJ. The axillary flap approach of the frontal recess. Laryngoscope 2002;112:494–499. Reprinted with permission.)

A Hajek Koeffler punch is used to remove the anterior wall of the agger nasi cell. The thickness of the bone depends upon the extent of the pneumatization of the agger nasi cell. If it is well pneumatized, this bone is thin and easy to remove and should be removed to the edge of the mucosal incisions (**Fig. 7–17**). If the agger nasi cell is small or absent, the bone can be thick and may only be able to be partially removed. If there are polyps in the agger nasi cell, these are removed with the microdebrider so that the extent of the cell can be clearly seen.

Now that the agger nasi cell has been entered and positively identified, the surgeon should review the 3-D reconstruction of the anatomy of the frontal recess that was previously performed (see Chapter 6). The location of the frontal drainage pathway should be sought with a probe or curette. The probe or curette should be gently slid up this drainage pathway and the obstructing cells removed by fracturing and removing the cells.

Once the frontal ostium has been visualized and is clear of any obstructing cells, the axillary flap is pulled forward and placed so that it partially rolls under the raw edge of bone of the residual anterior wall of the agger nasi cell (**Fig. 7–18**). This should provide cover for this area and prevent granulation tissue and subsequent adhesions from forming in this area.

Results of the Axillary Flap Technique

In a recently published series,[15] the axillary flap approach in conjunction with the 3-D building block concept provided visualization of 96% of the frontal sinus ostia in 118 consecutive

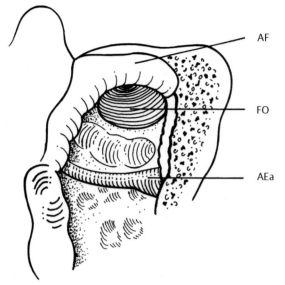

Figure 7–18 The axillary flap (AF) is rolled over the raw edge of the newly formed axilla. The frontal ostium (FO) and anterior ethmoidal artery (AEa) are visible. (From Wormald PJ. The axillary flap approach of the frontal recess. Laryngoscope 2002;112:494–499.)

frontal recess procedures. The remaining frontal ostia were identified with the aid of the mini-trephination technique described below. Of the 118 cases, six had significant adhesions present that required outpatient treatment.[15] Therefore, the axillary flap approach does not increase the risk of adhesion formation in the middle meatus.[13–16] **Figure 7–19** shows the typical appearance of the region of the axillary flap after such an approach to the frontal recess.

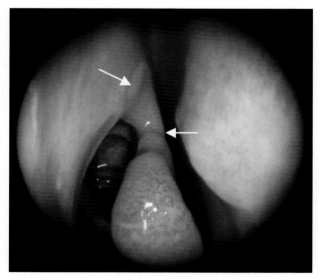

Figure 7–19 Postoperative appearance of the right axillary flap. The *white arrows* mark the incisions lines for the superior and inferior incisions.

Mini-trephination of the Frontal Sinus

The mini-trephination of the frontal sinuses is a very helpful technique when the drainage pathway of the frontal sinus is not easily seen. Placement of a cannula in the frontal sinus allows the sinus to be flushed with fluorescein-stained saline, and the pathway of this fluid in the frontal recess can be followed using a malleable frontal sinus probe* (Medtronic ENT). As the probe is passed up the fluorescein-stained pathway, the probe is used to gently widen this pathway until a curette can be placed along the pathway. The cells in the frontal recess can then be fractured (usually anteriorly or laterally) and removed to expose the frontal ostium (see video on accompanying DVD). In addition, the trephine can be used to ensure clearance of pus, mucus, or fungal material from the frontal sinus where the surgeon does not wish to place an instrument through the frontal ostium and risk damage to the mucosa of the frontal ostium. If a frontal sinus suction is nearly as large as the frontal ostium (often the case with a standard 3- or 4-mm olive tip suction), it may cause circumferential damage to the mucosa of the frontal ostium if it is forced through the ostium into the frontal sinus. This may in turn lead to stenosis or obstruction of the ostium. Clearance of the frontal sinus by irrigating through the mini-trephine cannula can avoid such injury. The mini-trephine cannula may be left in place for a variable period of time after the surgery so that the frontal sinus and frontal ostium can be flushed with saline. This flushing process can remove blood clot from the frontal ostium, which in turn may help maintain its patency as it heals. If the mucosa is significantly inflamed or polypoid, steroid drops may be placed into the frontal sinus for the period of time after surgery before the cannulae are removed. This in turn may help reduce the inflammation and potentially the formation of early scar tissue in the frontal ostia.

Technique of Placing the Mini-trephines

The CT scans should be reviewed to establish the presence and size of the frontal sinus. **Figure 7–20** shows absence of the right frontal sinus with a small left frontal sinus with a very narrow frontal ostium.

Note that the left frontal sinus does not extend above the eyebrow (bony rim of the orbit). The extent of superior pneumatization of the frontal sinus needs to be assessed on the CT scan before the mini-trephine is placed.

The landmark for placement of the skin incision is the medial aspect of the eyebrow. In most patients, the eyebrow is on the superior orbital rim and one should follow this medially on the CT scan to ensure that there is sufficient pneumatization of the frontal sinus above the superior orbital rim. Placement of the mini-trephine too high can result in intracranial penetration by the drill. If the frontal sinus is sufficiently pneumatized on CT, the skin landmarks for placement of the skin incision are as follows: draw an imaginary horizontal line from the middle of the medial end of one eyebrow to the medial end of the other eyebrow. Along this line pick the midpoint between the eyebrows and then estimate 1 cm from the midline along this imaginary line (**Fig. 7–21**).

Infiltrate with 1 to 2 mL of local anesthetic and adrenaline. A no. 15 scalpel blade is used to make the stab incision

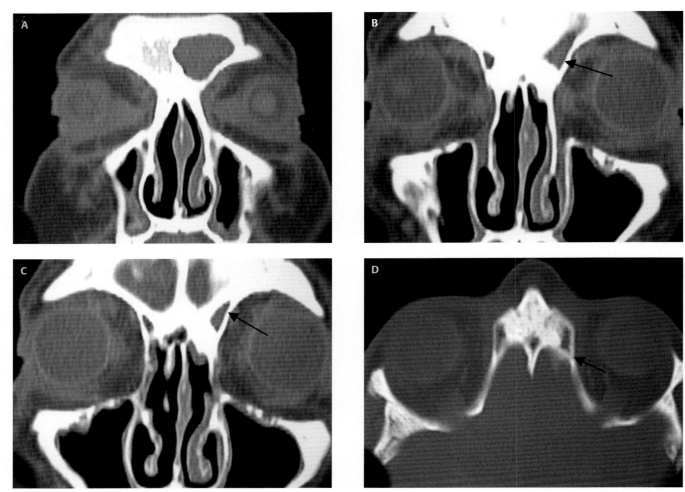

Figure 7–20 (A–D) The narrow left frontal ostium is marked with a *black arrow*.

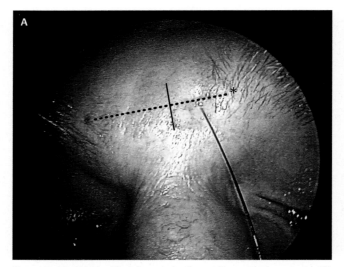

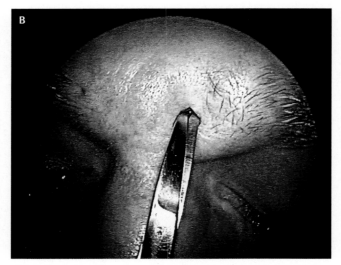

Figure 7–21 (**A**) The *black line* marks the midline with the asterisk (*) marking the medial aspect of the eyebrow. The *broken horizontal line* joins the ends of the eyebrows. The needle with local anesthetic is placed through a skin crease midway between these points. (**B**) After a stab incision, the wound is dilated with iris scissors.

through the skin onto bone. This incision can either be placed through a vertical frown line or, in the case of patients concerned about the possible aesthetic appearance of a scar, the incision can be placed through the medial hairs of the eyebrow. Although the latter two incisions may not be correctly placed between the medial aspect of the eyebrow and the midline, the skin of the frontal bone is mobile and after placement of the mini-trephine guide, this guide can be shifted by moving the skin until it is correctly placed on the bone as described above. If the bony trephine is placed too laterally, it may either endanger the supratrochlear neurovascular bundle or be outside of the frontal sinus. The stab incision is gently dilated with a sharp-pointed scissors. A drill guide is placed through this incision by first laying the guide flat on the skin and then rotating it into the incision. This is done with the incision being held open by tension placed with fingers on either side of the wound (**Fig. 7–22**).

If the guide is pushed into the incision without opening the wound, a small ellipse of skin can be caught and removed as the guide is pushed into the wound. If the skin incision has been placed through the hairs of the eyebrow, this point may be too lateral to perform the trephination. After placement of the drill guide, the skin is moved by pushing the guide to the point indicated by the above guidelines before the bone is trephined. The guide has teeth on the surface that comes in contact with the bone and these should be securely engaged onto the bone so that the guide does not move during the trephination process. The drill bit should be removed almost immediately it touches the bone. It should be completely withdrawn from the guide and the tip irrigated with saline or water. Failure to do this results in significant heating of the drill tip and can lead to a burn of the bone and the skin around the trephine. On the skin this can result in a circular wound that leaves an unsightly scar, and in the bone this can predispose toward osteitis. The trephine burr is designed to extend 11 mm beyond the guide and should not be able to penetrate the posterior table of the frontal sinus. On rare occasions in patients with small (underpneumatized) frontal sinuses and a

thick anterior table, the drill may not be long enough to penetrate the anterior table of the frontal sinus. Should this occur, the surgeon can move the trephine guide inferiorly (the bone of the anterior table tends to thin as one moves inferiorly) and reattempt frontal sinus trephination. The skin over the frontal sinus is mobile and easily moved by the guide. Do not attempt to move the trephine site superiorly as this can risk trephination of the intracranial cavity. The trephine is removed while the guide is held firmly in place. A wire stylet is placed through the guide into the trephine hole. The guide is removed and the frontal cannula is placed over the stylet into the frontal sinus (**Fig. 7–23**). The cannula is placed in a rotatory fashion and is not pushed too firmly into skin as the barrel widens and this can put pressure on the skin around the shaft of the cannula.

A syringe half-filled with saline and fluorescein is placed on the cannula and aspiration attempted. Aspiration of clear fluid indicates intracranial penetration and the cannula should be immediately removed and the wound sutured. Usually air, mucus, pus, or blood is withdrawn into the syringe. When the frontal ostium is completely blocked, only a vacuum will be created in the syringe. In this situation, the frontal ostium is observed while gentle pressure is placed on the syringe. Pus or mucus followed by fluorescein-stained saline should be seen. This area of emergence of the fluorescein can then be probed to identify the drainage pathway of the frontal sinus. Before any significant pressure is placed on the syringe, check the CT scan to ensure that there are no dehiscences of the posterior table of the frontal sinus. The saline and fluorescein mixture consists of 500 mL saline and 0.5 mL 5% fluorescein. This concentration should not cause meningeal irritation if inadvertently injected into the intracranial space.

Computer-Aided Surgery

Computer-aided surgery (CAS) utilizes new technology where the patient has undergone either a CT or magnetic resonance imaging (MRI) scan (or both) prior to surgery. These images

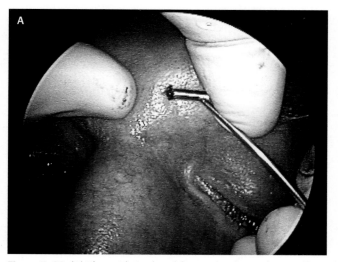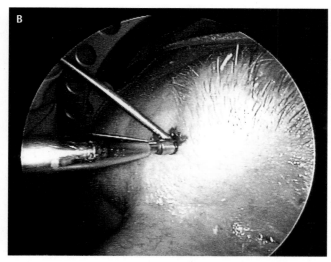

Figure 7–22 (A) The guide is placed flat on the skin and rotated into the wound to avoid coring an ellipse of skin. **(B)** The drill is placed through the guide.

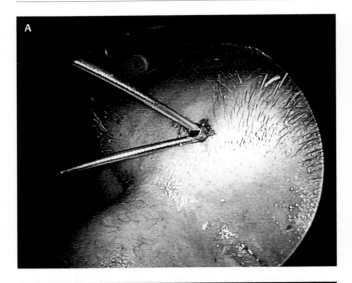

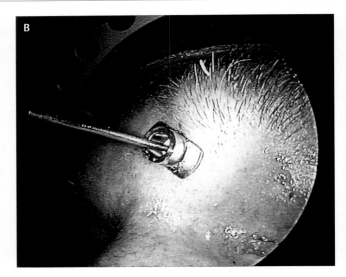

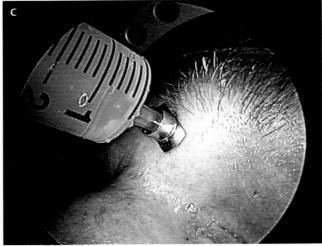

Figure 7–23 (A, B) The frontal cannula is slid over the stylet into the trephine hole and into the frontal sinus. **(C)** A syringe half-filled with fluorescein-stained saline is attached to the cannula and the frontal sinus aspirated before it is irrigated.

are downloaded onto a computer and the images presented to the surgeon in three planes (coronal, axial, and parasagittal). This is similar to the standard CT scans performed on our patients. The benefit with this system is that crosshairs can be placed on a cell and the crosshairs will appear in the same cell on the other two views (**Fig. 7–24**). The surgeon can identify a cell and see where that cell is in the other plane, and in the same way as described in Chapter 6 can build a 3-D image of the anatomy of the patient. Surgical planning can also be effectively performed on the machine prior to surgery.

There are two systems: the first is optical system where a camera tracks light-emitting diodes (LEDs) on the patient (headframe) and the instruments. The second system is electromagnetic where the computer tracks movement of electromagnetic markers on the patient (headframe) and on instruments. Both systems work well and have different advantages and disadvantages. To register the patient on the computer, landmarks are identified on the scans on the computer and then on the patient. The headframe monitors the movement of the patient's head. The instruments are tracked either optically or electromagnetically. In patients without intranasal

landmarks (absent middle turbinate, etc.), these systems allow important structures such as the skull base, orbit, optic nerve, and carotid to be identified. In addition, they allow residual cells within the frontal recess and sinus to be identified and removed. If a frontal sinus drainage pathway cannot be found, they can track an instrument tip so that the pathway can be identified and the instrument slid up the pathway and remaining cells removed from the frontal recess or sinus.

◆ **CHALLENGING SITUATIONS DURING FRONTAL RECESS AND FRONTAL SINUS SURGERY**

Narrow Frontal Ostium with Obstructive Cells with Thick Bony Walls

This situation is not uncommon but results in a difficult intraoperative situation. In this particular example, the patient has a thick beak with very underpneumatized agger

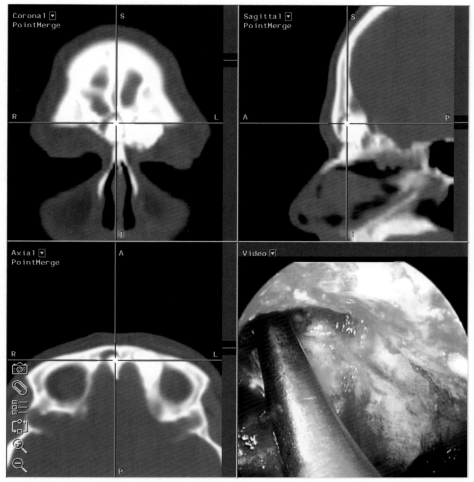

Figure 7–24 In this patient with a large frontal sinus osteoma, CAS was very helpful during endoscopic removal to identify and prevent injury to the skull base. The crosshairs indicate the roof of the frontal sinus after removal of the osteoma.

nasi cell and an intersinus septal cell (ISSC) with thick bony walls that cannot be easily fractured with standard instruments to enlarge the frontal ostium (**Fig. 7–25**). The agger nasi cell is very small and narrow and the bulla ethmoidalis pushes forward into the frontal recess squashing the frontal sinus drainage pathway anterolaterally (best seen on the axial scans; **Fig. 7–25**). The beak of the frontal process is very thick and although there is an ISSC, the wall of this cell is formed by thick bone that separates this cell from the frontal drainage pathway. It would be impossible to enlarge the frontal sinus drainage pathway without resorting to a drill. As discussed previously, drilling in this situation is more likely to result in postoperative scarring and obstruction of the frontal ostium with iatrogenic long-term frontal sinusitis that can be difficult to manage. The intraoperative management of this patient should include complete clearance of the opacified maxillary sinus with a canine fossa trephine and creation of a large middle meatal antrostomy, followed by an axillary flap with removal of as much of the axilla of the middle turbinate as possible. This will expose the small, thin agger nasi cell. Because the bulla pneumatizes anteriorly, this should be opened as well as the suprabullar cell allowing identification of the skull

base and anterior ethmoidal artery, which should be seen adjacent to where the posterior wall of this cell touches the skull base. The curette can now be slid up the frontal sinus drainage pathway behind the agger nasi cell and this cell fractured forward and removed. Next, the anterior wall of both the bulla and suprabullar cells should be removed up to the skull base. The ISSC will be seen with the frontal ostium pushed laterally. Because the frontal ostium is narrow and could not be enlarged, and because of the inflamed state of the mucosa around the frontal ostium, a frontal sinus mini-trephine was inserted and the frontal ostium irrigated for 3 days postoperatively with both saline flushes and prednisolone drops.

Postoperatively, the frontal ostium was edematous for some months before settling down. The patient remains asymptomatic and the ostium healed (**Fig. 7–26**). This emphasizes the importance of removing the obstructive cells from the frontal recess (agger nasi, bulla, and suprabullar cells) and clearing the drainage pathway. The author believes that any attempt to enlarge this ostium with a drill would not have had such a positive outcome.

That is not to say that all patients will respond in this manner, and some patients may develop chronic edema

97

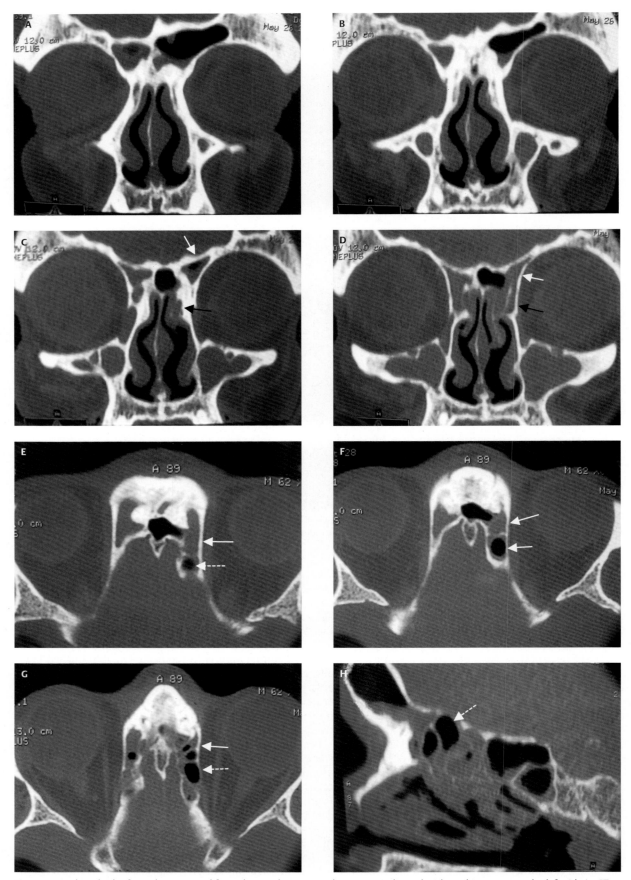

Figure 7–25 (A–H) The frontal ostium and frontal sinus drainage pathways are indicated with a *white arrow* on the left side in CT scans (**C–G**). The small agger nasi cell (*black arrow*) can be seen in scans (**C**) and (**D**). The suprabullar cell (*broken white arrow*) can be seen in scans (**E–H**).

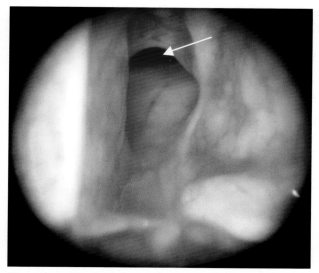

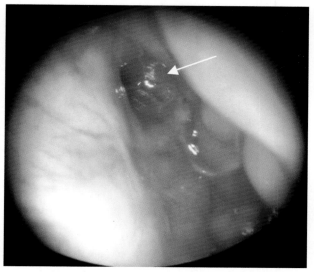

Figure 7–26 Postoperative picture of the left frontal ostium of the patient presented in **Fig. 7–25**. Note the healthy left frontal ostium (*white arrow*).

Figure 7–27 A patient who had a very narrow left frontal ostium with edema obstructing the ostium (*white arrow*). A thin suction could still be passed through this ostium, but despite ongoing medical treatment, the edema in this region has remained. If the patient remains symptomatic, further surgery is indicated.

with obstruction of a narrow ostium (**Fig. 7–27**). Such patients should be treated with systemic and topical steroids, douches, and regular office toilet, and if the symptoms persist, revision surgery is indicated (usually an endoscopic modified Lothrop procedure as described in Chapter 9).

Large Frontal Bulla Cell or T4 Cell Obstructing the Frontal Ostium

In some patients, there are cells that extend significantly into the frontal sinus through the frontal ostium and in

so doing compromise the ostium and the drainage and ventilation of the frontal sinus. These cells can be very difficult to manage, and the approach depends upon the size of the frontal ostium. If the patient has extensively pneumatized sinuses, then there is a reasonable chance the AP distance of the frontal ostium may be quite large, as is the case in this example (**Fig. 7–28**). Also note in this example that the anterior ethmoidal artery is on a mesentery. This commonly occurs when there is extensive pneumatization, and in these cases, this region should be

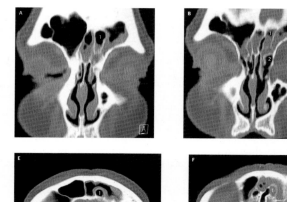

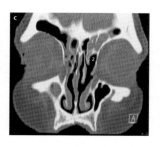

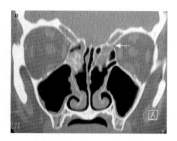

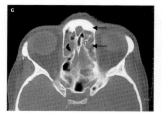

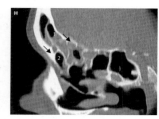

Figure 7–28 (A–H) The frontal bulla cell is numbered *1* and the roof of the agger nasi cell is numbered *2*. Note the large AP distance in the axial CT scans (**E–G**) and marked as the distance between the *parallel black arrows* on the axial CT scan (**G**) and the

parasagittal CT scan (**H**). Note the *broken white arrow* in scan (**D**) indicating the anterior ethmoidal artery on a mesentery and at risk of damage during surgery.

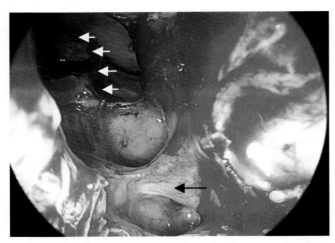

Figure 7–29 The left frontal ostium from the patient presented in **Fig. 7–28**. Note the attachment of the frontal bulla to the posterior wall of the frontal sinus indicated by the *short white arrows*. The anterior ethmoidal artery in its mesentery is indicated by the *black arrow*. Note the wide AP distance of the frontal ostium.

carefully scrutinized during surgery to avoid injury to this artery. In this case, the large frontal bulla cell is originating from the suprabullar region and hugging the skull base into the frontal sinus and progressing almost to reach the roof of the frontal sinus. If, as in this case, the AP distance is large, the cell can be reached through the natural frontal ostium and removed. In this case, it was possible to remove the entire cell from below without enlarging the frontal ostium. If the AP distance were small, however, then the cell would need ancillary measures for removal. In our department, this would usually be an endoscopic modified Lothrop procedure, but removal may also be performed by a combined approach (trephine into the frontal sinus through the eyebrow big enough to admit either an endoscope or an instrument). The instrument is introduced through the frontal sinus trephine and viewed through the frontal ostium or vice versa. Alternatively, an osteoplastic flap into frontal sinuses can be performed and the cell removed under direct visualization.

The intraoperative picture is seen in **Fig. 7–29** where the base of the frontal bulla cell can be seen on the posterior table of the frontal sinus through the natural ostium.

◆ POSTOPERATIVE CARE

Frontal Sinus Irrigation Regimes

The frontal sinus cannulae are left in place if there has been inadvertent trauma to the frontal ostium mucosa, if the natural frontal sinus ostium is very narrow (<3 mm), if there was evidence of osteitis with new bone formation in the frontal recess or ostium, and if there was extensive polyposis resulting in significant traumatized mucosa after the polyp removal. The frontal cannulae are flushed with 5 mL normal saline every 2 hours starting immediately after surgery. If

prednisolone drops are to be used, 0.5 to 1 mL is instilled with a syringe into the frontal sinus after every second douche. No nasal packing is used as this has not been found to reduce adhesion formation or to promote healing.[18]

Medications and Debridement

All patients are placed on a 5-day course of broad-spectrum antibiotics and requested to flush their noses and sinuses 4 to 6 times a day with saline after surgery. If significant polyps were found during surgery, patients are placed on a 3-week reducing course of oral prednisolone. Patients are reviewed in the office between 10 to 14 days after surgery. At this visit, all residual blood clots are removed and the sinus ostia inspected. A thin, curved suction is passed through the frontal sinus ostia and any secretions removed from the frontal sinus. All other sinus ostia are similarly checked. Any adhesions are divided. If these are significant, an early return visit is scheduled, but if all appears to be healing well, the patient is reviewed 4 to 6 weeks later.

References

1. Levine HL. Endoscopic sinus surgery: reasons for failure. Op Tech Otolaryngol Head Neck Surg. 1995;6:176–179
2. Kennedy DW, Senior BA. Endoscopic sinus surgery-a review. Otolaryngol Clin North Am 1997;30:313–330
3. Stammberger H, Kopp W, Dekornfeld TJ, Hawke M. Functional Endoscopic Sinus Surgery-The Messerklinger Technique. Special Endoscopic Anatomy. Philadelphia, PA: B.C. Decker Publishers; 1991:61–90
4. Stammberger H, Posawetz W. Functional endoscopic sinus surgery? Eur Arch Otorhinolaryng 1990;247:63–76
5. Thawley SE, Deddens AE. Transfrontal endoscopic management of frontal recess disease. Am J Rhinol 1995;9:307–311
6. Setliff RC III. Minimally invasive sinus surgery: rationale and technique. Otolaryngol Clin North Am 1996;29:115–129
7. Catalano PJ, Setcliffe RC III, Catalano LA. Minimally invasive sinus surgery in the geriatric patient. Op Tech Otolaryngol Head Neck Surg 2001;12:85–90
8. Catalano P, Roffman E. Outcome of patients with chronic sinusitis after minimally invasive sinus technique. Am J Rhinol 2003;17:17–22
9. Kuhn FA, Javer A, Nagpal K, Citardi M. The frontal sinus rescue procedure: early experience and 3-year follow-up. Am J Rhinol 2000;14:211–216
10. May M, Schaitkin B. Frontal sinus surgery: endonasal drainage instead of an external osteoplastic approach. Op Tech Otolaryngol Head Neck Surg. 1995;6:184–192
11. Schaefer SD, Close LG. Endoscopic management of frontal sinus disease. Laryngoscope 1990;100:155–160
12. Kuhn FA. Chronic frontal sinusitis: the endoscopic frontal recess approach. Operative techniques. Otolaryngol Head Neck Surg 1996; 7:222–229
13. Wormald PJ. Three-dimensional building block approach to understanding the anatomy of the frontal recess and frontal sinus. Op Tech Otolaryngol Head Neck Surg 2006;17:2–5
14. Wormald PJ. Surgery of the frontal recess and frontal sinus. Rhinology 2005;43(2):83–85
15. Wormald PJ. The axillary flap approach of the frontal recess. Laryngoscope 2002;112:494–499
16. Wormald PJ. The agger nasi cell. The key to understanding the anatomy of the frontal recess. Otolaryngol Head Neck Surg 2003;129:497–507
17. Kang SK, White P, Lee M, Ram B, Ogston S. A randomized control trial of surgical task performance in frontal recess surgery: zero versus angled telescopes. Am J Rhinol 2002;16:33–36
18. Wormald PJ, Boustred N, Le T, Hawke L, Sacks R. A prospective single blind randomized controlled study of use of hyaluronic acid nasal packs (Merogel) in patients after endoscopic sinus surgery. Am J Rhinol 2006;20:145–149

8

Surgery of the Bulla Ethmoidalis, Middle Turbinate, and Posterior Ethmoids and Sphenoidotomy, Including Three-Dimensional Reconstruction of the Posterior Ethmoids

If the embryology of the sinuses is reviewed, the middle turbinate forms from the third lamella and the superior turbinate from the fourth lamella. The ground lamella of the middle turbinate divides the ethmoid sinuses into anterior ethmoid sinuses (anterior to the ground lamella) and posterior ethmoid sinuses (posterior to the ground lamella). Anterior ethmoid sinuses are further subdivided into those associated with the frontal process of the maxilla, the frontal ethmoidal cells, and cells associated with the bulla ethmoidalis. The bulla ethmoidalis is a large ethmoid air cell that forms directly anterior to the ground lamella and behind the uncinate process. Cells directly above the bulla ethmoidalis are referred to as suprabullar cells. Posterior ethmoidal cells are found behind the ground lamella of the middle turbinate and lateral to the superior turbinate.

◆ SURGERY OF THE BULLA ETHMOIDALIS AND SUPRABULLAR CELLS (ANTERIOR ETHMOIDECTOMY)

The bulla ethmoidalis is either a single cell or group of cells that are visible directly behind the free edge of the middle and horizontal portions of the uncinate process. The gap between the anterior face of the bulla ethmoidalis and the free edge of the uncinate process is known as the hiatus semilunaris, which is the entrance to the ethmoidal infundibulum. When the anterior face of the bulla ethmoidalis extends to the skull base, it usually forms the posterior limit of the frontal recess. However, when its anterior lamella fails to reach the skull base, a suprabullar recess is created. The bulla ethmoidalis will usually have a posterior wall that is separate from the vertical portion of the ground lamella. The space between its posterior wall and the ground lamella is known as the retrobullar recess. The bulla ethmoidalis, like all sinuses, drains via a natural ostium. This can usually be found on its posteromedial aspect in the retrobullar recess.

To find the natural ostium, a double right-angled probe is passed medial to the bulla between the bulla and the middle turbinate. The tip of the probe is gently rotated laterally until it falls into the natural ostium (**Fig. 8–1**). As the probe is pulled forward, the medial and anterior walls are fractured. This fracture should be in continuity with the natural ostium.

To open the bulla ethmoidalis, the microdebrider is placed in this fractured area and the medial wall and anterior wall of the bulla removed. This allows the natural ostium to be enlarged and be a part of the opening created into the bulla. This follows the general philosophy of endoscopic sinus surgery (ESS) of including the natural ostium in any opening made into a sinus. If only a mini-ESS is being performed (uncinectomy and opening of the bulla), then 3 or 4 mm of the anterior and inferior edge of the bulla are retained. This 3 to 4 mm of the anterior face of the bulla form the posterosuperior part of the final common drainage pathway (see Chapter 5). This region is termed the *final common drainage pathway* as mucus from the frontal and anterior ethmoid cells and maxillary sinus is cleared to the nasopharynx along this pathway (**Fig. 8–2**).

If a posterior ethmoidectomy is to be performed in addition to opening the bulla, only 1 to 2 mm of the antermedial wall are retained. Removing more of the bulla gives improved access to the posterior ethmoid complex.

◆ SURGERY OF THE POSTERIOR ETHMOIDS

Three-dimensional Reconstruction of the Posterior Ethmoids to Prepare for Surgery

As described in Chapter 6, three-dimensional (3-D) reconstruction and planning of each surgical step is performed prior to dissection of the posterior ethmoids and sphenoid. In

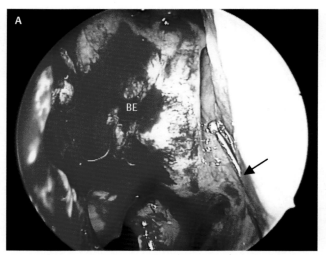
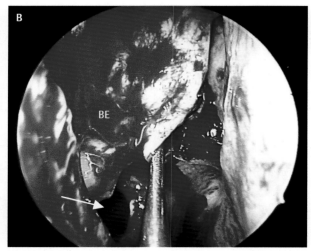

Figure 8–1 (**A**) The ball-probe (*black arrow*) is slid medial to the anterior face of the bulla ethmoidalis (BE). (**B**) The anterior face of the bulla is fractured creating an edge for the microdebrider. The maxillary sinus ostium is marked by *white arrow*.

a manner similar to when the agger nasi cell is used as the cornerstone of the dissection of the frontal recess, a cell or space in the posterior ethmoids needs to be identified that can be accurately correlated with the computed tomography (CT) scan. The space used in the 3-D reconstruction of the posterior ethmoids is the superior meatus. To be able to accurately identify the superior meatus on sequential CT scans, the transition from the anterior to the posterior ethmoids must be established on the CT scans. If the coronal CT scans are evaluated, the first landmark that is sought is the

superior turbinate. Each coronal sequential CT scan is evaluated until the superior turbinate is identified (**Fig. 8–3**).

Once the transition between the anterior and posterior ethmoids is established on the CT scans, the superior meatus (SM) should be sought. This is clearly marked in **Figs. 8–3C, D**. This space is directly above the horizontal part of the ground lamella and should be easily located on all CT scans. The ability of the surgeon to locate this space on both the CT scan and the patient is critical as it provides the starting point. Once penetration of the posterior ethmoids has taken place through the ground lamella, the superior meatus and superior turbinate are identified. The surgeon now has a landmark in the dissection that can be clearly placed on the CT scan. Each sequential cell in the posterior ethmoids is identified, and using the building block principle, a 3-D picture of the posterior ethmoids can be constructed. However, before a complete understanding of the anatomy of the posterior ethmoids is possible, a clear understanding of the transition between posterior ethmoids and sphenoid is necessary. This follows the theme of understanding the transition between the frontal sinus and anterior ethmoids, between the anterior and posterior ethmoids, and finally between the posterior ethmoids and sphenoid. The key to determining the transition from the posterior ethmoids to the sphenoid is identifying the first coronal CT scan in which the solid posterior bony choanae can be seen (**Fig. 8–4**).

In addition to the coronal CT scans, the parasagittal scan is helpful (**Fig. 8–5**). This scan is very useful in helping to place the cells either one on top of the other or anterior or posterior to the other cells of the posterior ethmoids. Cell number 3 is placed lateral to the parasagittal reconstruction and cannot be seen on scan (**C**). Each configuration of the posterior ethmoids is different and each side of every patient needs to be independently assessed and the 3-D picture built.

The following scans and diagram illustrate the building block 3-D reconstruction of the posterior ethmoids (**Fig. 8–5**). Although not all the posterior ethmoid and sphenoid scans can be shown, refer to **Figs. 8–3 and 8–4** for additional CT scans of the same patient if further

Figure 8–2 In this photo of the right nasal cavity, the final common drainage pathway is indicated by the *black arrow*. This also indicates the drainage pathway of the maxillary sinus. The *white arrow* indicates the drainage pathway of the frontal and anterior ethmoidal cells along the anterior face of the bulla ethmoidalis (BE). This portion of the BE forms the posterosuperior part of the final common drainage pathway. The residual portion of the uncinate process (UP) after uncinectomy and the natural ostium of the maxillary sinus (MO) are marked.

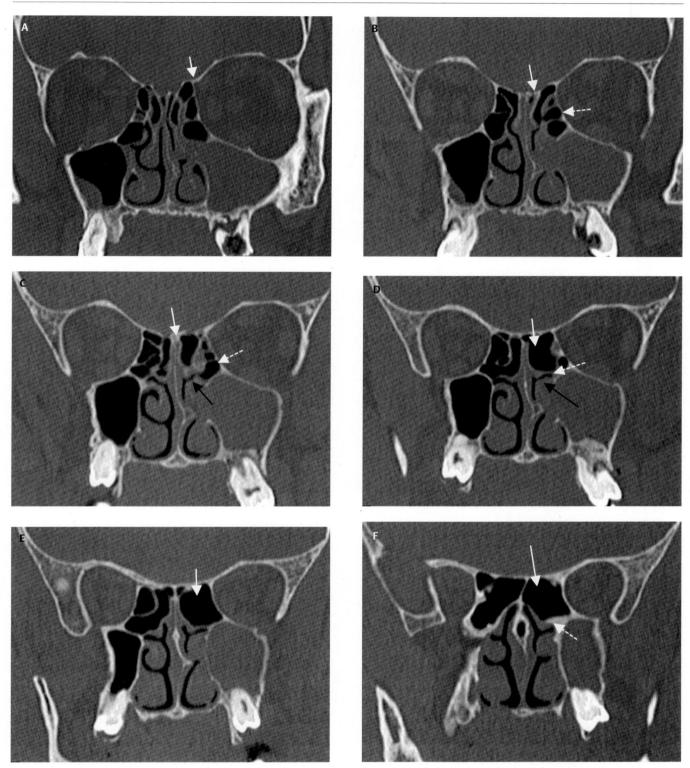

Figure 8–3 (A–F) These six sequential CT scans show the transition of the anterior to the posterior ethmoids. In (**A**), the anterior ethmoidal artery is marked with a *solid white arrow*. In (**B**), the superior turbinate is visible, and this scan marks the transition from the anterior to posterior ethmoids. The *broken arrow* marks the beginning of the superior meatus. In (**C**), the *broken arrow* again marks the superior meatus with the horizontal part of the ground lamella directly beneath the superior meatus (*black arrow*). In (**D**), the *solid white arrow* marks the single large posterior ethmoid cell with the superior meatus (*broken arrow*) and horizontal ground lamella (*black arrow*) visible. (**F**) This CT scan shows the single posterior ethmoid cell and the solid bone of the posterior choanae beginning to form (*broken white arrow*). This marks the beginning of the sphenoid sinuses.

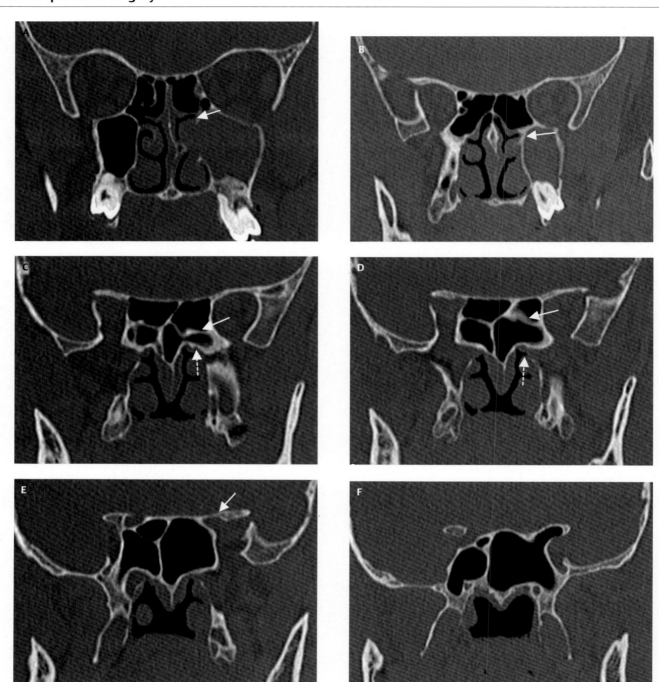

Figure 8–4 (A, B) These CT scans show the optic nerve (*solid white arrow*) without any posterior bony choanae. (**C**) In this scan, the solid bony choanae are first seen (*broken white arrow*) indicating the transition from the posterior ethmoids to the sphenoid. In most patients, the cell directly above the solid bone of the choana is the sphenoid sinus. (**D**) In this scan, a horizontal septation is seen (*solid white arrow*). This septation separates the sphenoid (always directly above the bony choanae) and the ethmoid cell pneumatizing over the top of the sphenoid.

clarification of the cells and reconstruction is needed. Note that once the superior meatus has been clearly identified in **Fig. 8–5A**, there is a single posterior ethmoid cell. This should be confirmed on both the parasagittal and coronal CT scans (**Figs. 8–5E, F, G**). Also note that the first CT scan in which the posterior bony choanae can be seen is **Fig. 8–5C** and there

is a horizontal septation seen in that scan (between cells *1* and *2*). Note on the two parasagittal scans (**Figs. 8–5F, G**) that the anterior face of the sphenoid is angled posteriorly allowing this wall to be cut by the CT giving the horizontal septation. On the left this is not carried significantly over the sphenoid, and the optic nerve is not seen in cell *1* and therefore

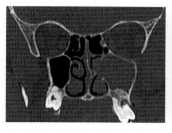
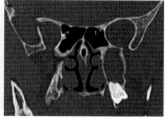
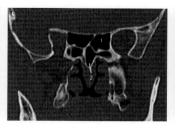
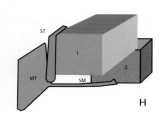

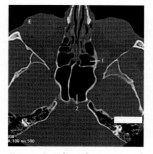
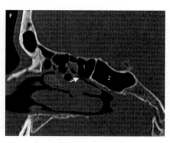
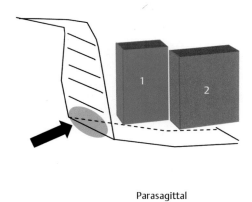
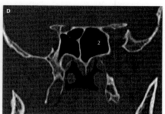

H

Figure 8–5 (A–D) A series of coronal CT scans followed by (**E**) an axial CT scan and (**F, G**) two parasagittal CT scans. Scan (**F**) is close to the midline whereas (**G**) is more lateral. Cells are numbered on the CT scan and in the 3-D reconstruction with cell *1* the single posterior

ethmoid and cell *2* the sphenoid sinus. MT, middle turbinate; ST, superior turbinate; SM, superior meatus. *Solid white arrows* in **F** and **G** indicate the horizontal part of the ground lamella.

this does not represent an Onodi (spheno-ethmoidal cell). The right side will be discussed later in this chapter. The 3-D reconstruction demonstrates this slight posterior angulation of the anterior face of the sphenoid and also gives the surgeon a clear indication of exactly what to expect once the surgeon has entered the superior meatus and clearly identified this space and the anterior end of the superior turbinate.

Surgical Plan for the Posterior Ethmoids

Once a 3-D reconstruction of the posterior ethmoids has been performed, a surgical plan is formulated as to how the dissection will be performed in the posterior ethmoids.

The first step is to enter the superior meatus through the ground lamella in a region that can be easily identified on the CT scans. To achieve this, the transition from the posterior horizontal ground lamella to the vertical ground lamella needs to be identified. To positively identify the horizontal ground lamella, slide the endoscope under the middle turbinate toward the back end of the middle turbinate. As the posterior end of the middle turbinate is approached, the horizontal portion of the ground lamella is directly above the endoscope. The endoscope is brought anteriorly following the horizontal ground lamella until it turns vertically. At the point where it turns vertically, in the area directly adjacent to the middle turbinate, the microdebrider or straight Blakesley is pushed through the ground lamella (**Fig. 8–6**).

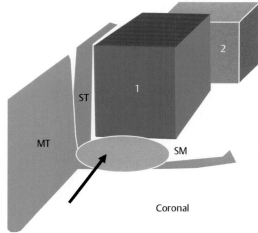

Coronal

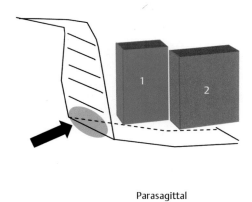

Parasagittal

Figure 8–6 The posterior ethmoids are entered at the junction of the horizontal and vertical portions of the ground lamella directly adjacent to the middle turbinate (as indicated by the

black arrow). Cell number *1* is the posterior ethmoid cell and *2* is the sphenoid. MT, middle turbinate; ST, superior turbinate; SM, superior meatus.

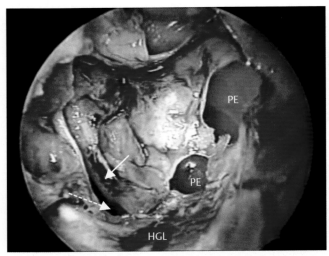

Figure 8–7 This intraoperative picture illustrates the opening of the superior meatus on the left side (*broken white arrow*). The superior turbinate can be clearly seen (*solid white arrow*) and the partially opened posterior ethmoid (PE) cells are seen.

This access area is widened horizontally until the superior meatus and anterior edge of the superior turbinate are identified with certainty (**Fig. 8–7**).

The surgeon can now place the point of dissection on the CT scans and knows how many and in what order the remaining cells are placed. These can then be sequentially entered and a complete dissection of the posterior ethmoids achieved. This low and medial entry into the posterior ethmoids minimizes the potential risk of damage to the skull base, which may occur if entry is made higher on the vertical portion of the ground lamella.[3]

The Middle Turbinate

In most patients, the middle turbinate is preserved. It is important during the surgery that the middle turbinate not be destabilized. The most common cause for destabilization of the middle turbinate is fracturing its anterior vertical insertion from the skull base. The axillary flap is designed to preserve this insertion but does remove some support from the anterior insertion of the middle turbinate. The horizontal portion of the ground lamella should also be preserved to give posterior stability to the middle turbinate. However, excessive manipulation of the middle turbinate can fracture the turbinate's insertion on the skull base and result in it becoming floppy. The manoeuvre that should be avoided is placing the endoscope and instruments medial to the middle turbinate. The combination of a 4-mm endoscope and a 4-mm instrument will usually be enough to fracture the middle turbinate. Therefore, the techniques of posterior ethmoidectomy and sphenoidotomy are described through the middle meatus lateral to the middle turbinate rather than medial to the middle turbinate. Despite all attempts to preserve the middle turbinate, there are some situations where partial or total resection of the middle turbinate is necessary.

Concha Bullosa

Patients with a concha bullosa need to have the lateral lamella of the middle turbinate removed to improve access to the middle meatus and, as this cell is often involved in the disease process, to clear the disease. To minimize damage to the lateral mucosa of the medial lamella, a scalpel is used to incise the anterior face of the concha bullosa vertically (**Fig. 8–8**).

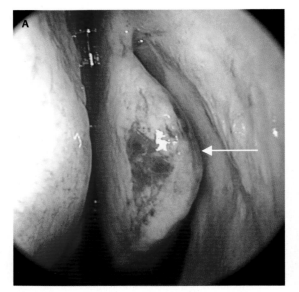
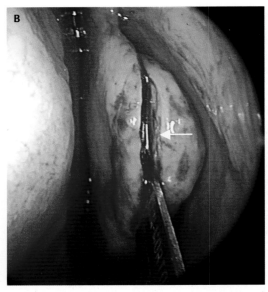

Figure 8–8 (**A**) In this scan, the concha bullosa is seen. Note the breadth of the middle turbinate (*white arrow*). (**B**) In this scan, the scalpel has been used to vertically incise (*white arrow*) the concha separating the medial and lateral lamella.

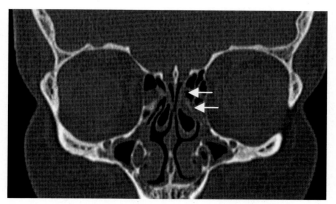

Figure 8–9 The upward continuation of the middle turbinate is indicated with *solid white arrows*. Note the opacity medial to this upward continuation of the lateral lamella of the middle turbinate.

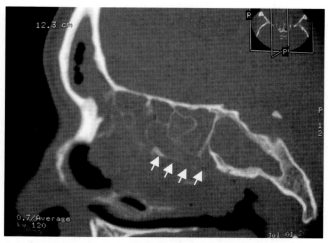

Figure 8–10 The horizontal portion of the ground lamella is indicated by a series of *solid white arrows*. If this structure is maintained in patients with extensive nasal polyps, it may result in underaeration of the posterior ethmoids and sphenoid.

A pair of 5-mm endoscopic scissors* (Medtronic, ENT) is used to continue the incision along the inferior margin of the middle turbinate to the lateral insertion of the turbinate on the lateral nasal wall. The scissors are used to continue the superior incision posterior as high as possible on the turbinate but progressively moving inferiorly as the posterior region of the turbinate is approached. Once the lateral lamella of the turbinate has been resected, it is removed. The residual upward continuation of the lateral lamella of the middle turbinate needs to be removed as part of the frontal recess and bulla ethmoidalis dissection. Failure to remove this upward continuation can result in residual disease in the medial compartment of the anterior ethmoids (**Fig. 8–9**).

Revision Surgery with Extensive Nasal Polyposis

The most common indication for middle turbinate resection is revision surgery with extensive polyposis. In patients who have previously undergone posterior ethmoidectomy, contracture of the horizontal part of the ground lamella may drag the middle turbinate laterally narrowing the ethmoidal space. This results in underventilation of the posterior ethmoid region and could precipitate secretion retention and polyp formation.[1,2] In patients with massive polyposis often from Sampter's triad (aspirin sensitivity, asthma, and polyps) or fungal sinusitis, increased aeration of the posterior ethmoid cavity may be necessary to reduce polyp recurrence.[1,2] In these patients, it may be necessary to partially resect the inferior portion of the middle turbinate and the horizontal portion of the ground lamella. This marsupializes the posterior ethmoids and sphenoid sinus (after a large sphenoidotomy) into the posterior nasal cavity with improved postoperative aeration of these sinuses (**Fig. 8–10**).

Lateralized Atrophic Middle Turbinate

In some patients, especially those with long-standing severe septal deflections into the nasal cavity, the turbinate may

be underdeveloped, very floppy, and lateralized (**Fig. 8–11**). In these patients, part of the turbinate may be resected at the time of surgery. When part of the middle turbinate is resected, then the horizontal portion of the middle turbinate should also be removed flush with the lateral nasal wall. This almost invariably exposes the middle turbinate branch of the sphenopalatine artery with resultant bleeding.

Lateral Displacement of the Middle Turbinate with Narrowing of the Frontal Recess

Particularly in patients who have had previous surgery or in patients with substantial olfactory fossa polyps,

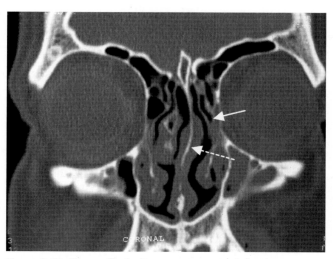

Figure 8–11 CT scan illustrating a severe septal deflection (*broken white arrow*) and corresponding underdevelopment and lateralization of the middle turbinate on the left (*solid white arrow*).

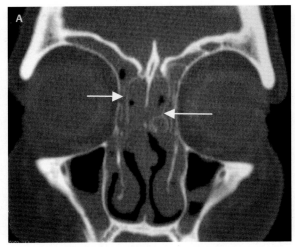

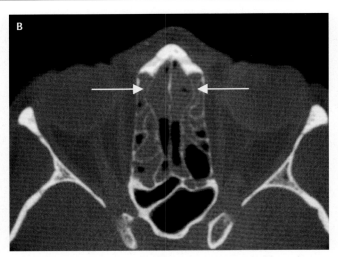

Figure 8–12 (**A**) Coronal CT scan shows significant lateralization of both middle turbinates (*white arrows*). (**B**) The extent of the lateralization of the middle turbinates is again seen on this axial CT scan (*white arrows*). The frontal recess is narrowed by at least 50% by this lateralization. Note opacified olfactory recesses in both scans.

lateral displacement of the middle turbinates may occur (**Fig. 8–12**). This narrows the outflow region of the frontal sinus substantially and creates two problems. The first is the very narrow lateral dimension of the frontal recess, which makes surgery in this region very difficult and increases the risk of damage to the lateral wall of the olfactory fossa. The degree of difficulty of the dissection increases if there is bleeding during the surgery. The lateralized portion of the middle turbinate is often thin and lacks rigidity and stability, and this may result in this segment of the middle turbinate becoming unstable during surgery with resultant increased likelihood of postoperative lateralization and obstruction of the frontal ostium. The second problem is that as the sinuses heal after surgery, the narrow lateral dimension increases the likelihood of blood clot with subsequent fibrosis, which leads to obstruction of the frontal ostium and consequent recurrent frontal sinusitis. If there are large polyps in the olfactory recess, these may need to be resected to remove the lateral pressure that the polyps place on the middle turbinate. Care should be taken to limit the amount of raw tissue in the olfactory fossa to prevent scar formation in the olfactory fossa. This is best achieved by keeping the opening of the microdebrider blade facing only superiorly thereby preventing any lateral or medial mucosal damage.

Posterior Attachment of Middle Turbinate

The horizontal ground lamella attaches to the lateral nasal wall posterior to the maxillary sinus. Branches of the sphenopalatine artery traverse this region supplying blood to the middle turbinate. If this part of the ground lamella is removed, these vessels may bleed. This region is always meticulously inspected at the end of surgery and any bleeders cauterized with the suction bipolar forceps. Although the vessel may clot during surgery, coughing or straining in the postoperative period may dislodge the clot with consequent significant postoperative epistaxis.

◆ ANATOMIC CONFIGURATIONS THAT PLACE THE PATIENT AT RISK DURING THE SURGERY

Certain anatomic variations need to be sought on the CT scans prior to the dissection taking place. Identification of these may help avoid possible complications during the dissection of the posterior ethmoids.

Low Skull Base

A low skull base narrows the vertical height of the posterior ethmoids significantly. This is important for the surgeon to recognize before surgery in the posterior ethmoids is commenced. If the surgeon is unaware that the skull base is low, he or she may think that there may still be superior cells due to low vertical height of the posterior ethmoids. Attempts to dissect further may injure the skull base. To illustrate the difference in vertical height, a CT scan with a normal skull base height and a patient with a low skull is shown in **Fig. 8–13**.

It is critical in a patient with a low skull base that the approach into the posterior ethmoids be low and medial. A high entry through the vertical portion of the ground lamella in a patient with a low skull base would certainly put the skull base at risk (**Fig. 8–14**).[3]

A Curved Posterior Skull Base

Normally, the posterior skull base is flat and the surgeon can dissect from the lamina papyracea medially along the skull base to the insertion of the superior turbinate with a minimum of risk. However, some patients may have a significant curve to the roof of the posterior ethmoids, and the surgeon should assess the CT scans prior to surgery to establish the status of the posterior ethmoid fovea ethmoidalis before surgery is

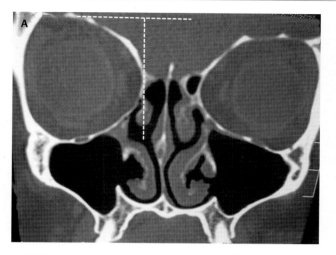

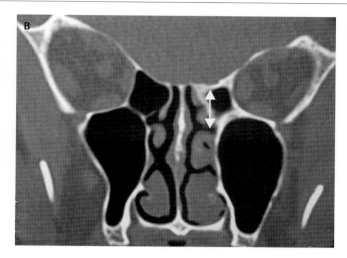

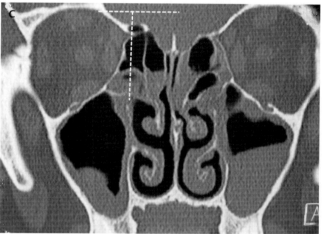

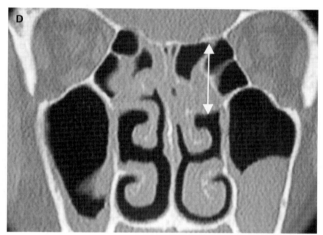

Figure 8–13 (A, B) In these scans, the skull base originates from a point almost half-way down the vertical height of the lamina papyracea of the orbit (*broken lines*) whereas in (**C, D**) the more normal configuration is seen with the fovea ethmoidalis taking

origin from the upper aspect of the lamina papyracea (*broken lines*). The vertical height of the ethmoid cavity (*solid double arrow*) is greater in (**C, D**) than in scans (**A, B**).

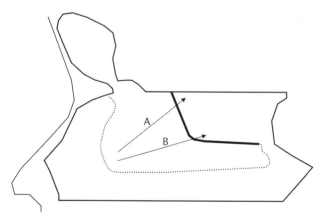

Figure 8–14 This parasagittal diagram of the ground lamella of the middle turbinate illustrates the potential danger of (*arrow A*) entering the posterior ethmoids high on the vertical portion of the ground lamella compared with the safety of (*arrow B*) entering the posterior ethmoids as low and medial as possible.

performed in this area (**Fig. 8–15**). Failure to recognize this curvature may result in the surgeon thinking that there is another cell situated medially on the skull base, and if removal is attempted, injury to the skull base can occur.

Spheno-ethmoidal Cell (Onodi Cell)

Previous descriptions of the spheno-ethmoidal (Onodi) cell state that it is a pneumatization of the posterior ethmoid cell laterally[3,4] and that the incidence can be as high as 42%.[5] However, in most cases this is not true as the spheno-ethmoidal (Onodi) cell is rather a posterior pneumatization of the ethmoid cell over the sphenoid pushing the sphenoid inferiorly. To accurately identify a spheno-ethmoidal (Onodi) cell, one must be able to recognize the transition from the posterior ethmoids to the sphenoid. This follows the theme of being able to recognize the transition from frontal sinus to anterior ethmoids (frontal recess), to recognize the transition from anterior

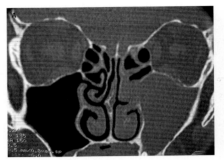
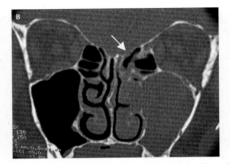
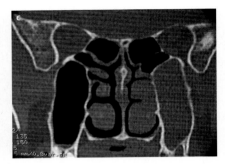

Figure 8–15 (A–C) The curved posterior ethmoid fovea ethmoidalis is indicated in (**B**) by the *white arrow*.

to posterior ethmoids, and finally to be able to recognize the transition from posterior ethmoids to sphenoid sinus. If coronal sequential CT scans of the posterior ethmoids are evaluated, the transition from posterior ethmoids to sphenoid starts on the first CT scan in which the posterior bony choanae can be seen (**Fig. 8–16**). Once the solid bony rim of the posterior choanae is identified, the cell sitting directly above this solid bone should be the sphenoid sinus. If there is any horizontal bony septation above this cell in this or subsequent more posterior coronal CT scans, this would cause suspicion that there may be a spheno-ethmoidal (Onodi) cell present (**Fig. 8–16**).

The posterior ethmoid cells should be followed in each sequential CT scan, and one should establish whether a posterior ethmoid cell pneumatizes over the sphenoid. The parasagittal scan should always be checked as this can be very useful in recognizing a spheno-ethmoidal (Onodi) cell. In **Fig. 8–16**, one can clearly see how the posterior ethmoid cell pneumatizes over the top of the sphenoid (SPH) which in turn creates the most useful characteristic of a spheno-ethmoidal (Onodi) cell—the horizontal septum (HS) seen on a scan that is taken through the sphenoid. Thus, the transition from the posterior ethmoids to the sphenoid is critical to establish before the horizontal septation is sought. This septation is created by the anterior face of the sphenoid being pushed into a more horizontal plane by the spheno-ethmoidal (Onodi) cell pneumatizing over the top of the sphenoid. The CT scans in **Fig. 8–17**, which include a parasagittal scan, illustrate the horizontal plane taken by the anterior face of the sphenoid when a spheno-ethmoidal cell is present. Axial scans are of little value in diagnosing a spheno-ethmoidal (Onodi) cell.

It is important to identify an Onodi cell as this cell has the optic nerve in its posterosuperior region where it is vulnerable to injury during dissection. If the cell is not recognized, the surgeon may not realize that the sphenoid sinus has been pushed inferiorly below the Onodi cell. If the access into the sphenoid is attempted through the Onodi cell, damage to the optic nerve, skull base, or carotid artery may result, as these structures are adjacent to this cell while the sphenoid is below and more medial. The relationship between the Onodi cell and optic nerve can be clearly seen in **Fig. 8–17C**.

◆ SPHENOIDOTOMY

After dissection of the posterior ethmoids and identification of the posterior ethmoid skull base, the sphenoid can be entered. The sphenoid ostium is located medial to the superior turbinate in 83% of patients.[6] If the sphenoid is normal (without disease visible on the CT scan), the spheno-ethmoidal recess can be inspected through the middle meatus by gently moving the superior turbinate laterally and visualizing the recess. If there is no disease in the spheno-ethmoidal recess, the sphenoid ostium should be visible in most patients. If the spheno-ethmoidal recess is diseased (inflamed hypertrophic mucosa or the presence of polyps), then consideration can be given to clearance of the recess usually with sphenoidotomy. If significant mucosal trauma is created in the recess by clearance of disease, then it is likely that the sphenoid ostium may be closed by scar tissue formation during healing, and a sphenoidotomy should be performed to prevent

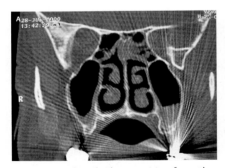
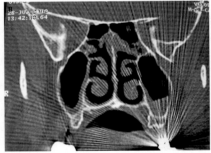

Figure 8–16 (A–C) The transition from the posterior ethmoids to the sphenoid occurs between CT scans (**B**) and (**C**). In (**C**), the bony posterior choanae (*broken white arrow*) are seen. At the point where a complete bony posterior choana is identified, the sinus directly above this bony choana should be the sphenoid sinus. The horizontal septation (*white arrow*) separates the sphenoid from the Onodi cell (OC) above it.

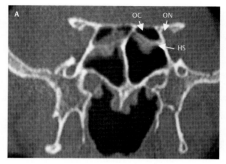
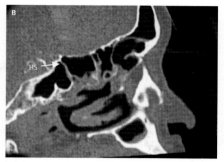
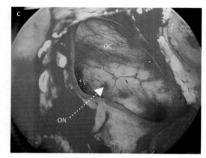

Figure 8–17 (A–C) Scans (**A, B**) indicate the value of the parasagittal scan in confirming the pneumatization of the spheno-ethmoidal (Onodi) cell (OC) over the sphenoid with the formation of a horizontal septum (HS) in (**A**) the coronal scan. In (**A**) and in (**C**), the adjacent operative picture, the optic nerve (ON) is identified and the relationship between this posterior spheno-ethmoid cell (OC) and the optic nerve (ON) can be seen.

this occurrence. If the sphenoid is diseased on the CT scan, it should be opened. It is preferable to open the sphenoid through the posterior ethmoids rather than by passing the instruments and endoscope medial to the middle turbinate as previously emphasized.[7] The already identified superior turbinate is used as the critical landmark for sphenoidotomy.[7,8] The lower one-third to one-half of the superior turbinate is removed either with a microdebrider or straight through-biting forceps. Once the turbinate is removed flush with the anterior face of the sphenoid, the microdebrider is used to palpate the face for the natural ostium of the sphenoid. It is usually found at the junction of the lower one-third and upper two-thirds but may be as high as the halfway point of the superior turbinate and is usually medial to the turbinate on the anterior face of the sphenoid (**Fig. 8–18**).[6]

In the majority of patients, the natural ostium will be located using the landmarks described above. However, in patients with a spheno-ethmoidal (Onodi) cell, the natural ostium may be lower and more medial as the sphenoid is compressed by the spheno-ethmoidal cell pneumatizing over the top of it. If the tip of the microdebrider does not fall into the natural ostium, a smaller straight suction is used to palpate this region. If the natural ostium can still not be located, then the CT scan is reviewed to confirm the position and size of the sphenoid sinus before proceeding further. If a sphenoid is present, then the following measurement technique should be followed to open the sphenoid. The bony rim of the posterior choana is located by passing the 4-mm microdebrider blade through the posterior ethmoids and into the nasopharynx. The tip of the microdebrider blade is pushed against the mucosa just above the bony choanae on the anterior face of the sphenoid. This creates a 4-mm indentation. Two further indentations are made above this one thereby measuring 12 mm from the bony rim of the posterior choana (**Fig. 8–19**).

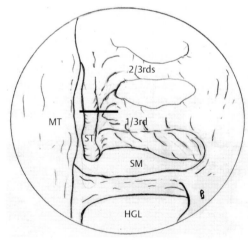

Figure 8–18 On the left side, the middle turbinate (MT), superior turbinate (ST), superior meatus (SM), and horizontal part of the ground lamella (HGL) is clearly identified before sphenoidotomy. In this figure, the posterior ethmoids have not as yet been opened. Once the posterior ethmoids have been sequentially opened, the superior turbinate is divided into thirds. The lower one-third is removed with either a straight through-biting Blakesley or powered microdebrider up to the anterior face of the sphenoid and the sphenoid ostium identified before it is opened.

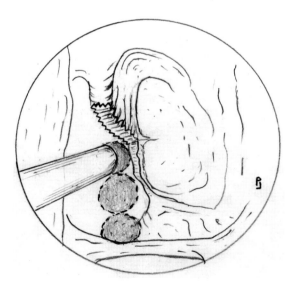

Figure 8–19 Three sequential indentations are made with the blunt end of the 4-mm microdebrider blade starting at the medial upper limit of the posterior bony choana and moving directly superiorly medial to the cut edge of the superior turbinate.

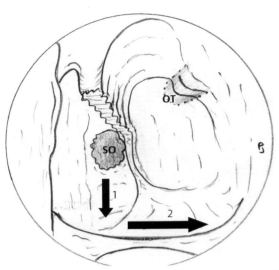

Figure 8–20 The sphenoid ostium (SO) is first opened inferiorly (*black arrow 1*) then laterally (*black arrow 2*). This should afford a clear view into the sphenoid sinus, and the remaining anterior face of the sphenoid can be removed up toward the optic tubercle (OT) but usually stopping short of the tubercle to lessen the potential risk to the optic nerve.

A Freer elevator is then used to push through the anterior face of the sphenoid directly above the third indentation. The tip of the instrument is pushed through the bone, and once it has penetrated the sphenoid cavity, it is twisted to enlarge the opening. A microdebrider or Kerrison punch is then used to further open the sinus. The natural ostium is opened with the punch or microdebrider initially inferiorly toward the floor of the sinus and then toward the lamina papyracea and into the posterior ethmoids (**Fig. 8–20**).

There should be at least 8 to 10 mm of anterior face of the sphenoid still above this lateral opening, and this newly created opening should therefore be well below the optic nerve. The opening can be further enlarged directly superiorly from the natural ostium, medially and inferiorly as well. Opening of the natural ostium of the sphenoid invariably creates a circumferential raw surface around the natural ostium, and therefore this opening needs to be enlarged into the posterior ethmoids to prevent postoperative stenosis. In patients with significant new bone formation, an inferiorly based mucosal flap can be elevated and the underlying bone drilled away before the flap is replaced.[9] This interrupts the circumferential raw area and prevents stenosis.

If the superior turbinate has been completely or partially removed by previous surgery, the measurement technique described above is used to locate the position of the natural ostium of the sphenoid sinus. Resection of part of the superior turbinate may possibly remove some olfactory neurons, but this has not been shown to adversely affect the sense of smell of the patient after surgery.[10] Sphenoidotomy for pituitary surgery is discussed in Chapter 13.

Complications of Sphenoidotomy

Epistaxis

Bleeding is very common from the posterior nasal artery as it traverses the anterior face of the sphenoid on its way to the posterior septum. The posterior nasal artery is a branch of the sphenopalatine artery and travels horizontally just above the posterior choana. It gives off a vertical branch that supplies the anterior face of the sphenoid. If this vertical branch is transected (and it often is as the sphenoid ostium is enlarged), a minor bleeder will be seen on the lower opening of the sphenoid. If the sphenoid ostium is further enlarged inferiorly toward the floor of the sphenoid sinus, the main trunk of the posterior nasal artery can be transected and result in a significant bleeder, which usually spurts in a horizontal and medial direction. This is best managed with the suction-bipolar forceps* (Medtronic USA) as the blood can be suctioned and cautery rapidly applied before the active bleeding results in the blood vessel being covered in blood and no longer visible for precise cautery. If a standard suction and standard bipolar forceps are used, the bleeder is usually so active that by the time that the suction is removed and the bipolar forceps positioned, the vessel can no longer be seen. Because the suction bipolar has integrated suction, this problem can be rapidly overcome.

Damage to the Optic Nerve and Cerebrospinal Fluid Leak

The most common cause of injury to the optic nerve during ESS is when a sphenoidotomy is attempted too high and too lateral and damage is caused to the orbital apex and optic nerve. In **Fig. 8–20**, a diagrammatic view of the posterior ethmoids and superior turbinate is presented. Attempted entry into the sphenoid in the superior lateral region will take the surgeon onto the orbital apex and optic nerve and even into the anterior skull base. This can result in a devastating complication of a damaged optic nerve with visual loss and a cerebrospinal fluid (CSF) leak with potential intracranial damage. In general, this situation begins when entry into the posterior ethmoids through the vertical portion of the ground lamella is made too high. The whole direction of surgery is then toward the skull base, and if the surgeon is inexperienced and does not recognize this, he or she may assume that the structure in front of them is a sloping anterior wall of the sphenoid sinus rather than the sloping wall of the skull base. If the skull base is thinner than usual, then entry into the anterior cranial fossa and/or damage to the optic nerve can occur. The key to preventing this devastating complication is to identify the superior meatus as the first step in the dissection of the posterior ethmoids immediately after the ground lamella is penetrated. This forces the surgeon to keep removing the ground lamella inferiorly until the superior meatus is clearly identified. If this dissection is continued and the anterior end of the superior turbinate is correctly identified, the surgeon is in the correct plane and place and so the risk of mistaking the skull base for the anterior face of the sphenoid should be minimized.

The other area that the optic nerve can be damaged is in the superolateral wall of the sphenoid sinus. The optic nerve is dehiscent in ~12%[5] of patients and inadvertent injury during surgery within the sphenoid sinus may lead to visual loss or blindness. It is tempting to use the microdebrider to remove polyps in the sphenoid, but great care needs to be taken using the microdebrider in this sinus. In general, the microdebrider should only be used along the floor and medial wall of the sphenoid and not in the superior or lateral region. Surgeons are also concerned when the sphenoidotomy is widened in a lateral direction. There are a few rules to follow during sphenoidotomy that can minimize the risk to the optic nerve. The natural ostium of the sphenoid is generally around the lower one-third of the superior turbinates insertion into the anterior face of the sphenoid. The forward-biting Hajek Koeffler punch is used to enlarge this natural ostium first inferiorly toward the floor and then laterally toward the orbit. As the orbit is approached, the instrument should be well below the orbital apex and optic nerve (**Fig. 8–20**).

The second rule is that if the distal part of the Hajek Koeffler punch can be placed behind a bony septation, it is generally safe to remove. Even a septation arising from the optic nerve can be safely removed onto the nerve by allowing the punch to rest on the nerve while the septation is engaged between the jaws of the punch and cleanly removed from the surface of the nerve. However, the superolateral region of the anterior face of the sphenoid is generally not removed to lessen any possible risk to the optic nerve (**Fig. 8–20**).

Damage to the Carotid Artery

The other major structure at risk during sphenoidotomy is the carotid artery. The bony wall covering the carotid is in most patients thin and is dehiscent in 5 to 8% of patients (**Fig. 8–21**).[5,11] This again emphasizes the risk of

using a microdebrider with the cutting gate toward the lateral wall of the sphenoid. It only takes milliseconds for a dehiscent carotid artery wall to be damaged by the very effective cutting mechanisms in microdebriders with potentially catastrophic results. There are two other ways that the carotid artery may be damaged. In some patients, the natural ostium of the sphenoid sinus is very small and the surgeon is unable to identify it and thus allow a safe entry into the sphenoid sinus. If a small or narrow instrument is pushed hard onto the face of the sphenoid in an attempt to penetrate the sphenoid, the bone may suddenly give way with the instrument then being driven into the sinus with considerable force. This instrument can then inadvertently penetrate the thin or dehiscent bone or dehiscent carotid with subsequent massive hemorrhage. In the operative technique previously described, a blunt Freer elevator is used to push through the anterior face of the sphenoid sinus. The entry into the sphenoid can be well controlled with this instrument, and the surgeon can easily feel as the bone is penetrated without risk of the instrument slipping inadvertently into the sinus. Also, the instrument has a large blunt surface that is less likely to injure the carotid.

The second situation where a carotid injury may occur is if the intersinus septum of the sphenoid is attached to the anterior face of the carotid artery (**Fig. 8–22**).

If this septum needs to be taken down as it is during pituitary surgery and its attachment is grasped and rotated, it may fracture and bony spicules may damage the carotid wall. This can be avoided by using a through-biting instrument to sharply remove the septum. If the septum is too thick, a diamond burr can be used.

Management of a carotid artery hemorrhage is discussed in Chapter 10.

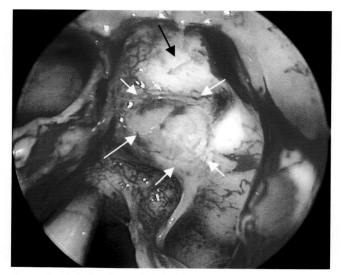

Figure 8–21 Left sphenoid with dehiscent carotid illustrated by *solid white arrows* and optic nerve illustrated with *solid black arrow*.

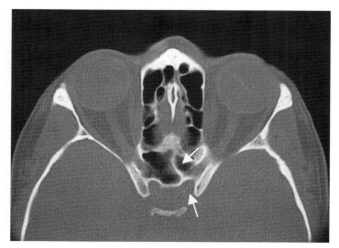

Figure 8–22 This axial CT scan shows the sphenoid sinus septum (*broken arrow*) inserting into the anterior face of the left carotid artery (*solid arrow*). Rotation of this septum during removal may result in a tear of the wall of the carotid artery.

References

1. Klossek JM, Peloquin L, Friedman W, Ferrier J, Fontanel J. Diffuse nasal polyposis: postoperative long-term results after endoscopic sinus surgery and frontal irrigation. Otolaryngol Head Neck Surg 1997;117:355–361

2. Dufour X, Bedier A, Ferrie J, Gohler C, Klossek JM. Diffuse nasal polyposis and endoscopic sinus surgery: long term results, a 65-case study. Laryngoscope 2004;114:1982–1987

3. Edelstein DR, Liberatore L, Bushkin S, Han JC. Applied anatomy of the posterior sinuses in relation to the optic nerve, trigeminal nerve and carotid artery. Am J Rhinol 1995;9:321–333

4. Elwany S, Elsaeid I, Thabet H. Endoscopic anatomy of the sphenoid sinus. J Laryngol Otol 1999;113:122–126

5. Kainz J, Stammberger H. Danger areas of the posterior rhinobasis. An endoscopic and anatomical-surgical study. Acta Otolaryngol 1992;112:852–861

6. Kim H-U, Kim S-S, Kang SS, Chung IH, Lee J-G, Yoon J-H. Surgical anatomy of the natural ostium of the sphenoid sinus. Laryngoscope 2001;111:1599–1602

7. Har-El G, Swanson R. The superior turbinectomy approach to isolated sphenoid sinus disease and to the sella turcica. Am J Rhinol 2001;15:149–156

8. Bolger WE, Keyes AS, Lanza DC. Use of the superior meatus and superior turbinate in the endoscopic approach to the sphenoid sinus. Otolaryngol Head Neck Surg 1999;120:308–313

9. Donald PJ. Sphenoid marsupialization for chronic sphenoidal sinusitis. Laryngoscope 2000;110:1349–1352

10. Orlandi RR, Lanza DC, Bolger WE, Clerico DM, Kennedy DW. The forgotten turbinate: the role of the superior turbinate in endoscopic sinus surgery. Am J Rhinol 1999;13:251–259

11. Unal B, Bademci G, Bilgili YK, Batay F, Avci E. Risky anatomic variations of sphenoid sinus for surgery. Surg Radiol Anat 2006;28: 195–201

9

Extended Approaches to the Frontal Sinus: The Modified Endoscopic Lothrop Procedure

Chronic frontal sinusitis has challenged surgeons for many years. In the past, frontal sinus obliteration through an osteoplastic flap (OPF) approach has been the gold standard for the management of recalcitrant frontal sinusitis.[1–3] Other external procedures such as fronto-ethmoidectomy have fallen into disfavor due to a failure rate of around 30%.[3] OPF and obliteration has a reported failure rate of around 10% but has a significant complication rate of around 65%.[3–6] The complications include cerebrospinal fluid (CSF) leak, frontal bossing, supraorbital neuralgia, chronic sepsis, mucocele formation, and chronic frontal bone osteitis with loss of the frontal sinus bone flap.[1–3,6] In recent years, the modified endoscopic Lothrop (MEL) procedure has been proposed as an alternative to the OPF with obliteration.[7–20] The MEL procedure is based on the technique originally described by Lothrop in 1914.[21] This technique involved removal of the upper portion of the septum, the floor of the frontal sinus, and the intersinus septum. Removal of the floor was accomplished with the aid of a small external incision (similar to a Lynch incision), which created a window through which the drill could be observed. Although this procedure was successful in 29 of 30 patients, the technique was considered too technically difficult for most surgeons to master, and it was not until Draf in 1991[7] and Gross in 1995[8,9] published series of patients using a modified version of the technique that interest was renewed. The major modification to the Lothrop technique is the absence of an external incision with the entire procedure performed endoscopically. The MEL can be used as an alternative to OPF with obliteration with recent publications[12] showing excellent short-term success rates with minimal complications. The indications for the MEL procedure should be the same as the indications for an OPF with obliteration, and these are detailed below.[12]

◆ INDICATIONS FOR MODIFIED ENDOSCOPIC LOTHROP PROCEDURE

Failed Endoscopic Sinus Surgery

The MEL procedure is indicated in patients who have failed standard endoscopic sinus surgery (ESS) techniques.[12] These include clearance of the frontal recess and removal of cells obstructing the frontal ostium.[20] In those very rare cases where patients have a very large cell obstructing the frontal ostium (i.e., a type 4 cell that extends into the frontal sinus by more than 50% of the vertical height of the frontal sinus), management may include a primary MEL procedure if the surgeon is certain that the cell is causing significant obstruction and that it is not possible to remove the cell with standard ESS techniques from below.[20] All patients should have had standard endoscopic sinus surgical approach with an attempt to remove obstructing cells from the frontal ostium and improve the drainage of the frontal sinus. It is only if such techniques fail that the MEL procedure should be considered for removal of a type 4 cell.[20] In **Fig. 9–1**, the patient had undergone five previous standard ESS procedures and was still left with significant frontal sinus symptoms and a large type 4 cell obstructing the frontal sinus ostium. This patient had a successful MEL procedure.

Neo-osteogenesis in the Frontal Recess and the Frontal Ostium

Significant new bone formation in the regions of the frontal recess after ESS indicates probable osteitis. This can be difficult to manage with standard ESS techniques. The neo-osteogenesis results in narrowed frontal sinus openings and increased

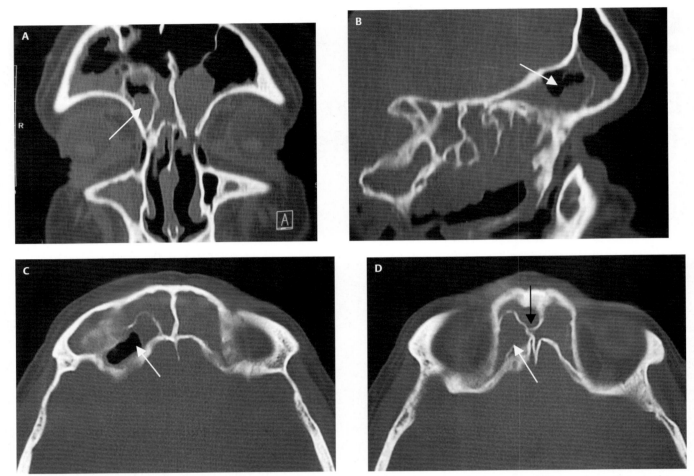

Figure 9–1 (A–D) CT scans of a patient with a type 4 cell (*white arrow*) who had undergone multiple previous ESS procedures. Note on the axial scan (**D**) the significantly narrowed frontal sinus drainage pathway (*black arrow*) caused by the type 4 cell (*white arrow*).

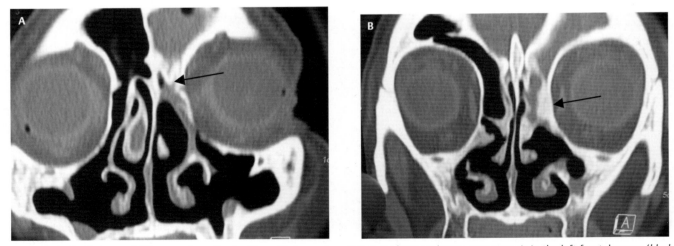

Figure 9–2 (A, B) Coronal CT scans of a patient with multiple previous ESS procedures with neo-osteogenesis in the left frontal recess (*black arrow*) with associated chronic frontal sinusitis.

vascularity in the region. Surgery to widen such narrowed ostia will often result in significant bleeding and loss of mucosa. The healing process may produce significant re-stenosis as ongoing low-grade osteitis and sinusitis continue to stimulate new bone formation and fibrosis. The MEL procedure overcomes this problem by drilling away a significant amount of the osteitic bone and creates the largest possible opening in the frontal sinuses. Even if some degree of re-stenosis occurs in the MEL procedure, this should not affect the function of the frontal sinuses.[22] Recent work done on the MEL procedure in our animal laboratory on the presence of neo-osteogenesis in a newly created frontal ostium suggests that most frontal ostia will restenose by an average of one third.[23, 24] This figure was not affected by the presence of neo-osteogenesis, which was found in 56% of animals. In addition, this re-stenosis did not affect the mucociliary drainage of the frontal sinuses as measured by the clearance of radioisotope from the frontal sinuses.[22] **Figure 9–2** shows a patient with significant neo-osteogenesis in the left frontal ostium. This patient had undergone six previous standard ESS procedures in an attempt to maintain a patent left frontal ostium. In all cases, the re-stenosis was rapid and associated with a return of frontal sinus symptoms.

Frontal Recess Adhesions

In patients who have previously undergone multiple ESS procedures, one will often find that the middle turbinates have been resected subtotally.[12] In this scenario, the middle turbinate remnant may lateralize and become adhesive to the lateral nasal wall in the frontal recess. This results in significant narrowing of the frontal drainage pathway and in some instances complete obstruction of the frontal ostium (**Fig. 9–3**). Standard ESS techniques will usually fail to re-create a mucosalized opening of sufficient diameter into the frontal sinuses and a MEL procedure or OPF with obliteration should be considered.

Disease Processes with Resultant Loss of the Posterior Wall or Floor of the Frontal Sinus

If the disease process results in bony erosion of either the posterior wall or floor of the frontal sinus, the mucosa of the sinus becomes adherent onto the dura or orbital periostium.[18] OPF with obliteration becomes extremely difficult in these patients as the mucosa cannot be safely or completely

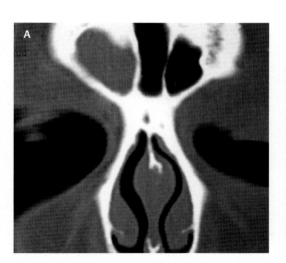

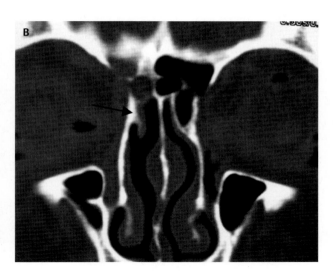

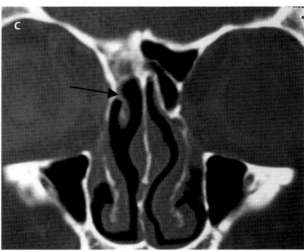

Figure 9–3 (A–C) This patient has had previous middle turbinate resection and the stump (*black arrow*) has lateralized blocking the frontal ostium. In addition, in CT scan (**C**), new bone formation can be seen above the middle turbinate.

removed from the dura or orbital periosteum and a recurrence of a mucocele is likely if the sinus is obliterated. These patients often have long-term severe chronic sinusitis and may have disease with a high incidence of recurrence such as fungal sinus disease. It is important to keep the frontal ostia open as obstruction of a frontal ostium may lead to either orbital or intracranial complications (**Fig. 9–4**).[18]

Failed Previous Osteoplastic Flap with Obliteration with Mucocele Formation[13]

Frontal sinus obliteration has been the gold standard for the management of recalcitrant frontal sinusitis for many years. However, severe mucosal disease such as that seen in patients with Sampter's triad (aspirin sensitivity, asthma, and nasal polyposis), allergic fungal sinusitis, and aggressive recurrent nasal polyposis is best managed endoscopically rather than with an OPF and obliteration.[14-18] There is now widespread agreement in the literature that the MEL procedure should be the operation of first choice in this difficult group of patients.[14-18]

One of the major problems with OPF and obliteration is the tendency for the adipose tissue placed in the frontal sinuses to resorb. Weber et al[14] in a large study of 82 patients who underwent OPF and obliteration showed that the majority of patients had less than 20% of the sinus obliterated after a median of 15.4 months.[14] In this patient group who aggressively form polyps, such space can be rapidly filled by even the smallest amount of residual mucosa inadvertently left in the frontal sinuses. In the postoperative period, this group tends to develop thick inspissated mucus among the regrowing polyps. Without a wide opening or marsupialization of the affected sinus, this mucus cannot be removed in the office. The inability to pass a large suction through the sinus ostium into the sinus cavity prevents this very tenacious mucus from being removed. A course of systemic prednisolone may loosen the mucus and lessens its tenacity facilitating its removal. Clearance of this toxic material allows shrinkage of the polyps and reestablishment of the nasal airway with control of polyp growth. In most patients, it is a relatively simple procedure to create a wide maxillary antrostomy, completely remove all ethmoid cells, and open widely the anterior face of the sphenoid sinus.

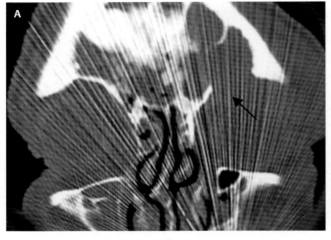

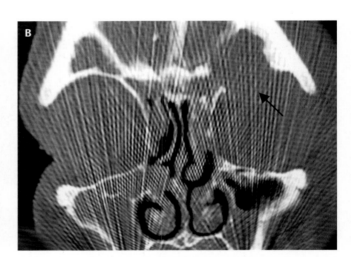

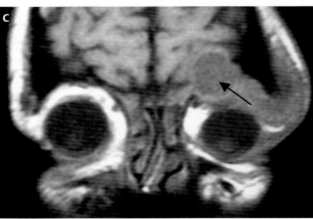

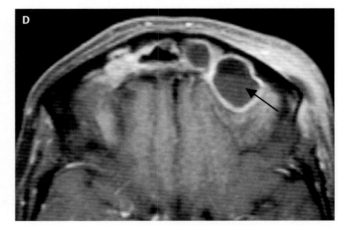

Figure 9–4 (A–D) This patient with chronic frontal sinusitis with loss of the roof of the orbit and loss of the posterior table of the frontal sinus developed an abscess (*black arrow*) with associated cellulitis around the orbit and depression of the left globe. In addition, this abscess had eroded the posterior table of the frontal sinus and compressed the anterior cerebral hemisphere (seen on MRI scans [**C**] and [**D**]). This was managed by a MEL procedure with the creation of a large communal frontal ostium.

However, the frontal sinuses are extremely difficult to access without the wide opening that the MEL procedure creates. Naturally sized frontal ostia tend to be quickly obstructed by thickened mucosa, and this results in a buildup of thick mucus in the frontal sinuses that may be resistant to aggressive prednisolone therapy and attempted suction clearance. One of the difficulties with OPF and obliteration in this group of patients is when there is loss of bone over the orbit or dura. Due to the aggressive nature of the polyposis and in some cases aggravated by repeated surgeries, there may be loss of the anterior or posterior bony frontal sinus wall. This brings the mucocele lining in direct contact with the orbital periosteum and/or dura and makes it impossible to remove all the mucosa from these structures without resection.[15] Even microscopic mucosal remnants left on the periosteum or dura will lead to the development of a mucocele in the obliterated cavity (**Fig. 9–5**).

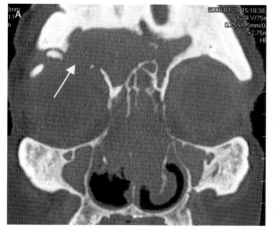
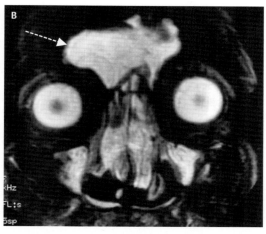
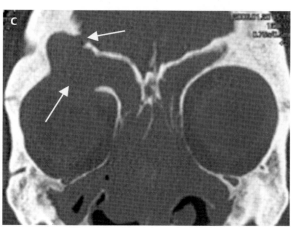
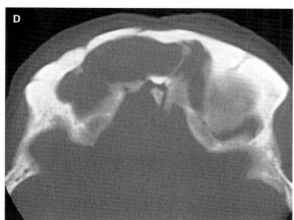
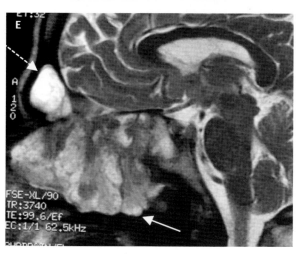

Figure 9–5 CT scan (**A**) shows frontal sinus opacification with an orbital roof dehiscence (*white arrow*). T2-weighted MRI scan (**B**) shows a frontal sinus mucocele (*broken white arrow*). CT scan (**C**) shows both orbital and posterior table dehiscences where the mucocele is in contact with the orbital periosteum and the dura. Axial CT scan (**D**) shows previous osteotomies in the anterior table of the frontal sinus, and MRI scan (**E**) shows the frontal sinus mucocele (*broken white arrow*) and the extensive nasal polyp formation in the nasal cavity (*solid white arrow*).

Another contraindication to OPF and obliteration is when the patient has very large pneumatized frontal sinuses.[15,18] In these patients, it is extremely difficult to eradicate all the mucosa from the lateral and posterior recesses of the frontal sinus, and this residual mucosa will form mucoceles that if left untreated will erode the bony walls of the sinus and may well give rise to either intracranial or orbital complications (**Fig. 9–6**). Mucoceles that form in a previously obliterated frontal sinus can be treated by an MEL procedure.[13,14,18] The mucocele should be sufficiently large that it can be accessed through the frontal recess and marsupialized into the frontal recess (**Fig. 9–6**).[13,18]

Patients who have previously had an OPF with obliteration often present with frontal pain, and it can be quite difficult to ascertain whether their pain is from a frontal sinus mucocele or from other causes. All these patients undergo magnetic resonance imaging (MRI) to ensure that there is indeed a mucocele present. If there is no mucocele present, surgery is usually not offered and the patient is given treatment for neuralgic pain or myofacial pain syndrome. To assess if the pain is neuralgic or myofacial in origin, a trial of low-dose amitriptyline (10 mg per night) is prescribed for 6 weeks. If neuralgia or myofacial pain syndrome is contributing to the patient's pain, there should be an improvement in symptoms with this treatment.[19] Most patients will also undergo radioisotope screening to exclude osteitis of the previous bone flap. If the radioisotope scan is positive, consideration may have to be given to removal of this bone flap.

Tumor Removal from the Frontal Sinus

The MEL procedure is useful for the removal of benign tumors from the frontal sinuses. These tumors include osteomas and inverting papillomas. Fairly large osteomas can be removed through the MEL opening.[12,15,18] **Figure 9–7** illustrates a patient with a large frontal osteoma that has blocked the pathway of the right frontal sinus and resulted in the formation

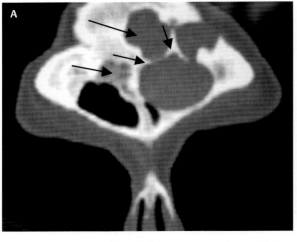
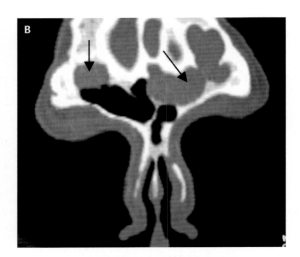
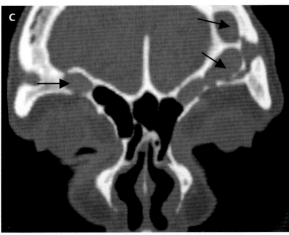
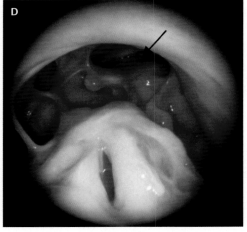

Figure 9–6 This patient has extensive pneumatization of the frontal sinuses. (**A–C**) OPF with obliteration failed with resultant superior and lateral mucocele formation. This was addressed with a MEL. (**D**) In this postoperative picture at 3 years, a *black arrow* indicates one of the opened mucoceles. (From Wormald PJ, Ananda A, Nair S. Modified endoscopic Lothrop as a salvage for the failed osteoplastic flap with obliteration. Laryngoscope 2003;113(11):1988–1992. Reprinted with permission.)

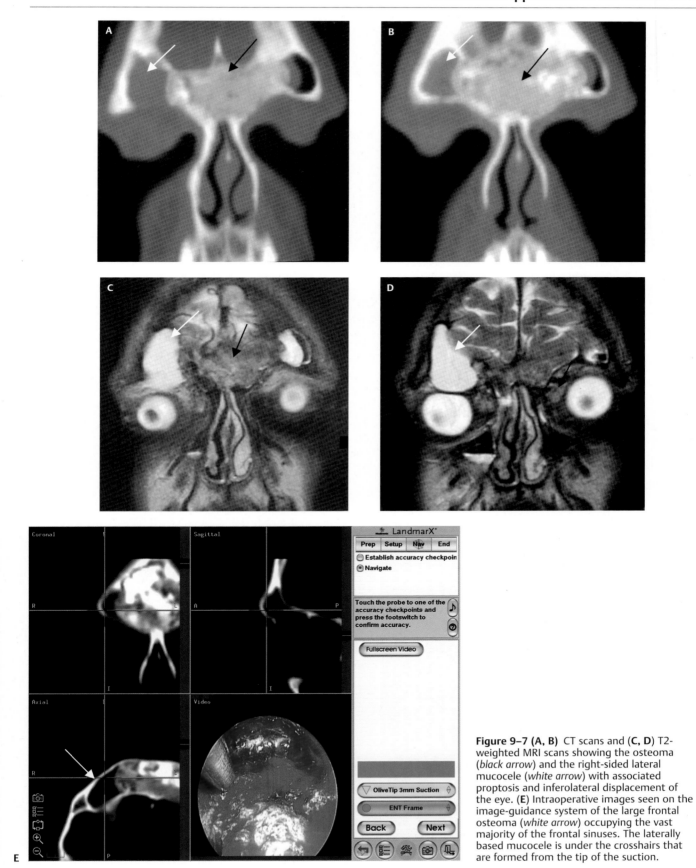

Figure 9–7 (A, B) CT scans and **(C, D)** T2-weighted MRI scans showing the osteoma (*black arrow*) and the right-sided lateral mucocele (*white arrow*) with associated proptosis and inferolateral displacement of the eye. **(E)** Intraoperative images seen on the image-guidance system of the large frontal osteoma (*white arrow*) occupying the vast majority of the frontal sinuses. The laterally based mucocele is under the crosshairs that are formed from the tip of the suction.

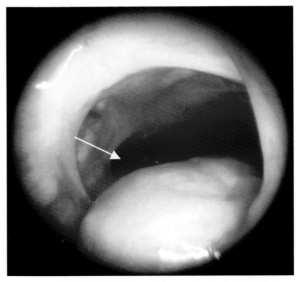

Figure 9–8 Endoscopic view of the frontal ostium created after removal of the large frontal osteoma shown in **Fig. 9–7**. The *white arrow* indicates the lateral pathway created into the laterally based mucocele indicated in **Fig. 9–7** on the CT scans.

of a large lateral mucocele. This mucocele had eroded the bone over the roof of the orbit with the lining of the mucocele in contact with a large proportion of the orbital periosteum (**Fig. 9–7**).

The patient had a MEL procedure with removal of 90% of the osteoma and drainage of the mucocele. A free mucosal graft was placed on the circumferential raw area created after removal of the osteoma. The patient is now 3 years postsurgery and has a nicely healed and patent right frontal sinus with free drainage of the lateral mucocele into the nose (**Fig. 9–8**).

The MEL procedure is also suitable for removing inverting papilloma from the frontal sinus.[12,15,20] **Figure 9–9** shows a recurrent inverting papilloma entering the frontal sinus on the left. This had previously been removed via a lateral rhinotomy procedure. The tumor is seen in the left frontal recess and sinus.

The entire tumor was removed after a MEL procedure until direct visualization. As a large area of frontal sinus mucosa was removed in association with the tumor, a free mucosal graft was placed. **Figure 9–10** shows the patient 1 year after the procedure. There still remains a little edema of the frontal ostium. Biopsies were negative for recurrence. Excellent

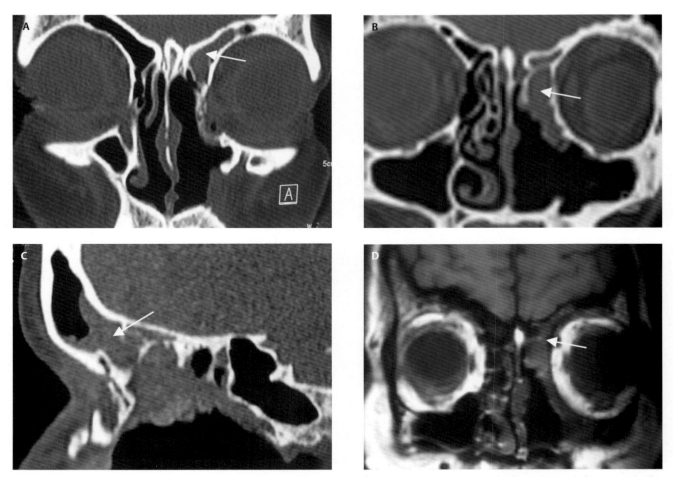

Figure 9–9 (A–C) The CT scans show recurrent inverting papilloma on the lamina papyracea entering the frontal sinus (*white arrows*). This is confirmed with (**D**) an MRI scan that shows the opacity within the frontal sinus is not just retained secretions.

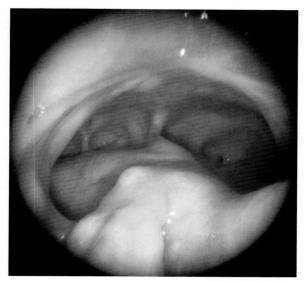

Figure 9–10 This endoscopic view shows the patient 4 years postoperatively with a nicely healed common opening into both frontal sinuses. The entire area of previous tumor involvement can be easily surveyed endoscopically for any recurrences.

visualization of the site of the tumor is provided by the large frontal ostium, and recurrences can be detected early.

◆ RELATIVE CONTRAINDICATIONS FOR THE MODIFIED ENDOSCOPIC LOTHROP PROCEDURE

Poorly Pneumatized Frontal Sinuses

In patients who have poorly developed (pneumatized) frontal sinuses, the bone of the frontal beak and the intersinus septum is very thick (**Fig. 9–11**).[12,18,20] This can make creation of a large frontal sinus ostium difficult as more bone needs to be taken away. In most cases, this results in a larger raw bony

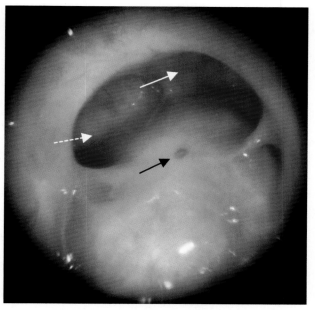

Figure 9–12 This is the postoperative picture taken of the patient shown in **Fig. 9–11** 3 years after surgery. The *black arrow* reveals a small granulation on the anterior skull base, which was subsequently removed. The *white solid arrow* indicates the frontal intersinus septum, and the *broken white arrow* indicates a small amount of mucus present in the right frontal sinus. The patient is currently asymptomatic.

surface as there is less residual mucosa in the region of the frontal sinus. In the postoperative period, there is a tendency for the frontal ostium to cicatrize. In **Fig. 9–11**, the patient has very underdeveloped frontal sinuses with a thick frontal beak and intersinus septum.

If the postoperative frontal ostium is viewed after 24 months (**Fig. 9–12**), the smaller than usual frontal ostium can be seen. This case illustrates the importance of creating the largest possible bony ostium at the time of surgery and that although underdeveloped frontal sinuses may be a relative

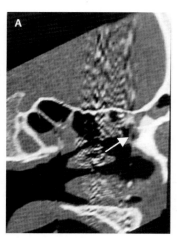
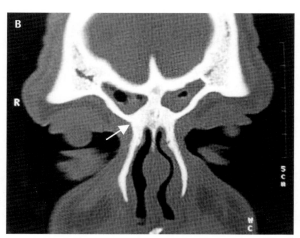
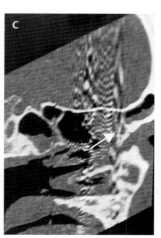

Figure 9–11 (A–C) Series of three CT scans ([**A**], right parasagittal, and [**C**], left parasagittal) illustrating the thick frontal beak resulting from underpneumatized frontal sinus (*white arrow*).

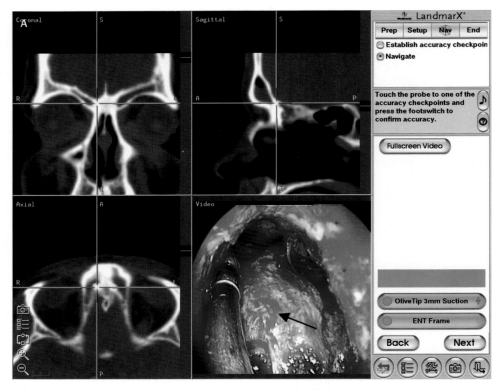

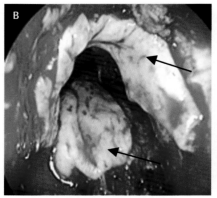

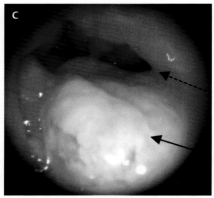

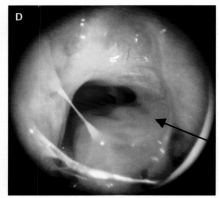

Figure 9–13 **(A)** This image taken from the computer-assisted surgical navigation (CAS) system shows the very narrow anteroposterior dimension of the frontal sinuses. The *black arrow* on the operative view indicates the relatively large area of bone removed from the forward extending anterior skull base. The only residual mucosa in this newly created frontal ostium is in the posterolateral regions. **(B)** The anterior and posterior free mucosal grafts (*black arrows*) that were put in place at the end of the surgery. **(C)** The frontal ostium after 3 months. The adhesion between the upper and lower grafts is indicated by the *black broken arrow*. **(D)** The frontal ostium at 5 years with the adhesion indicated by the *black arrow*. This adhesion can be seen in the early postoperative period in picture **(C)**, marked by the *broken black arrow*. The patient is currently asymptomatic.

contraindication, the patient can still have a successful MEL procedure if these principles are adhered to.

Narrow Anteroposterior Depth of the Frontal Sinus[12,18,20]

In some patients, the skull base comes further forward than normal and narrows the anteroposterior width of the frontal sinus. This in turn limits the anteroposterior width that can be created during surgery and increases the likelihood of postoperative scarring and closure of the frontal ostium. In **Fig. 9–13**, the patient has a very narrow anteroposterior diameter of the frontal sinus. This limits the opening that can be surgically created.

◆ SURGICAL TECHNIQUE[12,13,17,18,25–28]

It is currently our routine to use image-guidance equipment for all our MEL procedures.[12,13,18,20,26] Image-guidance helps to identify the olfactory fossa projections and aids in the creation of the largest possible frontal sinus ostium. This ability to create the largest possible opening is critical for the success of this procedure. Image guidance is set up before surgery. Once the accuracy of the system is verified, surgery begins. The first step is to surgically revise, as necessary, the maxillary, ethmoid, and sphenoid sinuses. It is important that this be done before the frontal sinus surgery as the frontal sinus component can be relatively time-consuming and the surgical field tends to worsen progressively as the operation proceeds. Visualization of the anatomy of the maxillary, ethmoid, and sphenoids can be difficult due to excessive bleeding if this is left to the end of the surgical procedure.

Infiltration with lidocaine and adrenaline is performed in the region above the axilla of the middle turbinate and the vault of the nose. The adjacent septum anterior to the middle turbinate is also infiltrated. A 0-degree scope is used for the majority of the dissection and a 30-degree scope is used when the floor of the frontal sinus is removed. The first step is to remove the mucosa above the middle turbinate up to the roof of the nose with a powered microdebrider exposing the underlying bone.[12] The mucosa of the septum anterior to the middle turbinate adjacent to the roof of the nose is removed over a 3 × 2 cm area (**Fig. 9–14**). This step is performed bilaterally. The cartilage and bone in the septal window is removed. An instrument should be able to be passed from the one side of the nose through the septal window and under the axilla of the middle turbinate on the other side.[12]

If this is not possible, the septal window should be lowered until this can be easily done. If there is a pathway between the frontal sinus and the frontal recess (i.e., there is

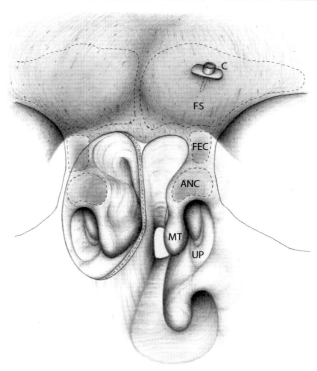

Figure 9–15 Drawing illustrating the positioning of the frontal cannula (C) through the skin of the forehead just medial to the eyebrow into the lumen of the frontal sinus (FS). A fronto-ethmoidal cell (FEC) and an agger nasi cell (ANC) are indicated in the diagram. (From Wormald PJ. Salvage frontal sinus surgery: the Modified Lothrop Procedure. Laryngoscope 2003;113:276–283. Reprinted with permission.)

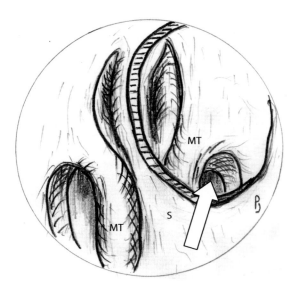

Figure 9–14 Drawing after creation of the septal window with the middle turbinates (MT) and septum (S) on view. The *arrow* indicates that the septal perforation needs to be lowered until an instrument can be passed from the one side of the nose (in this case, the right side) across the septal perforation under the axilla of the opposite middle turbinate (in this case, the left side).

no mucocele present with complete separation of the frontal sinus and frontal recess), a frontal sinus mini-trephine is placed in each frontal sinus. Flushing the frontal sinus mini-trephine will result in fluorescein-stained saline being seen under the axilla of the middle turbinate. This step is done early as it increases the safety of the dissection. Regular flushing of the frontal sinus will result in fluorescein flowing through the frontal ostium allowing the surgeon to have a constant posterior reference point and thus keep the dissection away from the skull base. The fluorescein-stained saline delineates the frontal ostium, and we can therefore dissect the bone anterior to the ostium (but not medial) knowing that the dissection is anterior to the skull base (**Fig. 9–15**).

The CT scans of both frontal recesses are viewed in three planes, and the anatomy of the frontal recess is reconstructed using the building block technique previously described.[27,28] The 3.2-mm cutting burr is used to remove the frontal process of the maxilla directly above the axilla (**Fig. 9–16**). In the initial stages of this dissection, the burr is swept from the frontal ostium anterior across the frontal process of the maxilla removing both anterior and lateral bone. This opens the access to the frontal ostium in a funnel shape. This process is analogous to performing a front-to-back mastoidectomy by removing the outer cortical bone and creating a funnel-shaped access to the antrum. As this lateral

A

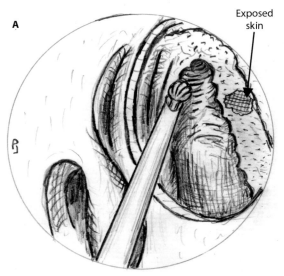

Exposed
skin

B

FS

MT

MT

Figure 9–16 (A, B) The 3.2-mm cutting burr is used to remove the bone above the axilla of the middle turbinate. In (**A**), the anterior wall of the agger nasi cell and the beak of the frontal process of

the maxilla are removed until the frontal sinus is entered. Note the small lateral area of exposed skin that marks the lateral extent of the dissection. In (**B**), the frontal sinus (FS) has been entered.

and superior bone removal continues anterior and superior to the axilla of the middle turbinate, a small amount of skin is exposed to define the lateral extent of the dissection.

Dissection is continued superiorly using regular flushes of the fluorescein to identify the anterior lip of the frontal ostium and to allow the bone anterior to the frontal ostium (the bone that forms the frontal "beak") to be removed. Care is taken to ensure that drilling is done in only a superior and lateral direction without drilling medially as this may endanger the skull base. It is important to accurately define the lateral extent of the dissection by exposing a small area of skin. As long as the exposure of the skin is done directly above

FS

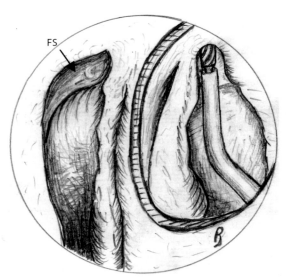

Figure 9–17 The frontal sinus (FS) has been opened bilaterally. The angled burr is used to remove the "beak" or anterior wall of the frontal sinus further enlarging the frontal ostium.

the axilla of the middle turbinate, the drill will be anterior to the orbit. This dissection is in the same coronal plane as the lacrimal sac, and the lacrimal sac may exposed if bone is removed laterally within 8 mm of the axilla of the middle turbinate. The skin exposure is done bilaterally to define the lateral limits of dissection and to ensure achievement of maximal ostial width. Drilling continues superiorly until the floor of the frontal sinus is entered and the frontal sinus can be seen. Further removal of this floor and of the beak of the frontal process of the maxilla (the anterior wall of the dissection) is facilitated by using an angled burr (**Fig. 9–17**). Once the floor of the frontal sinus is opened on one side, the endoscope and drill are transferred into the opposite nostril and the process repeated until the floor of the second frontal sinus is exposed. Note that up until this point no medial dissection has taken place. If the dissection is brought medially before the frontal sinus is entered, the surgeon is likely to damage the forward projections of the olfactory fossae and cause a CSF leak. Once the floor of the frontal sinus is entered, the straight burr is usually changed to an angled burr and the telescope to a 30-degree scope (**Fig. 9–17**).

The dissection is now brought medially from both sides until the frontal intersinus septum is seen (**Fig. 9–18**). Note that this medial dissection takes place at the upper limit of the opening of the frontal sinuses and that drilling in a medial direction lower down can still potentially endanger the skull base. This dissection is alternated from side to side thereby connecting the two frontal sinuses. The last structure to be removed is the intersinus septum. Once this is done, the frontal sinus opening is in the shape of a crescent (**Fig. 9–18**).

The aim of the surgery is now to transform this crescent opening into an oval opening thereby creating the largest possible anteroposterior and lateral diameters for the frontal ostium. The first step is to remove the intersinus septum as high as possible, right up to the roof of the frontal sinus. Once this is done, the anterior frontal bone is removed until

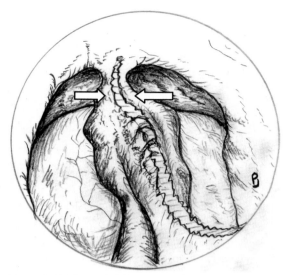

Figure 9–18 The medial dissection is done at the upper limits of the opened frontal sinuses as indicated by the *block arrows*. Once the intersinus septum is reached, the opening is in the shape of a crescent.

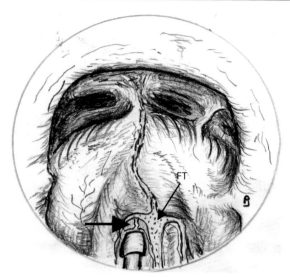

Figure 9–19 The maximum lateral opening has been created and the bony beak removed until there is a smooth transition from the frontal sinus anterior wall into the nose without bony ridges. The frontal "T" (FT) is formed by the junction of the middle turbinates and the septum. An olive-tipped suction pushes the mucosa posteriorly exposing the first olfactory neuron (*black arrow*).

there is no longer an anterior ridge or lip of bone separating the frontal sinus from the nasal cavity. When the anterior table of the frontal sinus is viewed with a 30-degree scope, the transition from the frontal sinus to nasal cavity should be smooth. Any bony ridges should be removed (**Fig. 9–19**).

The final and most dangerous step of the operation is to remove the bone over the forward projection of the skull base. This forward projection forms the frontal "T." The "T" is made up by the two middle turbinates attaching to the septum (**Fig. 9–18**). The frontal sinus intersinus septum, nasal septum, and associated middle turbinates are drilled posteriorly toward the skull base. At the "T," the olfactory fossae project forward from the skull base and great care needs to be taken so that the "T" is lowered as far as possible without exposing the dura of these olfactory projections. These projections can most clearly be seen on the axial scan (**Fig. 9–20**).

The position of these forward projections or horns can be identified in two ways. First, the image-guidance suction can be used to determine the exact position of these forward projections of the skull base. However, these should always

be clinically correlated by sliding a suction Freer elevator between the bone and mucosa in the roof of the nose and gently pushing the mucosa downward. The anterior ethmoidal nerve and first olfactory fibers are easily visible and indicate the most anterior position of the olfactory bulb (**Fig. 9–21**). It is important to clinically correlate findings of the image guidance as the headframe can shift with resultant inaccuracies.

Once the position of the forward projections of the anterior skull base are located, the bone over the anterior skull base is lowered to within 1 mm of the olfactory fibers. This is done either with a diamond burr or with the 3.2-mm straight cutting burr. If a cutting burr is used, the bone should be lightly brushed with the burr spinning at maximum revolutions (12,000 rpm). The technique is similar to that used when removing the final bone from the facial nerve during facial nerve decompression. Lowering this forward projection of the olfactory fossa is crucial for the largest possible opening

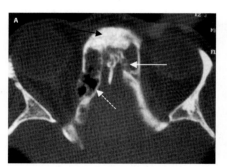
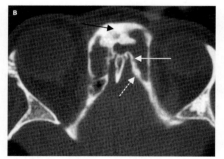
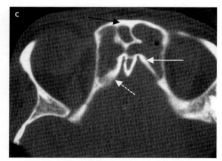

Figure 9–20 (A–C) Sequential axial CT scans illustrating the frontal beak (*black arrow*) and the forward projection of the olfactory fossa into the transition area between the frontal recess (**A**) and the frontal sinus (**C**). The skull base is indicated by the *broken white* *arrows*. For the maximum anteroposterior diameter to be created, the bone of the frontal beak should be drilled down to a thin layer and the bone overlying the forward projections of the olfactory fossae (*white arrow*) drilled back as close as possible to the skull base.

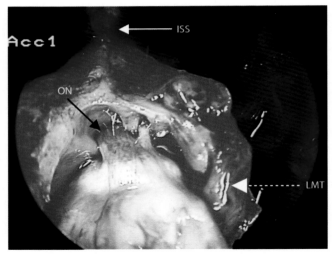

Figure 9–21 This intraoperative photo demonstrates the first olfactory neuron (ON) as the mucosa is peeled away from the skull base during widening of the frontal sinus ostium. The intersinus septum (ISS) and left middle turbinate (LMT) can be seen.

to be created into the frontal sinuses. Failure to remove this projection gives a narrow anteroposterior dimension and a crescent-shaped opening that has a greater tendency to stenose. Lowering the bone over the olfactory fossa gives the widest possible anteroposterior dimension to the new common frontal sinus ostium (**Fig. 9–22**).

In most patients, an oval-shaped frontal sinus ostium is created. The average dimensions should be ~18 mm in the

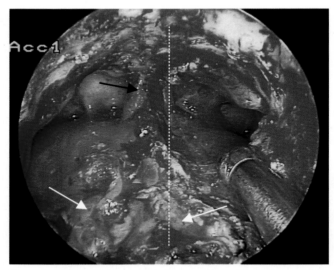

Figure 9–22 This intraoperative photo illustrates the wide frontal sinus ostium achieved at the end of the endoscopic modified Lothrop procedure. The *black arrow* indicates the frontal sinus septum and the *white arrows* the anterior extensions of the olfactory fossa. Note how the bone over the fossae has been lowered onto the skull base giving an oval-shaped opening rather than a crescent-shaped opening into the frontal sinuses. The *white broken line* indicates the large anteroposterior extent of the frontal ostium. The 4-mm olive-tipped suction is placed in the picture as a size reference.

anteroposterior plane and 20 to 24 mm from side to side. The size of the opening is determined by the patient's anatomy but should be made as large as possible.

At the end of the procedure, the suction bipolar forceps are used to achieve hemostasis. Particular attention is paid to the posterior edge of the septal window and anterior ends of the middle turbinates. If the middle turbinates are unstable, they are sutured with a dissolving suture through the septum. This allows their lateral surfaces to heal before the suture dissolves and they lateralize. This prevents adhesions from forming.

◆ POSTOPERATIVE CARE[12,13,18]

The frontal sinus cannulae are left in place for up to 5 days. Frontal sinus saline douches are started through the frontal cannulae within 2 hours of completion of the operation. This will wash any blood clot out of the frontal ostium. In addition, 0.5 mL of prednisolone solution is placed in each frontal sinus after every second frontal sinus douche. The aim of the prednisolone is to dampen the inflammatory response of the mucosa as we have shown in animal studies that a less inflamed mucosa heals faster. Immediately prior to removal of the frontal sinus cannulae, 5 mL of steroid and antibiotic cream (*not* ointment) is injected through each cannulae. This coats the newly created frontal sinus ostium and tends to decrease the amount of adherent crusts that form in this region in the postoperative period. The patients are reviewed again at 2 weeks when all crusts, residual cream, and blood clots are meticulously removed from the frontal sinus ostium. This process is crucial because if these adherent clots are left, they form the framework into which collagen is laid encouraging fibrosis of the frontal sinus ostium. In our animal model, postoperative douching of the frontal sinus after a MEL procedure tended to improve the mucociliary drainage of the frontal sinuses at 2 and 4 months after surgery.[22] This trend was not statistically significant.

◆ COMPLICATION: STENOSIS OF THE FRONTAL NEO-OSTIUM

In both studies done on the sheep animal model and on long-term review of 80 MEL patients, the frontal ostium narrowed to about a third of its original size.[23,24] It was also apparent that this narrowing occurred within the first 12 months after surgery and that thereafter the frontal ostium was stable.[24] The time course of how the frontal ostium narrowed is presented in **Fig. 9–23**.

The only significant factor in the patients who eventually developed frontal ostial stenosis was the size of the original ostium at the time of the initial surgery.[24] Other factors such as aspirin sensitivity, fungal sinusitis, and nasal polyposis were found not to influence the development of stenosis. This emphasizes the importance of creating the largest possible opening at the time of the original surgery and underlies the significant effort that is made to create the largest possible opening during surgery (exposure of skin on each side and complete removal of the frontal beak). These results also emphasize the success that the MEL has

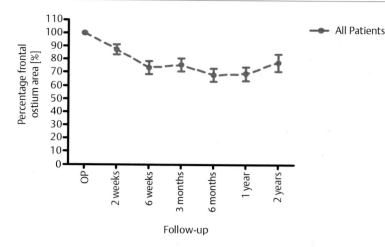

Figure 9–23 Time course for 80 patients in whom the frontal ostium was measured at the time of surgery and at regular time points in the postoperative period. All patients start with the biggest possible frontal ostium (100%), and each subsequent reading is a percentage of this original measurement. (From Tran K, Beule A, Singhal D, Wormald PJ. Frontal ostium restenosis after the endoscopic modified Lothrop procedure. Laryngoscope 2007 [in press]. Reprinted with permission.)

in the management of patients with these very difficult conditions. One would expect that aspirin triad and fungal sinusitis that aggressively form polyps would develop postoperative stenosis, as the high likelihood of polyp regrowth in these conditions would narrow the frontal ostium significantly, necessitating reoperation. In our most recent long-term study with significant follow-up, this was shown not to be the case with these conditions having no statistical influence on the development of postoperative stenosis.[24] It appears that MEL is one operation that can break the ongoing cycle of repeated polyp regrowth and revision surgery. This may be due to the surgeon's ability to remove the fungal mucin from the frontal sinuses and clear the frontal sinus in the office. If the patient is then given a course of prednisolone, the mucosa of the frontal sinus and ethmoids may return to

normal. Repeated suction clearance and prednisolone may be required, and as long as the patient is having four or fewer courses of prednisolone every 12 months, this regimen is continued and gives good control of the patient's symptoms. Once the patient requires more than four courses of prednisolone a year, revision surgery is offered.

◆ RESULTS

Our department has published studies of the largest series of MEL procedures to date.[12,13,18,24] The first study[12] involved 83 consecutive patients who underwent the MEL procedure for several indications.[12] Their presenting symptoms and etiology are shown in **Table 9–1**.[12]

Table 9–1 Summary of Pathology, Presenting Symptoms, Disease Severity, and Complications of Patients Having Endoscopic Modified Lothrop Procedure

Pathology	Number of Patients	Preoperative Frontal Pain	Preoperative Complications	Mean Lund and MacKay Score	No Communication between Frontal Sinus and Nose	Neo-osteogenesis in Frontal Ostium Region
Chronic sinusitis	10	10	1 orbital	1.5	0	7
Chronic fungal sinusitis	16	13	2 intracranial	2	0	3
Allergic fungal sinusitis	8	7	3 intracranial 1 orbital	2	0	0
Nasal polyps	3	3	0	1.5	0	0
ASA and polyps	15	13	0	2	0	0
Mucoceles	8	8	2 orbital	2	8	8
Previous osteoplastic flap with mucocele	17	17	2 intracranial 2 orbital	2	17	17
Frontal osteoma	2	2	0	1.5	0	2
Previous frontal sinus trauma	4	4	1 orbital 1 intracranial 1 CSF leak	1	2	2
Total	**83**	**77**	**17***	**1.72**	**27**	**39**

*One patient had two and one patient had three complications. Note Lund and Mackay of frontal sinus only.

Abbreviations: ASA, aminosalicylic acid (aspirin); CSF, cerebrospinal fluid.

Source: From Wormald PJ. Salvage frontal sinus surgery: the Modified Lothrop Procedure. Laryngoscope 2003;113:276–283. Reprinted with permission.

Of this group of 83 patients, six developed stenosis of the frontal ostium and required revision of the MEL procedure. In a subsequent study[24] with significantly longer follow-up, 10 of 80 (12.5%) patients required revision surgery indicating that the long-term stenosis rate remained low.[24] **Figure 9–24** shows a patient with frontal ostial stenosis.

The patency rate of the frontal ostium after MEL procedure was 93% at 21 months follow-up[12] and in the second study was 87.5% with a mean follow-up of 29.4 months. This second study measured the frontal ostium at surgery and at time intervals after surgery and showed that the size of the frontal ostium remained stable after 12 months. Three (4%) patients continued to deteriorate after 12 months. Thus, the overall incidence of frontal ostium stenosis (12.5%) is low if attention is paid to creating the largest possible frontal sinus opening at the time of surgery. **Figure 9–25** shows three examples of healthy frontal sinus ostia at more than 12 months after the MEL procedure.

As far as symptoms are concerned, the success rate was not as high as the patency rate. There were 21 of the 83 patients who continued to have symptoms from their sinuses. This

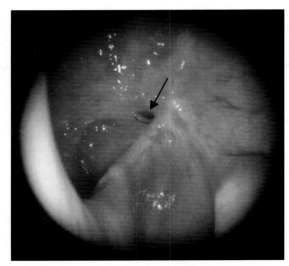

Figure 9–24 Patient has undergone significant frontal ostium stenosis until the residual ostium (*black arrow*) is only 2 × 4 mm. This will cause retention of secretions within the frontal sinuses and symptoms and needs to be revised.

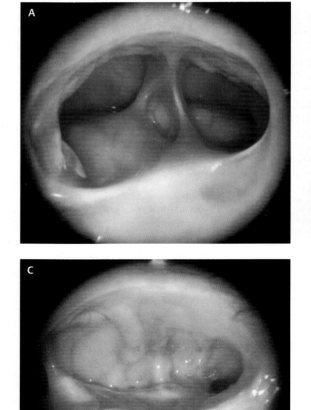

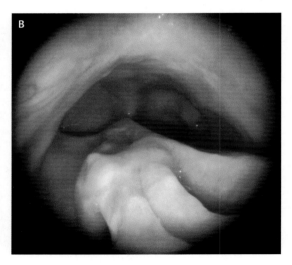

Figure 9–25 (A–C) Three patients after MEL procedure with oval-shaped frontal ostia and healthy frontal sinuses.

Table 9–2 Summary of the Outcomes of Patients Having Modified Endoscopic Lothrop Procedure

Pathology	Number of Patients	Intraoperative Complications	Postoperative Symptoms	Frontal Ostium Closed	Revision Lothrop Surgery	Average Follow-up (Months)
Chronic sinusitis	10	0	2 recurrent infections 1 continued frontal pain	2	1 at 4 months 1 at 8 months	22.9
Fungal sinusitis	16	0	3 recurrent fungus 1 continued frontal pain	1	1 at 7 months	21
Allergic fungal sinusitis	8	0	5 recurrent fungus	3	1 at 6 months 2 at 12 months	13.1
Nasal polyps	3	0	0	0	0	33
ASA and polyps	15	0	3 recurrent polyps 2 recurrent infections	0	0	24
Mucoceles	8	0	0	0	0	19.3
Previous osteoplastic flap with mucocele	17	0	1 recurrent infection 3 continued frontal pain	0	0	23
Frontal osteoma	2	0	0	0	0	23.5
Previous frontal sinus trauma	4	1 CSF leak from meningoencephalocele	0	0	0	17.5
Totals	**83**	**1**	**21**	**6**	**6**	**21.9**

Abbreviations: ASA, aminosalicylic acid (aspirin); CSF, cerebrospinal fluid.

Source: From Wormald PJ. Salvage frontal sinus surgery: the Modified Lothrop Procedure. Laryngoscope 2003;113:276–283. Reprinted with permission.

is summarized in **Table 9–2**.[12] It should be kept in mind that this group of patients is part of a highly recalcitrant group of patients who have undergone multiple previous operations and often have diseases such as aspirin sensitivity, polyps, asthma, and fungal sinusitis, which have high recurrence rates.

Note that there was one CSF leak. This occurred in a patient who had drainage of an orbital abscess associated with the superior rectus muscle in an already blind eye. Also associated with this abscess was a traumatic meningocele extending into the orbit from a fracture in the roof of the orbit. Once the abscess was drained, a flush of CSF was seen. This was repaired using a fat-plug and the "bath-plug" technique. To date, there have been no CSF leaks caused during the drill-out procedure or during lowering the bone over the projections of the olfactory fossae.

◆ **REVISION SURGERY**

Revision MEL procedure is conducted along similar lines to the primary surgery. Frontal trephine cannulae are placed early into the frontal sinuses and fluorescein in saline used to delineate the skull base. The frontal ostium is widened by removal of all scar tissue. If the repeat CT scan shows any areas of bone that are still significantly thick, then these are lowered until the maximum-sized frontal sinus ostium is created. Neuropatties soaked in 0.4% mitomycin C are applied to the region of the frontal ostium for 4 minutes. This area is extensively irrigated with saline. Postoperative care is similar to what has been described above other than all patients receive prednisolone drops after every second saline

douche. It is important to remove all crusts and blood clots at the 2-week postoperative visit. Failure to properly debride and clean the frontal ostium at this point can lead to the formation of adhesions, which may in turn contribute to long-term closure of the frontal ostium.

References

1. Casiano RR, Livingston JA. Endoscopic Lothrop procedure: the University of Miami experience. Am J Rhinol 1998;12:335–339
2. Becker DG, Moore D, Lindsey WH, Gross WE, Gross CW. Modified transnasal endoscopic Lothrop procedure: further considerations. Laryngoscope 1995;105:1161–1166
3. Wormald PJ. The axillary flap approach to the frontal recess. Laryngoscope 2002;112:494–499
4. Close LG, Lee NK, Leach JL, Manning SC. Endoscopic resection of the intranasal frontal sinus floor. Ann Otol Rhinol Laryngol 1994;103:952–958
5. Alsarraf R, Kriet J, Weymuller EA Jr. Quality-of-life outcomes after osteoplastic frontal sinus obliteration. Otolaryngol Head Neck Surg 1999;121:435–440
6. Catalano PJ, Lawson W, Som P, Biller HF. Radiographic evaluation and diagnosis of the failed frontal osteoplastic flap with fat obliteration. Otolaryngol Head Neck Surg 1991;104:225–234
7. Draf W. Endonasal micro-endoscopic frontal sinus surgery, the Fulda concept. Op Tech Otolaryngol Head Neck Surg 1991;2:234–240
8. Gross WE, Gross CW, Becker D, Moore D, Phillips D. Modified transnasal endoscopic Lothrop procedure as an alternative to frontal sinus obliteration. Otolaryngol Head Neck Surg 1995;113:427–434
9. Gross CW, Gross WE, Becker D. Modified transnasal endoscopic Lothrop procedure: frontal drillout. Op Tech Otolaryngol Head Neck Surg 1995;6:193–200
10. Schlosser RJ, Zachmann G, Harrison S, Gross CW. The endoscopic modified Lothrop: long-term follow-up on 44 patients. Am J Rhinol 2002;16:103–108

11. Ulualp SO, Carlson TK, Toohill RJ. Osteoplastic flap versus modified endoscopic Lothrop procedure in patients with frontal sinus disease. Am J Rhinol 2000;14:21–26

12. Wormald PJ. Salvage frontal sinus surgery: the modified Lothrop procedure. Laryngoscope 2003;113:276–283

13. Wormald PJ, Ananda A, Nair S. Modified endoscopic Lothrop as a salvage for the failed osteoplastic flap with obliteration. Laryngoscope 2003;113(11):1988–1992

14. Weber R, Draf W, Keerl R. Osteoplastic frontal sinus surgery with fat obliteration: technique and long tern results using magnetic resonance imaging in 82 operations. Laryngoscope 2000;110:1037–1044

15. Javer AR, Sillers M, Kuhn F. The frontal sinus unobliteration procedure. Otolaryngol Clin North Am 2001;34:193–210

16. Hosemann W, Kuhnel T, Held P, Wagner W, Felderhoff A. Endonasal frontal sinusotomy in surgical management of chronic sinusitis: a critical evaluation. Am J Rhinol 1997;11:1–9

17. Weber R, Draf W, Kratzsch B, Hosemann W, Schaefer S. Modern concepts of frontal sinus surgery. Laryngoscope 2001;111:137–146

18. Wormald PJ, Ananda A, Nair S. The modified endoscopic Lothrop procedure in the management of complicated chronic frontal sinusitis. Clin Otolaryngol 2003;28:215–220

19. West B, Jones NS. Endoscopy-negative, computed tomography-negative facial pain in a nasal clinic. Laryngoscope 2001;111:581–586

20. Wormald PJ, Chan SZX. Surgical techniques for the removal of frontal recess cells obstructing the frontal ostium. Am J Rhinol 2003;17:221–226

21. Lothrop HA. Frontal sinus suppuration. Ann Surg 1914;50:937–957

22. Rajapaksa SP, Ananda A, Cain T, Oates L, Wormald PJ. The effect of the modified endoscopic Lothrop procedure on the mucociliary clearance of the frontal sinus in the animal model. Am J Rhinol 2004;18(3):183–187

23. Rajapaksa SP, Ananda A, Cain TM, Oates L, Wormald PJ. Frontal ostium neo-osteogenesis and restenosis after modified endoscopic Lothrop procedure in an animal model. Clin Otolaryngol Allied Sci 2004;29(4):386–388

24. Tran K, Beule A, Singhal D, Wormald PJ. Frontal ostium restenosis after the endoscopic modified Lothrop procedure. Laryngoscope 2007 (in press)

25. Gross CW. Surgical treatments for symptomatic chronic frontal sinusitis. Arch Otolaryngol Head Neck Surg 2000;126:101–102

26. Loehrl TA, Toohill RJ, Smith TL. Use of computer-aided surgery for frontal sinus ventilation. Laryngoscope 2000;110:1962–1967

27. Wormald PJ. The agger nasi cell. The key to understanding the anatomy of the frontal recess. Otolaryngol Head Neck Surgery 2003;129:497–507

28. Wormald PJ. Surgery of the frontal recess and frontal sinus. Rhinology 2005;43(2):83–85

10

Sphenopalatine Artery Ligation and Vidian Neurectomy

Epistaxis may be classified clinically into anterior and posterior bleeds.[1] If the vascular supply of the nose is reviewed, it is apparent that anterior epistaxis would originate from the vascular anastomosis of vessels around Little's (or Kiesselbach's) area or from the anterior ethmoidal artery. Little's plexus is formed by branches from the sphenopalatine artery (via the posterior nasal artery branch) anastomosing with branches from the greater palatine, nasolabial (a branch of the facial artery), and anterior ethmoidal artery. Bleeding from Little's area is usually easily visible and managed by either local cautery or an anterior nasal pack. Bleeding from the anterior ethmoidal artery is rarely spontaneous and usually seen after trauma with associated skull base fractures or intraoperative injury. Posterior bleeding is often seen from under the inferior turbinate where branches of the sphenopalatine artery (SPA) anastomose with branches from the pharyngeal artery. This area is termed Woodruff's area. Bleeders in this region can be difficult to visualize due to their location under the posterior end of the inferior turbinate. Other posterior bleeders may arise from the lateral nasal wall, posterior choana, or posterior septum.

◆ POSTOPERATIVE EPISTAXIS

Significant postoperative epistaxis (as opposed to the blood-stained ooze usually seen in the first 24 hours after nasal surgery) typically occurs when a vessel of significant diameter bleeds. Logically, this would be either in the region of the sphenopalatine or anterior ethmoidal artery. Intraoperative damage to the anterior ethmoidal artery is almost always visible during surgery and would in most patients need to be dealt with immediately, as the resultant bleeding usually obscures the surgical field, making further surgery difficult if not impossible. However, vessels divided in the region of the SPA may bleed for a short period of time and then undergo spasm and thrombose. As these vessels are located posteriorly, the blood will drain into the nasopharynx and not come to the notice of the surgeon, who may then not seek out the bleeding vessel and cauterize it. By the time the surgery is completed, the vessel may either be in spasm or thrombosed. If the patient strains or becomes hypertensive in the immediate postoperative period, significant epistaxis can result, which may necessitate the placement of a nasal pack or return to the theater to cauterize the bleeding vessel. On occasion, epistaxis may occur days or even weeks postoperatively. In this situation, the patient has likely developed a postoperative infection with increased vascularity, and if the blood clot detaches from the vessel or is dislodged by coughing or straining, epistaxis may result.

To prevent postoperative epistaxis, close inspection of the region of the SPA is performed at the end of surgery. Particular attention is paid to the region of the horizontal insertion of the ground lamella into the lateral nasal wall, especially if the ground lamella has been resected, and to the lateral nasal wall in the superior meatus (**Fig. 10–1**). In addition, close inspection is made of the antero-inferior region of the sphenoid where the lower edge of the sphenoidotomy. If the sphenoid has been widely opened, then the posterior nasal artery or its vertical branch may have been divided (**Fig. 10–1**). Bipolar cautery is applied with the suction bipolar forceps* (Medtronic) until the field is dry. If the patient is still hypotensive at this stage, the anesthesiologist is asked to raise the blood pressure into the normal range before the patient is awakened. During this time, this region is inspected regularly on both sides, and any vessels that bleed as the pressure is raised are cauterized.

Comorbidities for Spontaneous Epistaxis

The majority of patients (69%) presenting with severe epistaxis have associated comorbidities.[1] These usually include hypertension, cardiovascular disease, and clotting

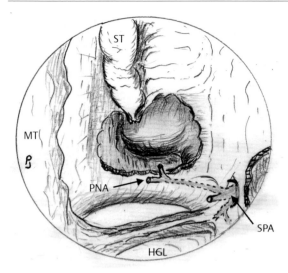

Figure 10–1 The vessels branching from the sphenopalatine artery (SPA) commonly bleed after ESS. Branches supplying the horizontal portion of the ground lamella (HGL) and the anterior wall of the sphenoid (posterior nasal artery [PNA]) need to be cauterized using a suction bipolar at the end of surgery to ensure that no bleeding occurs in the postoperative period. MT, middle turbinate; ST, superior turbinate.

abnormalities. More than 60% of patients managed in our series were either on aspirin or on warfarin as part of their ongoing medical treatment.[1] As the effects of aspirin and aspirin-like drugs are not immediately reversible, no specific treatment is given for these clotting abnormalities. However, in patients who are on warfarin, this is stopped and if necessary a transfusion of fresh-frozen plasma is given to rapidly lower the INR (below 2) before proceeding to surgery.

◆ SPHENOPALATINE ARTERY LIGATION

Indications for Sphenopalatine Artery Ligation

Before SPA ligation is considered, it needs to be established that the bleeding is coming from the posterior region of the nose. Patients assessed for possible SPA ligation are asked to forcefully blow their nose to expel all blood clots from the nose. The nose is then sprayed with a combination of lidocaine and epinephrine. The patient keeps his or her head forward after the nose blowing allowing blood to drip into a kidney dish held below the nose. A rigid nasal endoscope and suction are then passed into the nose to assess where the bleeding is coming from. If the vessel is clearly visible, cautery is attempted.[2] If the vessel is not visible but bleeding is confirmed to be posterior, then an inflatable or expanding posterior nasal pack is placed and the patient prepared for surgery.

Surgical Technique

This procedure can be performed under either local anesthetic or general anesthetic. The first step is to put the bleeding vessel into spasm. A pterygopalatine block is placed transorally. The greater palatine canal is located by palpation of the hard palate. A finger is passed along the hard palate until the junction of the hard and soft palate is felt. The finger is slowly slid anteriorly along the midpoint between the midline and teeth. The depression created by the greater palatine foramen is felt. This is usually opposite the second molar tooth (**Fig. 10–2**).[1,3]

With the finger still on the mucosal depression, an endoscope is slid into the mouth and the location of the depression endoscopically confirmed. The finger is then removed while the endoscope position is maintained. A 2-mL

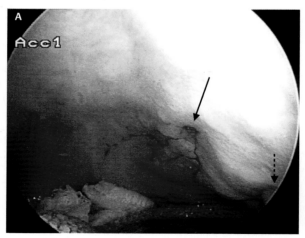

Figure 10–2 (**A**) The location of the left greater palatine canal is indicated with a *solid black arrow*. A bloodstain from the pterygopalatine injection is visible in this region. The second molar tooth is indicated with a *broken black arrow*. (**B**) The

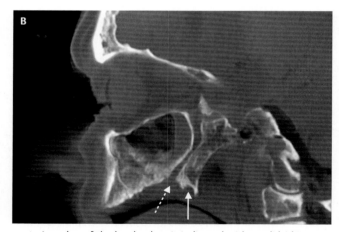

posterior edge of the hard palate is indicated with a *solid white arrow*. This is the first landmark. The finger is slid anteriorly until the depression of the greater palatine canal is felt (*broken white arrow*).

A

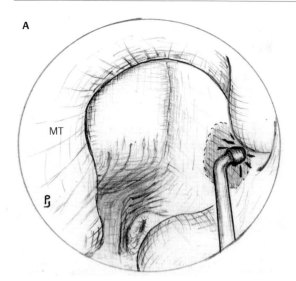

B

Figure 10–3 **(A)** The right-angled curved suction palpating the posterior fontanelle of the maxillary sinus. **(B)** The U-shaped incision extending from the inferior surface of the horizontal part of the middle turbinate to just above the insertion of the inferior turbinate. MT, middle turbinate.

syringe with 1:80,000 lidocaine and adrenaline is attached to a 25-gauge needle that has been bent at 25 mm from the tip at a 45-degree angle. The detailed anatomy of the greater palatine canal is presented in Chapter 2. The greater palatine canal is on average 18 mm long and the overlying soft tissue has an average depth of 7 mm. Therefore, bending the needle at 25 mm ensures that the needle does not enter the pterygopalatine fossa for any significant distance.[3] This lessens the risk of damage to the maxillary nerve or artery by the needle. The foramen and canal are located with the tip of the needle and the needle slid up into the canal to the bend. After aspiration has been performed, 2 mL of lidocaine and adrenaline are injected. Spasm of the SPA with cessation of active bleeding was achieved in all the patients in our published series who were actively bleeding at the time of surgery.

The nasal cavity is decongested using the combination of cocaine- and adrenaline-soaked neuropatties. The lateral wall of the nose anterior to the posterior end of the middle turbinate is infiltrated with lidocaine and adrenaline. A right-angled suction is used to palpate the membranous posterior fontanelle of the maxillary sinus and the junction of the membranous portion to the palatine bone. Once the palatine bone is identified, a U-shaped incision is made onto bone. The incision is started under the horizontal portion of the ground lamella, down the palatine bone, and continued along the insertion of the inferior turbinate posteriorly (**Fig. 10–3**).[1]

The suction Freer elevator is used to elevate the mucosal flap. It is important to establish the subperiosteal plane at the point of incision as this allows a relatively bloodless dissection and also allows the periosteum to be stripped off the underlying bone in a manner similar to that used in raising a subperichondrial flap during a septoplasty. The initial elevation is done in the inferior region of the flap just above the

insertion of the inferior turbinate on the lateral nasal wall (**Fig. 10–4**).[1]

Keeping the dissection low initially keeps the surgeon under the SPA. This dissection should be carried posteriorly until the anterior face of the sphenoid is reached. This is an important landmark as it allows the surgeon to be sure that the dissection has been carried far enough posterior before the dissection is taken superiorly. As the flap is lifted

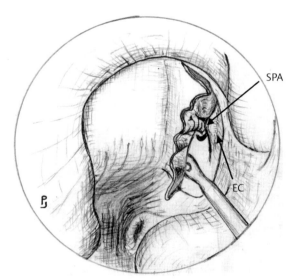

Figure 10–4 A suction Freer elevator is used to elevate the mucosal flap in the subperiosteal plane keeping the initial dissection low just above the insertion of the inferior turbinate until the anterior face of the sphenoid is reached. As the dissection is taken superiorly, the ethmoidal crest (EC) and sphenopalatine artery (SPA) are seen.

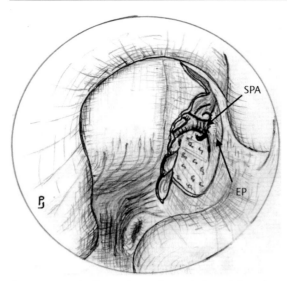

Figure 10–5 The flap is elevated superiorly and the sphenopalatine artery (SPA) is tented as it exits the sphenopalatine foramen. The ethmoidal process (EP) of the palatine bone has been curetted to further expose the sphenopalatine foramen and SPA.

superiorly, the SPA is visualized exiting the sphenopalatine foramen. It is tented by the flap (**Fig. 10–5**).[1]

An additional landmark that can be sought is the ethmoidal bony process of the palatine bone.[4,5] This bony projection is seen directly anterior to the sphenopalatine foramen (**Fig. 10–4 and Fig. 10–5**). It can be curetted away to improve visualization of the foramen. The artery is contained within the tissues exiting the foramen. Dissection with the suction Freer elevator is performed above the pedicle and the artery identified within the pedicle. Once it is clearly delineated, two Ligar clips are placed on the artery. Care should be taken to ensure that the clip is placed all the way across the pedicle. The artery may divide before exiting the foramen, and it is not uncommon for there to be a posterior branch exiting the foramen behind the anterior branch.[5] This posterior branch may exit through its own foramen in up 16% of patients.[5] This branch (called the posterior nasal artery) travels across the posterior choana to the posterior aspect of the septum to supply the majority of the blood to the septum (**Fig. 10–1**). Endoscopic Ligar clip applicators should be used as they are easier to manipulate in the posterior region of the nasal cavity. The Ligar clip should be placed across the pedicle and the front of the clip applicator pushed until it touches the anterior face of the sphenoid. As the clip is closed, the tips are moved slightly anterior to the sphenoid face so that they do not rub against the bone during closure. If, despite this maneuver, the clip does not sit properly across the pedicle, then further dissection may be needed before further clips are applied. When the pedicle is first exposed, there is too great a volume of tissue to be clipped, and the vessels should be dissected out and clipped individually. A malleable suction Freer elevator or standard suction Freer elevator can be of value for this as the pedicle tends to ooze during this dissection before the clip is applied. Continuous

suction through the instrument allows dissection to continue despite any oozing of blood.

Clipping is recommended in spontaneous epistaxis as the caliber of the SPA is large in these patients and bipolar cautery alone may not be as effective. However, the vessel is usually cauterized after clipping to make sure no bleeding results if the clip is dislodged during the dissection for the posterior nasal artery (PNA). The PNA is sought in all patients as it may significantly contribute to a spontaneous posterior bleed and if not sought may contribute to failure of the procedure. Such dissection may dislodge the clip from the SPA and if the artery had not been cauterized in addition to being clipped, it may result in a significant bleed that can be difficult to manage. Once the PNA is identified, it is cauterized with the suction bipolar. It is difficult to clip as it sits on the anterior face of the sphenoid and so the clip will often not sit over the vessel properly. The mucosal flap is replaced and held in place by a 2 × 2 cm piece of fibrillar Surgicel. This is used as a considerable proportion of patients are either on aspirin or warfarin and it helps control oozing from the incision. No other packing is placed in the nose. The patient is discharged soon after recovery if no further bleeding is noted.

Results

In a recently published series of 13 consecutive patients,[1] four patients underwent SPA ligation under local anesthetic and nine under general anesthetic. The four who had local anesthetic were considered to be at risk if given general anesthetic. The average age was 55.9 years (range, 23 to 79 years) with an approximate equal sex distribution (males 7, females 6). All patients presented with intractable posterior epistaxis and had SPA ligation. One patient developed further epistaxis during the 12-month follow-up period resulting in a 92% primary success rate in the treatment of the epistaxis.[1] The patient who re-bled was on aspirin and had a platelet abnormality with widespread ecchymosis on his arms and legs.

To date, a further 26 patients have had SPA in our department. Similar incidences of comorbidities and anticoagulation were seen. The success at 12-month follow-up remains in the region of 90%.

◆ BLEEDING FROM A LARGE VESSEL IN THE NOSE OR SINUSES

Controlled Bleeding

A spurting artery in the region of the frontal recess will usually indicate damage to the anterior ethmoidal artery. The region should be packed with neuropatties soaked in adrenaline and cocaine. After waiting several minutes, the area can be checked. If the bleeding is from the skull base or from the region of the orbital periosteum associated with the skull base, suction bipolar cautery can be used to control the bleeding. Unipolar diathermy should not be used as it can arc to exposed dura and cause a cerebrospinal fluid (CSF) leak. If the bleeding is from the medial region of the frontal recess, Surgicel and Gelfoam soaked in thrombin should be placed over the artery and the area firmly packed. Our preference is to use ribbon gauze soaked with bismuth iodoform paraffin paste (BIPP). This allows pressure to be placed over the Gelfoam and Surgicel. The BIPP gauze can be removed after a day or two. Cautery (bipolar or unipolar) should be avoided as there is a significant risk that any cautery (higher risk with unipolar) may burn a hole through the dura and cause a CSF leak.

Arterial spurting from the region of the SPA should be controlled with suction bipolar forceps* (Medtronic ENT). If this is not available, a pterygopalatine fossa block will usually put the vessel in spasm and allow bipolar diathermy (without suction) to be used to control the bleeder (see Chapter 2). Arterial bleeding is usually from the PNA or the SPA (**Fig. 10–1**).

Uncontrolled Bleeding

Bleeding from the internal carotid artery in the sphenoid is a major and potentially lethal complication. The volume of blood is enormous, and often standard suctions will not keep pace with the bleeding. The anesthetist needs to rapidly obtain large-caliber vascular access and get emergency replacement blood. In addition, the anesthetist should rapidly lower the patient's blood pressure to around 50 or 60 mm Hg systolic to allow the nasal suction to cope with the bleeding. A second surgeon should be immediately called and a suction placed down the other nostril so that the bleeding is sufficiently controlled to allow the primary surgeon to place a ribbon gauze pack into the sphenoid and to tightly compress the bleeding vessel. Once the bleeding is controlled, a neck incision is made over the sternomastoid muscle and muscle harvested. With both surgeons working together, the nasal pack is removed and the muscle placed over the bleeding vessel. The ribbon gauze is replaced over the muscle and the sphenoid and nasal cavity tightly packed. Be aware that ribbon gauze packs impregnated with substances such as BIPP are not suitable because the BIPP may embolize into the ruptured blood vessel and then intracranially. Additionally, the radiologist cannot evaluate the area due to the iodine in the ribbon gauze pack. Saline-soaked gauze is preferred. The vascular surgeon and interventional radiologist are called immediately, and usually the first step is to perform an angiogram to assess the damage to the vessel. If possible, the radiologist can place a stent in the damaged region of the vessel, or if this is not possible, occlusion or bypass of the artery may need to be performed.

Long-term Management

The management of intractable epistaxis can either be with a nasal pack and postnasal balloon or ligation of the artery. If packing is used, the balloon will usually occlude the nasopharyngeal airway.[6] In elderly patients, this may produce hypoxic

episodes that may in turn precipitate fatal arrythmias.[7–10] The alternative to endoscopic SPA ligation is ligation of the maxillary artery through a Caldwell Luc approach.[11–13] Although this has a good success rate (87 to 90%), there are significant associated morbidities, with cheek and teeth pain and paresthesia being the most common (28%).[11–13] The nonsurgical option of management is to embolize the bleeding vessel.[13] Again, this is usually a successful procedure but has significant associated morbidities including hemiplegia, facial pain and facial paresthesia, ophthalmoplegia, and blindness.[11,13] The overall complication rate of this procedure is 29%. The advantages of endoscopic SPA ligation are that it can be done under either local or general anesthetic and it is relatively quick and straightforward with minimal associated morbidity and a good success rate. Our policy is that the nose should not be packed after the procedure and if possible that the patient should be discharged from the hospital within 12 hours of the procedure. This dispenses with the need to keep patients in the ward with a packed nose, resulting in a better utilization of hospital resources.

◆ VIDIAN NEURECTOMY

Vidian neurectomy was established by Golding-Wood in the 1960s for the management of intractable vasomotor rhinitis, allergic rhinitis, and for nasal polyposis.[14] The Vidian nerve supplies the nasal cavity with parasympathetic secretomotor fibers, and sectioning of this nerve was found to improve symptoms of rhinorrhea, sneezing, postnasal space discharge, and nasal obstruction.[14–16] The initial enthusiasm for this technique was tempered by recurrence of symptoms after a 2-year follow-up and by complications. The surgical technique for severing the nerve has varied[14–16] and in some cases the nerve was never accurately identified before it was either cut or cauterized.[16] It is interesting that even though there have been several reports regarding the success of this technique over many years[13–18] in the management of chronic rhinorrhea and in some cases of nasal polyposis, this technique has not been widely adopted. One of the reasons for this may be the lack of a reliable and safe surgical technique for identifying and sectioning the nerve.

Anatomy of the Vidian Canal

The Vidian canal is formed just anterior to the foramen lacerum where the carotid artery turns vertically up toward its vertical segment in the sphenoid sinus. The greater superficial petrosal nerve and fibers from the sympathetic plexus around the carotid artery join to form the Vidian nerve, which enters the Vidian canal just anterior to the foramen lacerum. To aid understanding of the course of the Vidian canal, a series of coronal computed tomography (CT) scans are presented starting in the foramen lacerum and progressing forward allowing the Vidian canal to be identified and followed anteriorly to where the canal opens in a funnel fashion into the pterygopalatine fossa (**Fig. 10–6**). If the parasagittal CT

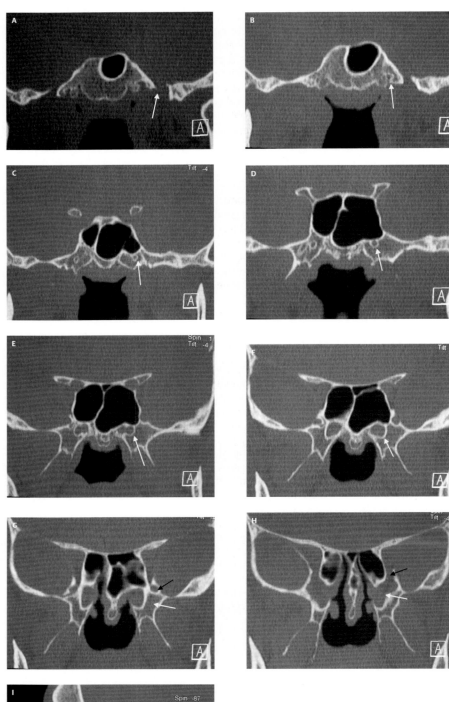

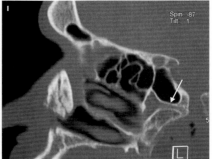

Figure 10–6 (A–I) The series of coronal CT scans begins with scan (**A**) through the foramen lacerum (*white arrow*) and as the scans move anteriorly (**B–H**), the Vidian canal can be followed along the floor of the sphenoid (*white arrows*) into the pterygopalatine fossa (**G, H**). Note the foramen rotundum (*black arrow*) in scan (**G**) and the infraorbital fissure (*black arrow*) in scan (**H**). Scan (**I**) is a parasagittal scan and shows the Vidian canal from the foramen lacerum to the pterygopalatine fossa (*white arrow*). Note how the canal funnels outward as it enters the fossa.

scan of this region is viewed, the Vidian canal can be clearly seen traversing the base of the sphenoid sinus into the pterygopalatine fossa.

Understanding the anatomy of the Vidian canal is very important in the endoscopic management of tumors infiltrating the pterygopalatine fossa and particularly in the management of juvenile nasopharyngeal angiofibromas (JNAs). JNAs tend to track down the Vidian canal and widen the canal toward the carotid artery. If this is not looked for both on the imaging and during surgical removal of JNA, residual tumor can be left in the canal and may form the nidus for tumor regrowth. The following cadaver dissection illustrates the relationship between the Vidian canal, floor of the sphenoid sinus, and carotid artery (**Fig. 10–7**). In this specimen, the carotid artery has been drilled out. The roof of the Vidian canal has been thinned and the canal can be seen as it travels along the floor of the sphenoid from the carotid artery to the Vidian canal foramen.

Surgical Technique

The nasal preparation and injection of the pterygopalatine fossa through the mouth is performed as previously described (see Chapter 2). The mucosal incisions for Vidian neurectomy are the same as for SPA ligation. The artery is localized and cauterized with the suction bipolar diathermy forceps. Cautery is preferred as the clips tend to slip off or are knocked off as the surgery progresses to the area behind the sphenopalatine foramen. The SPA is significantly larger in patients with active epistaxis than in patients undergoing elective surgery (Vidian neurectomy), and therefore bipolar cautery is effective for obtaining hemostasis in the latter cases.

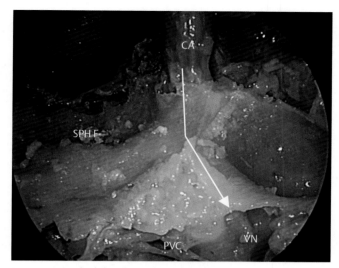

Figure 10–7 The left sphenoid sinus has been widely opened and the carotid artery (CA) drilled out. The Vidian canal is indicated with a *solid white arrow*. The Vidian nerve (VN), palatovaginal canal (PVC), and floor of sphenoid (SPH F) can be seen.

Once the SPA foramen is identified, the mucosal flap is raised behind the foramen until the face of the sphenoid sinus is identified (**Fig. 10–8**). One of the first structures seen as this flap is elevated is a nerve emanating from the anterior face of the sphenoid and progressing laterally into the pterygopalatine fossa. This nerve can easily be mistaken for the Vidian nerve. It is the pharyngeal nerve, a branch of the pterygopalatine ganglion, traveling into the palatovaginal canal and then onto the pharynx to provide sympathetic and parasympathetic fibers to this region (**Fig. 10–8**).

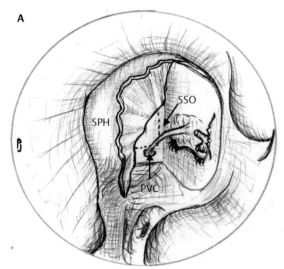

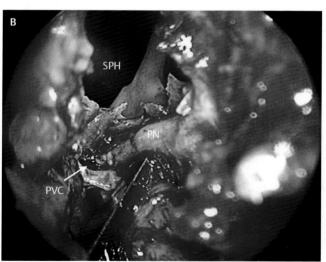

Figure 10–8 (A) In this diagram, the anterior face of the sphenoid sinus (SPH) is exposed and the outline of the sinus marked (SSO) with *dotted lines*. The palatovaginal canal (PVC) is seen with the posterior pharyngeal branch of the pterygopalatine ganglion entering the canal. **(B)** In this intraoperative photograph, the sphenoid sinus (SPH) has been opened and the pharyngeal nerve (PN) is seen entering the palatovaginal canal (PVC).

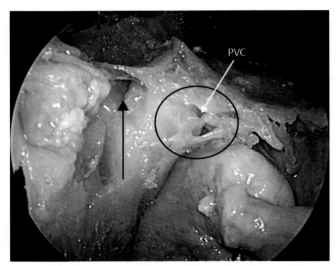

Figure 10–9 The palatovaginal canal (PVC) is circled on the right side. Note its more medial position and smaller diameter than the Vidian canal with Vidian nerve (*black arrow*).

If a successful Vidian neurectomy is to be performed, it is vitally important to understand the relationship between the palatovaginal canal (PVC) and the Vidian canal. These two canals both transmit sizable nerves and both emanate from the anterior face of the sphenoid and are separated by only a few millimeters. Important differences allowing accurate identification of each of these structures are the more medial position of the PVC, the relatively smaller nerve passing through the PVC, and the significantly smaller diameter of the PVC compared with the Vidian canal (**Fig. 10–9**).

The posterior pharyngeal nerve is divided and the anterior face of the sphenoid is identified and perforated with a Freer elevator (**Fig. 10–10A**). This opening is enlarged until a clear view into the sphenoid sinus is obtained and the floor of the sphenoid sinus identified. This gives certainty regarding the horizontal location of the Vidian canal as it always runs along the floor of the anterior aspect of the sphenoid sinus (**Fig. 10–10B**). The key landmark is the palatine bone. If a line is drawn vertically up the posterior aspect of the palatine bone and the intersection of this line with a line drawn through the floor of the sphenoid sinus, the intersection of these two lines marks the Vidian canal (**Fig. 10–10B**). Check the coronal CT scans in **Fig. 10–6** and the cadaver dissection in **Fig. 10–9** to confirm this.

To expose the Vidian canal, the posteroinferior margin of the sphenopalatine foramen needs to be removed (**Fig. 10–11**). This is best done with either a straight through-biting Blakesley forceps or a forward-biting 2-mm Kerrison punch. This will remove the medial wall of the pterygopalatine fossa and allow the Vidian canal to be clearly identified. Note that the periosteum overlying the pterygopalatine fossa is still intact, and if this is torn the yellow fat within the fossa should be visible. This should be expected and should not be confused with orbital fat.

A sickle knife is used to incise the periosteum from the anterior face of the sphenoid in a horizontal manner toward the anterior lip of the SPA foramen. The fat of the pterygopalatine fossa is exposed and the sickle knife is used to probe the fat and expose the Vidian nerve. Note that the funnel shape of the Vidian canal should be sought and note that the nerve is large (3 to 4 mm in diameter). Also note that the Vidian canal travels directly posteriorly toward the vertical part of the carotid artery. If there are

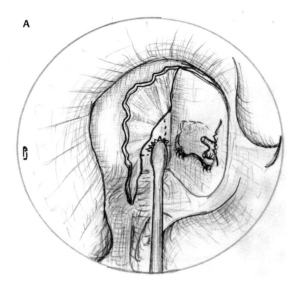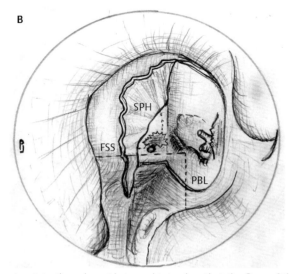

Figure 10–10 (A) In the drawing on the left side, the Freer elevator is used to perforate the anterior face of the sphenoid sinus just above the floor of the sinus. This opening is enlarged and a clear

view into the sphenoid sinus obtained so that the floor of the sphenoid sinus (FSS) can be clearly seen. (B) A line is drawn in continuation with the posterior margin of the palatine bone (PBL).

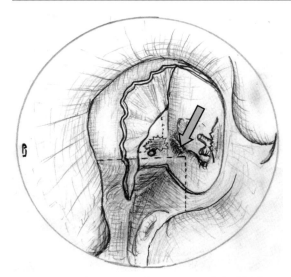

Figure 10–11 The posteroinferior region of the SPA foramen needs to be removed to identify the Vidian canal (*black arrow*).

additional septations within the sphenoid sinus, these septations will in most cases attach to the roof of the Vidian canal in the floor of the sphenoid sinus (providing an additional landmark). The nerve is usually immediately visible after it exits the Vidian canal at the level of the floor of the sphenoid sinus. It is dissected free until it is seen to move laterally toward the pterygopalatine ganglion in the pterygopalatine fossa (**Fig. 10–12**).

Extensive lateral dissection can allow the maxillary nerve to be visualized but this is not recommended for the standard Vidian nerve section. Once the nerve is identified,

confirmation that it is the Vidian nerve is made by following the nerve into the Vidian canal. This canal runs in an anteroposterior direction and the nerve can be visualized exiting the canal. A 2- to 3-mm section of the nerve is removed and the remaining nerve exiting the Vidian canal is cauterized with bipolar diathermy. Unipolar diathermy is not recommended as the infraorbital canal and maxillary nerve are in relative close proximity and damage can occur with injudicious usage of unipolar diathermy in this region. Optic nerve injury has also been described after blind attempts were made to cauterize the Vidian nerve. Therefore, we advocate clear visualization and positive identification followed by section of the nerve and bipolar diathermy of the nerve root (**Fig. 10–13**). The mucosal flap is replaced. If it tends to fall away from the lateral nasal wall, a small piece of Gelfoam is placed under the middle turbinate over the flap to hold it in place. No other packing is placed in the nose.

Results

Over the past 5 years, nine patients have undergone 14 operations. The mean follow-up was 25 months. Most of the patients suffered intractable rhinorrhea (80%) with nasal obstruction (72%), postnasal drip (64%), and sneezing (57%) also prominent. Postoperatively, there was a significant improvement in rhinorrhea and nasal obstruction at the last follow-up (mean greater than 2 years). In three patients, there was a worsening of sneezing postoperatively. In addition, 35% of patients suffered a variable amount of dry eye and 28% had nasal crusting. Half of the Vidian neurectomies were deemed to be highly successful by the patients at a mean follow-up time of 2 years.[19]

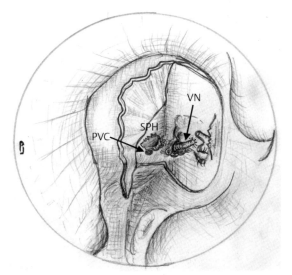

A

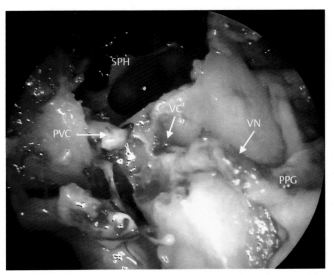

B

Figure 10–12 (A) In this drawing, the Vidian nerve is seen exiting the Vidian canal running toward the sphenopalatine foramen before moving laterally toward the maxillary nerve in the pterygopalatine fossa. **(B)** This is a magnified view from a cadaver dissection of the Vidian nerve (VN) exiting the Vidian canal (VC) and running laterally to join the pterygopalatine ganglion (PPG) hanging from the maxillary nerve (V2). The palatovaginal canal (PVC) and sphenoid sinus (SPH) can be seen.

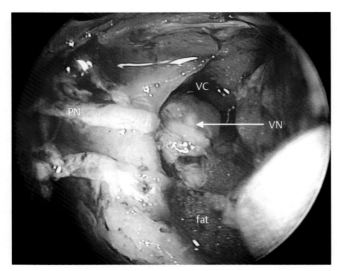

Figure 10–13 The left Vidian nerve (VN) has been cut, and the entire bone of the Vidian canal (VC) around the nerve can be seen. The stump of the nerve should then be cauterized with a bipolar forceps. The pharyngeal nerve (PN) and fat of the pterygopalatine fossa can be seen.

Conclusion

Vidian neurectomy has been shown to result in significant histologic changes in the nasal mucosa including mast cell depletion.[20] The exact mechanism by which Vidian neurectomy results in improvement in symptoms postoperatively is unknown. As most previous studies have not histologically confirmed the sectioning of the nerve, there may be patients who have not actually had their Vidian nerve sectioned but have been included among patients who have undergone Vidian neurectomy. A significant amount of research on the outcomes after Vidian nerve neurectomy needs to be performed before the role of Vidian nerve neurectomy in endoscopic sinus surgery is properly defined.

References

1. Wormald PJ, Wee DTH, van Hasselt CA. Endoscopic ligation of the sphenopalatine artery for refractory posterior epistaxis. Am J Rhinol 2000;14:261–264

2. Sharp HR, Rowe-Jones JM, Biring GS. Endoscopic ligation or diathermy of the sphenopalatine artery in persistent epistaxis. J Laryngol Otol 1997;111:1047–1050

3. Mercuri LG. Intraoral second division nerve block. Oral Surg Oral Med Oral Pathol 1979;47(2):109–113

4. Snyderman CH, Goldman S, Carrau R, Ferguson B, Grandis J. Endoscopic sphenopalatine artery ligation is an effective method of treatment for posterior epistaxis. Am J Rhinol 1999;13:137–140

5. Wareing MJ, Padgham ND. Osteologic classification of the sphenopalatine foramen. Laryngoscope 1998;108:125–127

6. McGarry GW, Aitken D. Intranasal balloon catheters: how do they work? Clin Otolaryngol 1991;16:388–392

7. Jacobs JR, Dickson CB. Effects of nasal and larnygeal stimulation upon peripheral lung function. Otolaryngol Head Neck Surg 1986;95:298–303

8. Shaheen OH. Epistaxis in the middle aged and elderly [thesis]. London: University of London

9. El-Guindy A. Endoscopic transseptal sphenopalatine artery ligation for intractable posterior epistaxis. Ann Otol Rhinol Laryngol 1998;107:1033–1037

10. Papsidero MJ. The role of nasal obstruction in obstructive sleep apnea syndrome. Ear Nose Throat J 1993;72:82–84

11. Metson R, Lane R. Internal maxillary artery ligation for epistaxis: an analysis of failures. Laryngoscope 1988;98:760–764

12. Premachandra DJ, Sergeant RJ. Dominant maxillary artery as a cause of failure in maxillary artery ligation for posterior epistaxis. Clin Otolaryngol 1993;18:42–47

13. Strong EB, Bell DA, Johnson LP. Intractable epistaxis: transantral ligation vs. embolization: efficacy review and cost analysis. Otolaryngol Head Neck Surg 1995;113:674–678

14. Golding-Wood PH. Observation of petrosal and Vidian neurectomy in chronic vasomotor rhinitis. J Laryngol Otol 1961;75:232–247

15. Kamel R, Saher S. Endoscopic transnasal Vidian neurectomy. Laryngoscope 1991;101:316–318

16. Fernandes CM. Bilateral transnasal Vidian neurectomy in the management of chronic rhinitis. J Laryngol Otol 1988;102:894–895

17. Greenstone MA, Stanley PJ, Makay IS. The effect of Vidian neurectomy on the nasal mucociliary clearance. J Laryngol Otol 1988;102:894–895

18. Krajina Z. Critical review of Vidian neurectomy. Rhinology 1989;27:271–276

19. Robinson SRR, Wormald PJ. Endoscopic vidian neurectomy. Am J Rhinol 2006;20(2):197–202

20. Konno A, Togawa K. Vidian nerve neurectomy for allergic rhinitis. Arch Otorhinolaryngol 1979;225:67–77

11

Powered Endoscopic Dacryocystorhinostomy

Endoscopic dacryocystorhinostomy, (DCR) was initially described by Caldwell in the 19th century.[1] It fell into disrepute, however, as surgeons experienced problems with visualization of the surgical site. In the early 20th century, Toti described the external DCR procedure, and with a few modifications this procedure remains largely unchanged from those early descriptions.[2] As the technique has developed, so the success rate for the external procedure improved until today in the hands of properly trained oculoplastic surgeons, success rates of between 90 and 95% can be expected.[3] As endoscopic sinus surgery became popular in the late 1980s, there was renewed interest in endoscopic DCR, with the initial descriptions having appeared in the late 1980s and early 1990s.[4-6] As could be expected of a new and developing technique, the initial success rates were lower than that of external DCR and varied between 65 and 90%.[4-6] Laser endoscopic DCR was promoted in the mid-1990s but success rates were disappointing and tended to be at the lower end of the spectrum (around 75%).[7-9] This was probably due to the technique creating only a small opening into the posterior inferior lacrimal sac through the thin lacrimal bone. It is well recognized currently in the literature on external DCR that a small ostium does not achieve the same success rates as a large opening of the lacrimal sac.[10]

The original endoscopic DCR technique was described as follows: a mucosal flap anterior to the middle turbinate was raised and the junction between the lacrimal bone and frontal process of maxilla established. A Hajek Koeffler punch was used to remove what bone one could over the lacrimal sac.[4] In the early 1990s, the author reviewed his own results with this technique and found a disappointing long-term patency rate of only 83%.[11] On review of the literature on external DCR, the critical factor necessary for achieving the 90 to 95% success rate was a wide bone removal so that the entire lacrimal sac was exposed.[10,12-14] Following this, the mucosa of the lacrimal sac and nasal mucosa were anastomosed with sutures allowing primary intention healing without significant granulation. This raised the question, could the external DCR technique be duplicated by a similar intranasal tech-

nique? If this were to be done, the first step was to define the intranasal anatomy of the lacrimal sac.[13] The early descriptions of the intranasal anatomy of the sac placed the sac anterior to the middle turbinate with minimal extension of the sac above the insertion of the middle turbinate, on the lateral nasal wall (the so-called axilla of the middle turbinate as it resembles an armpit).[13,15,16] To investigate the precise location of the sac, a series of CT dacryocystograms (DCGs) in patients undergoing DCR were performed and the relationship of the lacrimal sac and the axilla of the middle turbinate evaluated.[13] This study showed that the anatomy of the sac on the lateral nasal wall was significantly different to what had been previously described in the literature (**Fig. 11–1**). The sac was not only anterior to the middle turbinate but also a significant proportion was located above the axilla of the middle turbinate. On average, the sac extended 8 mm above the axilla of the middle turbinate.[13] Therefore, if the external DCR principles were to be applied to endoscopic DCR, a different technique was required. This led to the design of a new technique (powered endoscopic DCR), which is presented below.[14,17,18]

◆ PREOPERATIVE ASSESSMENT

Examine the Eye for Other Causes of Watery Eye

Excess Tear Production

- *Conjunctival disease* Patients with conjunctivitis present with sticky secretions or pus in the eye that is often worse when they awake in the morning. Antibiotic eye drops are used to treat bacterial infections and prevent colonization in patients with viral conjunctivitis.
- *Dry eye* Patients may have significant dryness that will irritate the eye and produce tearing. Application of artificial tears is usually all that is necessary.
- *Lid malposition* Ectropion or entropion cause the puncta to not be properly positioned in the tear lake. A floppy

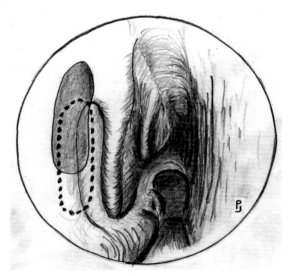

Figure 11–1 The *broken line* indicates the location of the sac prior to our studies on the intranasal anatomy of the lacrimal sac. The shaded area is the actual intranasal position of the lacrimal sac on the lateral nasal wall. Note it extends between 8 to 10 mm above the axilla of the middle turbinate. (From Wormald PJ. Powered endoscopic DCR. Otolaryngol Clin North Am 2006;39:539–549. Reprinted with permission.)

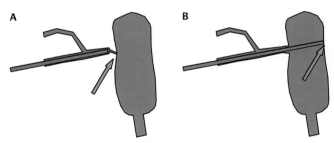

Figure 11–2 **(A)** A soft stop is felt as the probe rests against a common canaliculus stricture or obstruction. **(B)** A hard stop is felt as the probe comes to rest against the bone encasing the lacrimal sac.

lower eyelid (increased lid laxity) may also place the puncta in a position where tear collection is impaired. Surgical repositioning or tightening of the lid is required.

♦ *Blepharitis* Blepharitis causes a mucoid discharge from the eye. In this condition, there is an alteration in the bacteriology of the mucous glands in the hair follicles of the eyelashes resulting in a mucoid discharge from the eye. The vision will be blurred and the eye often burns. Treatment is to rub the eyelid margin with gauze soaked in warm soapy water twice a day. This will need to be done for about 3 months before the condition resolves.

♦ **Epiphora**

♦ *Punctal stenosis* Obliteration or narrowing of the superior or inferior punctum.
♦ *Canalicular stenosis or obstruction* Superior or inferior canalicular stenosis or obstruction, which may follow trauma or viral infection.
♦ *Nasolacrimal duct blockage* Usually from an unknown cause.

Examine for Nasolacrimal Duct Obstruction

In epiphora caused by nasolacrimal duct obstruction (NLDO), tears will frequently run down the cheek. This is more noticeable in conditions that stimulate tear formation such as walking in a cold wind. During examination, the position and size of the puncta should be assessed. The lid laxity and positioning of the puncta in the tear lake should be determined. To assess the patency of the inferior, superior, and common canaliculi, the upper lacrimal system should be probed

(**Figs. 11–2**). The punctum is dilated with a punctum dilator. A Bowman lacrimal probe is then used to probe the inferior canaliculus and common canaliculus.

Differentiating between a soft and a hard stop on probing helps assess the patency of the canalicular system. If a common canaliculus stricture is present, it should be diagnosed preoperatively so appropriate steps can be taken to correct it during surgery and the patient can be informed that the likelihood of a successful procedure is significantly less than in the case with a DCR performed for nasolacrimal duct obstruction.

Syringing of the lacrimal system will also help assess the patency of the nasolacrimal system. In NLDO, there will be significant reflux through the upper punctum with no saline penetration into the nose. In partial NLDO, there will be reflux through the upper punctum with saline penetration into the nose but only with increased syringing pressure. Penetration into the nasal cavity without reflux through the upper punctum indicates a patent (but not necessarily functional) lacrimal system. It is sometimes confusing to determine exactly where the saline is refluxing as some may reflux from the punctum that has been injected or from the other punctum or from a combination.

Examine the Nasal Cavity

Rigid nasal endoscopy is performed on all patients presenting with epiphora. A significant proportion (15%) of patients required surgery for nasal pathology at the same time as the DCR was performed. Mostly this was for associated chronic sinusitis. All patients need to be questioned regarding nasal symptoms and endoscopy performed to assess the nasal cavity. If there is evidence of nasal and sinus disease, appropriate investigations are performed and treatment instituted. If medical therapy fails to resolve the problem, surgery is performed at the same time as the DCR.

Perform Dacryocystogram and Lacrimal Scintillography

We routinely perform a DCG to assess the patency of the canalicular system and penetration of dye into the nasolacrimal sac.[17] If the patient has a hard stop on probing with a blocked system on syringing, this investigation can be

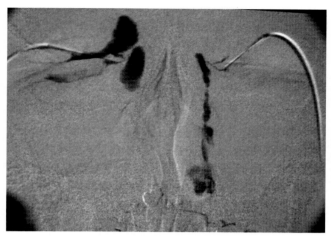

Figure 11–3 Right nasolacrimal duct (NLD) obstruction with reflux through the superior punctum into the conjunctiva with patent left NLD system.

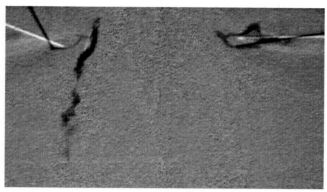

Figure 11–4 Obstruction of the left common canaliculus–sac junction with reflux of dye into the conjunctival region.

omitted. Filling of the sac but failure of the dye to penetrate the nasal cavity confirms the diagnosis of NLDO (**Fig. 11–3**).

Patency of the NLD system without reflux through the canalicular system normally indicates an anatomically patent system (**Fig. 11–3**, left side). Failure of the dye to penetrate the lacrimal sac may indicate a common canalicular obstruction (**Fig. 11–4**).

To assess the function of the NLD system, lacrimal scintillography is performed. DCG assesses anatomy but not function. A radioisotope is placed in the conjunctival fornix and regular scanning performed for 30 minutes. If the isotope penetrates the lacrimal sac and not the nasal cavity, NLDO exists (**Figs. 11–5**).

In some patients, the DCG may show no filling of the lacrimal sac, whereas scintillography shows filling of the sac (**Figs. 11–6**). This may occur when the sac is full of mucus and the distended sac kinks the common canaliculus just before it enters the sac.

Scintillography also helps identify a functional obstruction when the DCG is normal (patent) in a symptomatic patient. If the scintillography confirms lack of nasal cavity penetration of the isotope, then a functional NLDO exists (**Figs. 11–7**). These patients can be managed by performing an endoscopic DCR but the outcome is not as successful as with anatomic obstruction of the NLD system (see Results of Functional NLDO).

◆ SURGICAL TECHNIQUE[14,17–19]

After nasal decongestion with neuropatties and infiltration with lidocaine and adrenaline, a no. 15 scalpel blade is used to make the initial mucosal incisions (see accompanying DVD). It is important that these incisions be correctly placed as they form the borders for the subsequent bone removal and lacrimal sac exposure. The first incision is made horizontally 8 to 10 mm above the axilla of the middle turbinate, starting ~3 mm posterior to the axilla and coming forward ~10 mm onto the frontal process of the maxilla (bony prominence in the lateral nasal wall just anterior to the middle turbinate). The blade is then turned vertically and a vertical incision made to about two-thirds of the vertical height of the middle turbinate, stopping just above the insertion of

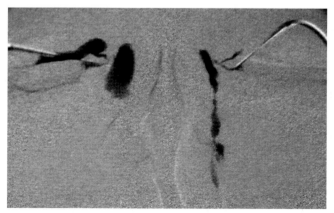

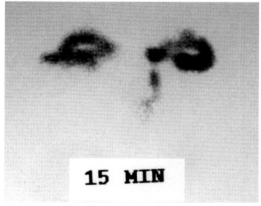

A   B

Figure 11–5 (**A**) DCG shows NLDO on the right side. (**B**) The scintillography shows penetration of the radioisotope on the left into the nasal cavity but shows holdup on the right with no nasal cavity penetration. This confirms the diagnosis of NLDO.

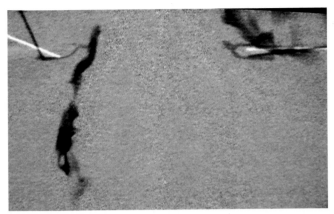
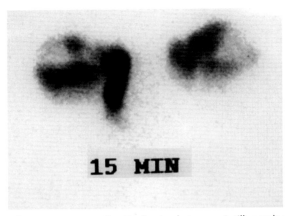

A

B

Figure 11–6 (**A**) Obstruction of left common canaliculus on DCG (**B**) with radioisotope penetrating the lacrimal sac on scintillography, indicating likely distention of sac kinking common canaliculus–sac junction.

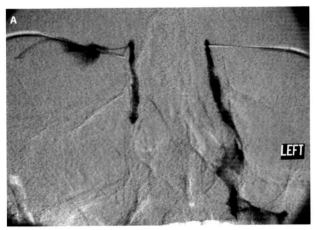
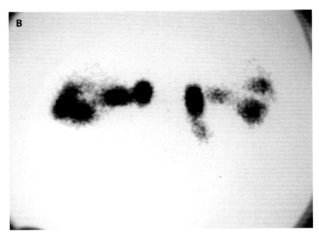

Figure 11–7 (A, B) This is the same DCG and scintillogram as seen in **Fig. 11–6**. If the right side is examined on the DCG, the system appears normal. On the scintillogram, however, no penetration of the nasal cavity occurs, though the sac fills nicely with radioisotope.

Later time points need to be checked to ensure that this continues to be the case. This is a functional nasolacrimal obstruction on the left side and an anatomic obstruction on the right side.

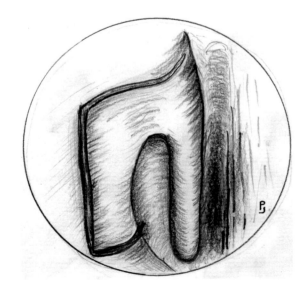

Figure 11–8 Mucosal incisions 8 to 10 mm above and anterior to the axilla of the middle turbinate. (From Wormald PJ. Powered endoscopic DCR. Otolaryngol Clin North Am 2006;39:539–549. Reprinted with permission.)

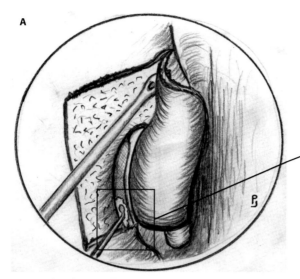

Figure 11–9 (A) This drawing illustrates elevation of the flap with a suction Freer elevator. Note the round knife removing the thin lacrimal bone in the inferior region of the dissection. **(B)** This intraoperative photo is an enlargement of the frontal process

lacrimal bone junction (*black arrow*) with a clear view of both these structures. ([A] From Wormald PJ. Powered endoscopic DCR. Otolaryngol Clin North Am 2006;39:539–549. Reprinted with permission.)

the inferior turbinate into the lateral nasal wall. The blade is turned horizontally and the inferior incision is started at the insertion of the uncinate process and brought forward to meet the vertical incision (**Fig. 11–8**).

A suction Freer elevator is used to elevate the mucosal flap while ensuring that the tip of the instrument always maintains contact with the bone (**Figs. 11–9**). Be particularly careful to keep the tip of the suction Freer on bone as it rides over the prominence of the frontal process of the maxilla as the bone contour can fall away abruptly and contact with the bone and surgical plane can be lost. At this point, the bone should be palpated so that the junction of the soft lacrimal bone and hard bone of the frontal process can be identified. This is a key landmark and must be sought in all primary surgeries. Note that the lacrimal bone is sought at the bottom of the region from which the mucosal flap has been raised, just above the insertion of the inferior turbinate. The thin lacrimal bone is 2 to 5 mm wide before the insertion of the uncinate process is reached. Dissection stops at the uncinate, and the uncinate insertion should not be disturbed. A round knife (Storz, Germany) (from the standard ear tray of instruments) is used to flake the soft lacrimal bone away from the posteroinferior region of the sac. If this is difficult, the frontal process can be removed first before the lacrimal bone is flaked away.

Once the lacrimal bone has been removed, a forward-biting Hajek Koeffler punch (Storz) is used to remove the lower portion of the frontal process of the maxilla. The tip of the punch is used to push the lacrimal sac away from where the bone is to be removed. The punch is engaged in the hard bone of the frontal process and this bone removed. The lacrimal sac may be inadvertently grasped as the punch is closed. The punch should be opened after the initial bite to allow any sac wall that may have been pinched in the jaws of the punch to be released. After this maneuver, the punch is closed over the loose bone and this

bone removed. This avoids tearing the sac with the punch. Bone removal continues both anteriorly and superiorly until the punch can no longer be seated on the bone. Removal of the frontal process of the maxilla uncovers the antero-inferior portion of the lacrimal sac (**Fig. 11–10**) and only stops when the bone becomes too thick for the punch to engage. At this point, a 25-degree curved 2.7-mm rough diamond burr (Medtronic ENT, Jacksonville, FL, USA) is attached to the microdebrider and used to remove the rest of the bone

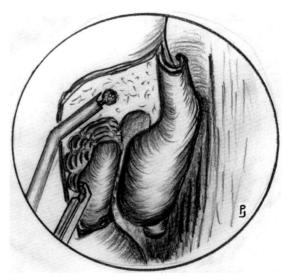

Figure 11–10 (A, B) Removal of the bone of the frontal process of the maxilla by Hajek Koeffler punch (*lower end*) and DCR diamond burr (*upper end*). (From Wormald PJ. Powered endoscopic DCR. Otolaryngol Clin North Am 2006;39:539–549. Reprinted with permission.)

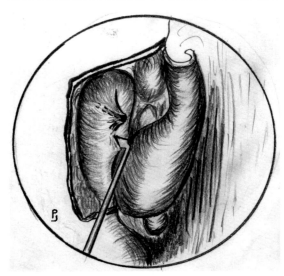

Figure 11–11 Bowman lacrimal probe tenting the flap to facilitate incision with the DCR spear knife. This incision should be made along the posterior third of the tented sac wall to ensure the largest possible anterior flap. (From Wormald PJ. Powered endoscopic DCR. Otolaryngol Clin North Am 2006;39:539–549. Reprinted with permission.)

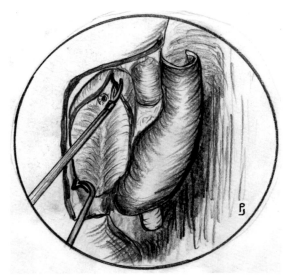

Figure 11–12 The mini-sickle knife is used to make the inferior and superior releasing incision on the anterior mucosal flap to allow the flap to be rolled out onto the frontal process of the maxilla. The superior and inferior releasing incisions are cut in the posterior flap with the scissors from the skull base set. (From Wormald PJ. Powered endoscopic DCR. Otolaryngol Clin North Am 2006;39:539–549. Reprinted with permission.)

up to the superior mucosal incision. In the vast majority of cases, an agger nasi cell is present and the mucosa of this cell will be exposed as the sac is followed superiorly above the axilla of the middle turbinate. The diamond burr can be brought into light contact with the lacrimal sac lining without damaging the sac. Significant pressure by the diamond burr on the sac will cause damage. A cutting burr will remove the bone faster; however, it does cause significant damage to the sac wall and will often result in a hole in the sac wall. The bone is removed until the entire sac is exposed. The sac should stand proud of the lateral nasal wall so that when the sac is incised and the mucosal flaps are rolled out, they will lie flat on the lateral nasal wall. Thus the sac will be marsupialized into the wall rather than an ostium being created in the sac.

Next, the inferior punctum is dilated with a punctum dilator, and a Bowman lacrimal probe is passed into the sac. When the probe is moved up and down in the sac, its tip should be able to be seen moving behind the sac wall. This confirms that the probe is indeed within the sac (**Fig. 11–11**). Movement of the sac without visualization of the tip of the probe usually indicates that the probe is still at the common canaliculus–sac junction and the lateral wall has been pushed onto the medial wall with some movement of the medial wall. Cutting down on the probe if it is not in the sac lumen can result in damage to the common caniliculus opening. With the tip of the probe visible through the sac wall, a DCR spear knife* (Medtronic ENT) is used to make a vertical incision as far posteriorly as possible through the sac wall. This results in the largest possible anterior flap. The tip of the spear knife is pushed into the tented sac wall just underneath the region of the probe and the sac wall is cut using a rotating motion (**Fig. 11–11**). Do not place the entire blade of the spear knife into the sac but rather cut with the

anterior two-thirds of the blade. The sac is slit from top to bottom. The DCR mini-sickle knife* (Medtronic Xomed, Jacksonville, FL, USA) is used to make upper and lower releasing incisions in the anterior flap so that the flap can be rolled out on the lateral nasal wall (**Fig. 11–12**).

Three-millimeter soft-tissue scissors from the Skull Base Set (Medtronic ENT) are used to make upper and lower releasing incisions in the posterior flap, and this flap is also rolled out. The sac should now be completely marsupialized and lie flat on the lateral nasal wall (**Fig. 11–12**).

To determine the width of the mucosal flaps, the amount of raw bone above and below the sac is estimated. The original mucosal flap is repositioned over the opened sac so that the areas of raw bone can be measured up against the original flap. Once the width of flap is determined, the flap is trimmed with a pediatric through-biting Blakesley forceps, leaving the upper and lower limb of this flap the same thickness as the raw area above and below the marsupialized sac (**Fig. 11–13**). Most of the middle section of the original flap is removed to allow the posterior wall of the flap and mucosal edge of the mucosal flap to be approximated. The posterosuperior region of lacrimal and nasal mucosa is difficult to approximate because the middle turbinate holds the nasal mucosal flap away from the side wall. In this region, the agger nasi cell is opened and the mucosa from this cell approximated to this region of the lacrimal mucosa. This results in a U-shaped flap, and the surgeon should aim to achieve approximation of lacrimal and nasal mucosa superiorly, posteriorly, and inferiorly. This mucosal flap can be difficult to fashion with standard through-biting Blakesley forceps so the pediatric Blakesley forceps are kept for DCR surgery alone and only used on this flap. This keeps them sharp and allows the mucosa to be cut without tearing of

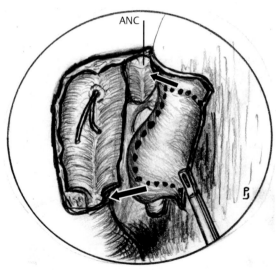

Figure 11–13 The mucosal flap is trimmed with the pediatric through-biting forceps. The superior and inferior mucosal flaps are matched to the raw bone above and below the opened lacrimal sac (*block arrows*). The agger nasi cell (ANC) mucosa is exposed and opened to allow apposition in this area. (From Wormald PJ. Powered endoscopic DCR. Otolaryngol Clin North Am 2006;39:539–549. Reprinted with permission.)

the mucosa and losing the flap. Approximating the lacrimal and nasal mucosa should result in a first-intention healing rather than a secondary-intention healing and should reduce the formation of granulation tissue and scarring and therefore lessen the potential risk of closure of the sac and failure of the surgery (**Fig. 11–13**).

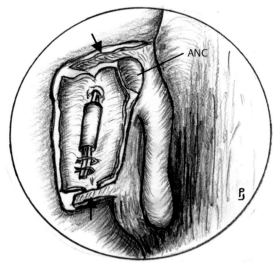

Figure 11–14 Placement of the silastic O'Donoghue lacrimal intubation tubes with a silastic sleeve space and Ligar clips to hold the tubes in place. The superior and inferior mucosal flaps are indicated with *black arrows*. (From Wormald PJ. Powered endoscopic DCR. Otolaryngol Clin North Am 2006;39:539–549. Reprinted with permission.)

The puncta are dilated and silastic lacrimal intubation tubes (O'Donoghue tubes) are placed through the upper and lower puncta and retrieved endonasally. A square of Gelfoam® (Pharmacia NSW, AUS) or Merogel® (Medtronic ENT) is slid up the tubing onto the lacrimal sac. A 10 mm piece of 4 mm silastic tubing is slid over the tubes pushing the Gelfoam on the flaps and holding the flaps in place. This tubing acts as a spacer below which Ligar clips are placed to secure the tubes (**Fig. 11–14**). Before placing the clips, ensure a loop of tubing is pulled in the medial canthus of the eye so that the tubes are not tight. If the loop is tight the tubes can cheese-wire through the puncta.

The silastic tubing is cut and the Gelfoam/Merogel gently lifted off the flaps and the position of the flaps checked before it is replaced. The post-nasal space is cleared of blood.

◆ POSTOPERATIVE CARE

Saline nasal spray is started within 3 to 4 hours after surgery. This aids in clearing any residual blood clots and keeping the nasal cavity moist and clear of secretions. Gentle blowing of the nose is allowed without closing the nasal vestibule. The patient is placed on broad-spectrum antibiotics for 5 days and antibiotic eye drops are used for 3 weeks. The O'Donoghue tubes are removed in the clinic after 4 weeks and the patency of the nasolacrimal system checked by placing a drop of fluorescein in the conjunctiva and endoscopically monitoring the flow of fluorescein from the conjunctiva to the nose. It is rare to see any granulations, but if they are present they should be removed. The patient is reviewed for a further 18 months before discharge.

◆ RESULTS

The results of this technique have been published in peer-reviewed journals.[14,17–21] When discussing the success rate of DCR, it is important to clearly define "success." In many previous studies, "success" has been defined as either a symptomatic improvement, a complete absence of symptoms, or as an anatomically patent nasolacrimal system after surgery. For a DCR to be called successful, both criteria (symptoms and anatomic patency) need to be fulfilled: the patient should be completely asymptomatic and there should be an endoscopically confirmed patent nasolacrimal system. The lacrimal sac should be marsupialized and well healed forming part of the lateral nasal wall (**Fig. 11–15A**). Once fluorescein has been placed in the conjunctiva, it should be visualized immediately in the marsupialized sac (**Fig. 11–15B**).

One of the recent published series included 162 consecutive DCRs with a minimum follow-up of 12 or more months.[18] Patients who had a nonfilling lacrimal sac on DCG possibly suggesting a common canaliculus problem but had otherwise normal canaliculi were included. Only patients who had a 3- to 4-mm-long obliteration of the common canaliculus on both DCG and probing were excluded. There were four patients who were excluded for significant common

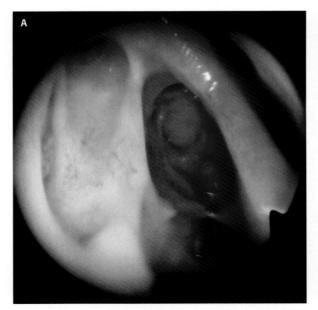
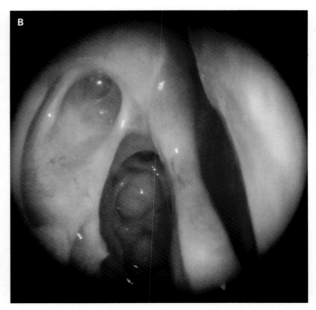

Figure 11–15 (**A**) Lacrimal sac marsupialized into the lateral nasal wall in a patient that had ESS. (**B**) Fluorescein seen draining freely into the opened lacrimal sac.

canaliculus stenosis/obstruction. Patients who have a non-filling lacrimal sac on DCG may have a large or distended lacrimal sac that may cause the common canaliculus to kink at its insertion to the sac. These patients can be successfully managed with an endoscopic DCR. To examine the results of this technique, the patients have been divided into those who had a primary DCR (no previous surgery), revision DCR, and those who filled the criteria for a pediatric DCR (less than 10 years old).

Results in Primary Dacryocystorhinostomy[14,17,18,20]

In one of the larger series[18] with 162 patients, 126 were primary DCRs, 19 revision DCRs, and 18 pediatric DCRs. In the primary DCR group, there were 115 patients who had a successful outcome (90%). Of the 11 patients considered failures, six had an anatomically patent nasolacrimal system with a free flow of fluorescein from the conjunctiva to the nose (such as demonstrated in **Fig. 11–15B**). This gives an anatomic patency rate of 96% (121/126). However, symptomatic patients are still classified as failures even if the surgery was technically successful. The primary DCR patient group can be further divided into anatomic or functional obstruction according to their preoperative investigations (DCG and scintillography). In the anatomically obstructed group, the success rate was 95% whereas in the functional group it was 81%. This functional group still had a 95% anatomic patency but a few patients still had symptoms and were therefore classified as failures. If success is defined as complete absence of symptoms with anatomic patency, functional obstruction of the lacrimal system does not have as good a prognosis as anatomic obstruction, and this should be kept in mind when consenting

patients with functional obstruction. An important caveat to this is that all patients who had symptoms in the functional group stated that the symptoms were significantly improved after the DCR.

Results and Technique Modifications in Revision Dacryocystorhinostomy[14,17,18]

There were 19 revision DCRs performed in this series. The success rate was 83% but increased to 89% with a second revision operation. The surgical technique for revision DCR is the same as for primary DCR with a few minor modifications. A variably sized bony ostium was created at the time of the primary DCR. The sac remnant may be significantly smaller and scarred than is the case with a primary DCR, and this may make the creation of nasal mucosa and lacrimal sac mucosa apposition more difficult. The initial mucosal incisions are still placed as previously described with the reservation that the anterior vertical incision must be placed anterior to the previously created bony ostium. If you are unsure where the anterior limit of the previous bony ostium is, palpate the frontal process of the maxilla. Start anteriorly on the frontal process and move posteriorly until the junction of the hard bone and soft ostium can be palpated. Once the initial mucosal incisions have been made, use the suction Freer elevator to elevate the mucosal flap from the bone anteriorly, above and below the previous bony ostium. The plane of the already elevated mucosa should be continued posteriorly using a scalpel. Sharp dissection is necessary as the mucosa is attached to the underlying sac by fibrous tissue. Once the mucosal flap is raised, bony removal and the rest of the DCR technique is as previously described.

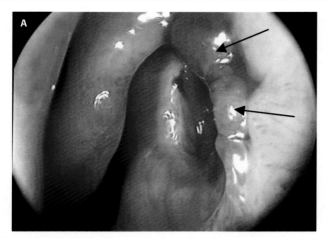

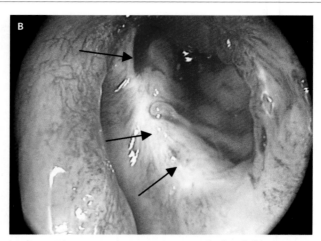

Figure 11–16 (A) The lacrimal ostium after 4 weeks in an 18-month-old patient with granulations on the anterior lip of the ostium (*black arrows*). (B) The lacrimal ostium after removal of these granulations. The posterior region of primary intention healing without granulation tissue is marked with *black arrows*. The patient continued to heal well and was asymptomatic at follow-up.

Results and Technique Modifications in Pediatric Dacryocystorhinostomy[14,17–22]

In the most recent series, there were 21 consecutive pediatric DCRs. The success rate was 92%. Patients included in this group were under the age of 14 years. In the pediatric age group, especially the patients in the 18-month-old to 6-year-old age group, there are important anatomic differences that the surgeon needs to be aware of. The nasal vestibule is much smaller and there can be some initial difficulty getting a 4-mm endoscope and an instrument in the nasal cavity simultaneously. The same-sized scopes and instruments are used for the pediatric and adult endoscopic DCRs. However, as surgery continues, the nasal vestibule stretches and its narrowness was never more than an initial concern. The other anatomic variation is the underdevelopment of the turbinates with a relatively small vertical height of the nasal cavity. This puts the axilla of the middle turbinate in relative close proximity to the skull base and increases the risk to the skull base. The initial mucosal incisions remain similar to those described in adults and the superior incision is still placed ~8 mm above the axilla. This will be just below the skull base in a 2-year-old so the surgeon must be aware of this proximity while removing bone from over the sac. The remainder of the procedure is the same as was previously described. Pediatric DCR is a very successful operation with 100% anatomic success rate in our series[20] (patency of the lacrimal ostium on endoscopy). Only 92% of these patients were completely symptom free, however.[20] The postoperative management for patients under 10 years of age is different than that previously outlined. We electively do a postoperative evaluation under general anesthesia after 4 weeks. The intranasal lacrimal ostium is evaluated and the O'Donoghue tubes are removed. There may be granulations around the ostium, especially on the anterior wall as this is the region where lacrimal and nasal mucosa are most difficult to approximate and there is often a little exposed bone after draping of all the mucosal flaps (**Figs. 11–16**). These granulations should be removed, and this region should subsequently heal well. In some patients, there may be minor adhesions between the lateral nasal wall and septum, and these are also divided. This occurs because the nasal cavity is small, and we do not perform a septoplasty unless there is significant septal deviation. In those patients with significant septal deviation, a Killian incision is performed and the septum mobilized from the maxillary crest and from the bony septum. No cartilage or bone is excised. This mobilization is usually sufficient and allows surgery to proceed in the previously obstructed nasal cavity. Mobilization without tissue resection also lessens the risk of disturbing the septum's further growth and consequently altering facial features.

◆ RATIONALE FOR THE ROUTINE INSERTION OF O'DONOGHUE TUBES

O'Donoghue tubes are placed after endoscopic DCR in an attempt to dilate the common canaliculus opening into the lacrimal sac. The tubes are not placed in an attempt to keep the sac open as the sac is so widely marsupialized with lacrimal and nasal mucosa apposition it would be unnecessary. The aim of the O'Donoghue tube insertion is to dilate the common canaliculus opening by placing silastic tubes for 4 weeks. Over many years of observing the Bowman lacrimal probe entering the lacrimal sac, it was apparent that the mucosal fold that forms the valve of Rosenmuller was tight in more than 50% of patients and that this may contribute to symptoms in some patients. It did not make sense to create a large lacrimal ostium but fail to address a potentially more proximal obstruction. Unfortunately, we have found it difficult to preoperatively diagnose tight valves. We do think it more likely in patients who on DCG do not have penetration of the dye into the sac but on scintigraphy have

151

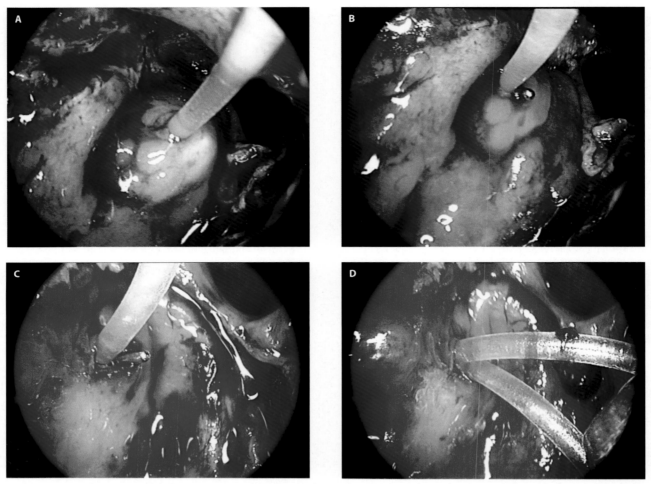

Figure 11–17 In the first patient, (**A**) the common canaliculus grips the single O'Donoghue tube tightly and (**B**) the tip of the probe is tightly held by the valve. In the second patient, (**C**) the silastic tube and probe are tightly held by the valve and (**D**) the two tubes are seen to dilate the valve.

penetration of the radioisotope into the sac. The radioisotope has more time to slowly penetrate the valve than the dye does and may indicate a tight common canaliculus opening. In an attempt to exclude this factor from affecting our success rates, we have made placement of these tubes a routine part of endoscopic DCR. In **Fig. 11–17**, we present two examples of tight valves of Rosenmuller and it can clearly be seen how the mucosal fold grips the end of the probe.

◆ ANCILLARY PROCEDURES

Septoplasty was necessary in 47% of patients. This was done endoscopically through a Killian incision. The area of obstructing septal deflection directly adjacent to the anterior end of the middle turbinate was removed while the anterior cartilage was kept intact. In 15% of patients, endoscopic sinus surgery was necessary for ongoing nonresponsive chronic sinusitis or nasal polyposis.

◆ COMPLICATIONS

Complications in powered endoscopic DCR are very rare. There were three cases of postoperative hemorrhage giving a complication rate of 1.9%. No other complications occurred. Serious complications can occur if the surgeon losses anatomic landmarks. These include damage to the orbit and orbital contents and damage to the anterior cranial fossa with a cerebrospinal fluid (CSF) leak. If the landmarks described above are kept in mind and the surgeon stays anterior to the insertion of the uncinate, penetration of the orbit is unlikely. Dissection posterior to the uncinate, however, will usually result in orbital fat exposure. Should this occur, it should be left alone and not manipulated in any way. As the bone is removed above the middle turbinate, the mucosa of the agger nasi cell will be exposed. The diamond burr should be kept in contact with the bone directly above the sac and bone removal should continue to the mucosal incision. If there is any doubt as to exactly which part of mucosa is sac wall and which is skin or agger nasi cell mucosa, a DCR light pipe* (Medtronic ENT) is introduced into the sac and the sac transilluminated. If the surgeon stays in close proximity to the sac while removing the bone, the likelihood of damage to the skull base with a subsequent CSF leak is very small.

◆ KEY POINTS

It is beneficial when starting to do endoscopic DCRs that the sinus surgeon develops a close liaison with an ophthalmologist.[11] Both have expertise in different areas and the combination of this expertise helps in both the workup for surgery and during the surgical procedure. Our team consists of an ENT surgeon and an oculoplastic surgeon. We assess patients together in the lacrimal clinic. The oculoplastic surgeon helps with the assessment of other causes of epiphora such as blepharitis, entropion, ectropion, lid laxity, and so forth, and will be able to teach the sinus surgeon how to syringe and probe the lacrimal system. The sinus surgeon is able to endoscopically assess the nasal cavity, septum, and any ancillary sinus disease that may be present. At surgery, the sinus surgeon has the endoscopic skills to deal with the septum and expose the lacrimal sac. The oculoplastic surgeon has the expertise in probing the lacrimal system and passing O'Donoghue tubes and dealing with lid laxity, entropion, or ectropion. Both surgeons should learn to be comfortable with all aspects of assessment and surgery, and we routinely alternate our roles during surgery.

The key to success in powered endoscopic DCR is to be able to picture the anatomy of the lacrimal sac as it will be encountered when the sac is approached from the nasal cavity. Understanding the anatomic relationships allows complete exposure of the sac and marsupialization of the sac into the lateral nasal wall. In addition, preservation of mucosa with fashioning of mucosal flaps allows the nasal and lacrimal mucosa to be apposed with first-intention rather than second-intention healing. This decreases the risk of granulation tissue and scar formation and gives a reliable and reproducible result.

References

1. Caldwell G. Two new operations for obstruction of the nasal duct, with preservation of the canaliculi, and with an incidental description of a new lacrymal probe. Am J Ophthalmol 1893;10:189–193
2. Toti A. Nuovo metodo conservatore dicura radicale delle suppurazione croniche del sacco lacrimale (dacricistorhinostomia). Clin Moderna (Firenza) 1904;10:385
3. Hartikainen J, Jukka A, Matti V. Prospective randomized comparison of endonasal endoscopic dacryocystorhinostomy and external dacryocystorhinostomy. Laryngoscope 1998;108:1861–1866
4. McDonogh M, Meiring J. Endoscopic transnasal dacryocystorhinostomy. J Laryngol Otol 1989;103:585–587
5. Metson R. Endoscopic surgery for lacrimal obstruction. Otolaryngol Head Neck Surg 1991;104:473–479
6. Steadman M. Transnasal dacryocystorhinostomy. Otolaryngol Clin North Am 1985;18:107–111
7. Gonnering RS, Lyon D, Fisher J. Endoscopic laser-assisted lacrimal surgery. Am J Ophthalmol 1991;111:152–157
8. Massaro BM, Gonnering R, Harris GJ. Endonasal laser dacryocystorhinostomy. Arch Ophthalmol 1990;108:1172–1186
9. Woog JJ, Metson R, Puliafito C. Holmium: YAG endonasal laser dacryocystorhinostomy. Am J Ophthalmol 1993;116:1–10
10. Linberg JV, Anderson R, Busted R, Barreras R. Study of intranasal ostium external dacryocystorhinostomy. Arch Ophthalmol 1982;100:1758–1762
11. Wormald PJ, Nilssen E. Endoscopic DCR: the team approach. Hong Kong Journal of Ophthalmology 1998;1:71–74
12. Welham RA, Wulc AE. Management of unsuccessful lacrimal surgery. Br J Ophthalmol 1987;71(2):152–157
13. Wormald PJ, Kew J, Van Hasselt CA. The intranasal anatomy of the nasolacrimal sac in endoscopic dacryocystorhinostomy. Otolaryngol Head Neck Surg 2000;123:307–310
14. Wormald PJ. Powered endonasal dacryocystorhinostomy. Laryngoscope 2002;112:69–71
15. Unlu HH, Govsa F, Mutlu C. Anatomic guidelines for intranasal surgery of the lacrimal drainage system. Rhinology 1997;35:11–15
16. Rebeiz EE, Shapshay S, Bowlds J, Pankratov M. Anatomic guidelines for dacryocystorhinostomy. Laryngoscope 1992;102:1181–1184
17. Wormald PJ, Tsirbas A. Investigation and treatment for functional and anatomical obstruction of the naso-lacrimal duct system. Clin Otolaryngol 2004;29:352–356
18. Tsirbas A, Wormald PJ. Endonasal dacryocystorhinostomy with mucosal flaps. Am J Ophthalmol 2003;135(1):76–78
19. Wormald PJ. Powered endoscopic DCR. Otolaryngol Clin North Am 2006;39:539–549
20. Leibovitch I, Selva D, Tsirbas A, Greenrod E, Pater J, Wormald PJ. Pediatric endoscopic endonasal dacryocystorhinostomy in congenital nasolacrimal duct obstruction. Graefes Arch Clin Exp Ophthalmol 2006;244:1250–1254
21. Mann BS, Wormald PJ. Endoscopic assessment of the dacryocystorhinostomy ostium after endoscopic surgery. Laryngoscope 2006;116:1172–1174
22. Tsirbas A, Davis G, Wormald P. Revision dacryocystorhinostomy: a comparison of endoscopic and external techniques. Am J Rhinol 2005;19(3):322–325

12

Cerebrospinal Fluid Leak Closure

The traditional management of anterior skull base cerebrospinal fluid (CSF) leaks was via an anterior craniotomy and intracranial repair of the CSF leak. This was usually done by elevating the frontal lobes in the region of the suspected site of the leak and laying a sheet of fascia lata over this area. The success rate of this technique was around 70% but usually left the patient with some loss of smell. In addition, frontal lobe retraction is associated with the risk of postoperative epilepsy. In the late 1980s and early 1990s, endoscopic closure of CSF leaks was first reported. Since then, many published series have reported success rates of above 90%.[1–3] This high success rate and the very low associated morbidity are the major advantages of the endoscopic technique.[1] A variety of materials have been used to close these leaks.[3,4] Free mucosal grafts, pedicled mucosal grafts, fat, fascia, muscle, and synthetic materials such as hydroxyapatite have all been described with similar success rates.[3,4] In a recent review, Hegazy et al[3] felt that the type of material did not appear to make a significant difference to the success rate of the closure. Whereas this may indeed be the case in small CSF leaks, the purely on-lay technique may not be as suitable for larger leaks.[3,4] The techniques proposed in this chapter (the bath-plug closure and fascia lata repair) have been used in a large series of patients and have been found to be reliable for both large and small leaks.[5,6] In our experience, if the on-lay technique alone is used for medium or large defects with a free flow of CSF, the graft tends to be pushed away from the skull base and hence from the dural defect and the flow of CSF resumes. Although the leak may be sealed at the end of the operation, coughing or straining in the postoperative period may raise the CSF pressure sufficiently to cause the leak to start again. An analogy of patching these high-flow CSF leaks with on-lay technique alone is like trying to patch a plastic bag of water by applying a patch to the outside of the bag.[5,6] The bath-plug technique allows the plug to be placed on the inside of the bag and uses the pressure from the water to increase the seal on the plug. The other

technique presented (underlay alone or underlay and on-lay fascia grafting) and the indications for this technique also overcome this problem of the CSF pressure pushing the graft away from the skull base as the fascia is placed intracranially and the CSF pressure again helps create the seal. This chapter does not attempt to describe all the alternative techniques but will concentrate on the bath-plug and underlay fascia techniques, as we have considerable experience in a wide variety of situations with these techniques and have found them to be both versatile and reliable.[5,6]

◆ ETIOLOGY OF CEREBROSPINAL FLUID LEAKS

Anterior skull base CSF leaks can be divided into four broad categories according to their etiology. In a recent large series from our department, there was a fairly even spread between leaks caused by skull base trauma, spontaneous leaks, leaks associated with meningoencephaloceles, and iatrogenic leaks.

Traumatic Cerebrospinal Fluid Leaks

Traumatic CSF leaks usually follow an anterior skull base fracture. The initial management is conservative as most of these leaks will cease within 10 days of the injury. However, leaks that persist longer than 10 days should be closed. One of the major causes of continued CSF leakage is rotation of a bony spicule that continues to hold the edges of the torn dura apart. If the bone fragment is freely mobile, then this should be removed at the time of closure of the leak (**Fig. 12–1**).

More common than traumatic CSF leaks of the sphenoid are those seen in the fovea ethmoidalis or at the fovea ethmoidalis–olfactory fossa junction (**Fig. 12–2**).

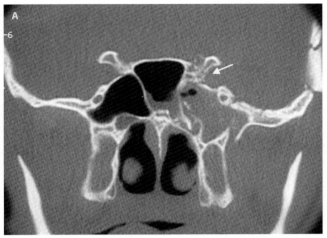
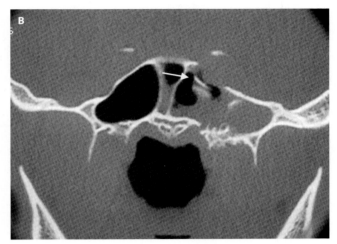

Figure 12–1 CT scans of patient with a fracture through the clinoid (*white arrow* [**A**]) with a displaced bony fragment (*white arrow* [**B**]) and a CSF leak. Note the fluid level in the sphenoid.

Less frequent are fractures in the posterior table of the frontal sinus. Fortunately, these leaks rarely need closure but if they persist, access is usually only possible with an endoscopic modified Lothrop procedure or an osteoplastic flap. The endoscopic modified Lothrop procedure allows most of the posterior table of the frontal sinus to be accessed, and the CSF leak can be closed under direct visualization (**Fig. 12–3**).

Spontaneous Cerebrospinal Fluid Leaks

Spontaneous CSF leaks are usually seen either in the cribriform plate or lateral wall of the sphenoid sinus. Cribriform fossa leaks often result from a dilation of the dural sheath around the olfactory fibers. A small prolapse of dura may result that may leak CSF (**Fig. 12–4**).

Spontaneous CSF leaks in the sphenoid sinus are usually seen in well-pneumatized sphenoid sinuses where the sinus pneumatizes into the clinoid process under the maxillary nerve. This brings this region of the sphenoid sinus into contact with the temporal lobe region of the middle cranial fossa with only thin bone separating the two. One theory as to why the skull base becomes eroded in this region is that arachnoid granulations in the floor of the middle cranial fossa often do not have a venous connection. When these arachnoid sacks fill with CSF and pulsate, they may gradually erode the bone, eventually leading to a prolapse of dura and arachnoid into the sphenoid with an associated leak.[7–10] In addition, it is thought that several of these patients may have undiagnosed benign raised intracranial pressure as part of the etiology. In **Fig. 12–5**, a defect is seen in this lateral aspect of this well-pneumatized sphenoid with an associated opacity (prolapsing meninges and CSF).

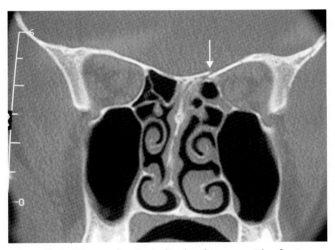

Figure 12–2 CT scan of patient after head trauma with a fracture through the fovea ethmoidalis (*white arrow*) and with associated CSF leak. Note the fluid level in the adjacent ethmoid sinus.

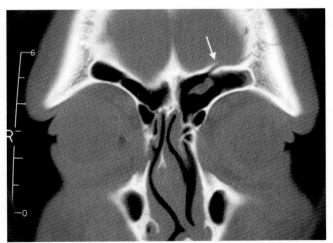

Figure 12–3 CT scan of a patient with a fracture through the posterior table (*white arrow*) of the frontal sinus with an associated CSF leak.

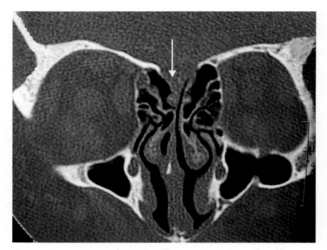

Figure 12–4 A coronal CT scan illustrating a triangular dilatation of the cribriform plate around an olfactory neuron (confirmed at surgery).

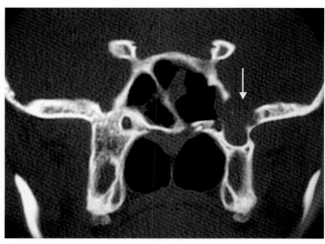

Figure 12–5 Defect in left lateral wing of sphenoid with prolapse of dura through the defect.

Meningoencephaloceles with Associated Cerebrospinal Fluid Leaks

Meningoencephaloceles may either be spontaneous (congenital or acquired) or associated with a previous traumatic event. Congenital meningoencephaloceles usually present within the first few years of life. The meningoencephalocele consists of meninges and dura containing CSF with a variable amount of brain tissue prolapsing through the skull base defect into the nasal cavity or sinuses. The brain tissue within the encephalocele is usually nonfunctional and is usually resected as the first step of the procedure. Posttraumatic meningoencephaloceles often have a funnel-shaped defect in the skull base, and this needs to be recognized during the repair process as this affects the ability of the surgeon to

properly visualize the edges of the bony skull base defect as well as the intracranial cavity. The funnel-shaped bony defect is caused by the intracranial contents protruding through the defect and pushing the edges of the bony defect downward into the nasal cavity/sinuses (**Fig. 12–6**).

Iatrogenic Cerebrospinal Fluid Leaks

Iatrogenic leaks will frequently be seen on the lateral wall of the olfactory fossa and fovea ethmoidalis. The lateral wall of the olfactory fossa forms the medial limit of the dissection of the frontal recess. It can be very thin varying from 0.1 to 1 mm in thickness and is perforated by the anterior ethmoidal artery. Damage to this lateral wall of the olfactory

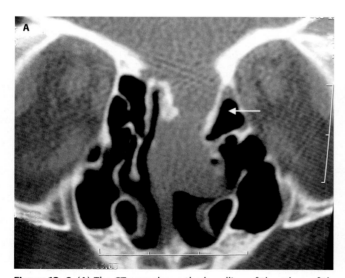

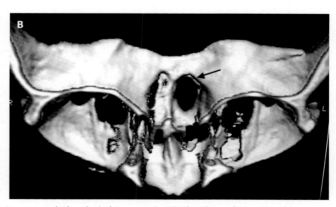

Figure 12–6 (**A**) The CT scan shows the bevelling of the edges of the meningoencephalocele (*white arrow*). (**B**) The three-dimensional reconstruction illustrates the funnel shape of the skull base defect through which the meningoencephalocele protrudes (*black arrow*).

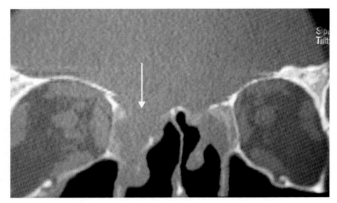

Figure 12–7 Intraoperative iatrogenic injury to the anterior fovea ethmoidalis (*white arrow*) on the right side.

fossa may occur if the dissecting instruments are turned medially during surgery in this region. Laceration of the anterior ethmoidal artery with bleeding may prompt the use of diathermy in an attempt to obtain hemostasis. Unipolar diathermy, if used to cauterize a bleeding vessel, may burn through the bone and dura causing a CSF leak. The remaining skull base (fovea ethmoidalis) may be damaged if the surgeon loses orientation and fails to recognize that the dissection has reached the skull base. If cells are assumed to be present on the skull base, an attempt to remove these "cells" may damage the skull base with an associated CSF leak (**Fig. 12–7**). Generally, these leaks are readily apparent at the time of surgery and can be fixed with the described bath-plug technique.

◆ PREOPERATIVE ASSESSMENT

This is performed if the patient presents with a suspected CSF leak. Intraoperative CSF leaks should be dealt with at the time of the surgery. The most reliable method of confirming a CSF leak is to test the clear watery secretions from the nose for β2-transferrin (β2-transferrin is only present in CSF).[4,5,7,11] Once the CSF leak has been confirmed, the site of the leak is sought by performing a high-resolution fine-cut computed tomography (CT) scan of the sinuses.[5,11] On this scan, dehiscences of the anterior skull base are sought. Depending upon the suspected cause, different areas in the anterior skull base are thoroughly scrutinized for bony defects. An additional clue may be the presence of fluid in the sinuses indicating that the leak is in the region of the opacified sinuses. Patients with spontaneous CSF leaks without evidence of any bony dehiscences on CT scan and without any opacification of any sinuses should have the cribriform plate region carefully examined intraoperatively for the CSF leak, as it has been our experience that this is the most likely source of the leak (**Fig. 12–4**).

If the site of the leak is not apparent on the CT scan, a high-resolution T2-weighted magnetic resonance imaging (MRI) scan may allow visualization of fluid within the sinuses, and if the patient is leaking at the time of the MRI, it may allow identification of the site of the leak.[5,11] All patients with suspected meningoceles or meningoencephaloceles should have a preoperative MRI. This allows brain tissue within the meningoencephalocele to be identified, and the opinion of the neurosurgeon should be sought whether the resection of this tissue transnasally is considered reasonable and safe (**Fig. 12–8**).

Although in the past there have been other investigations used to identify CSF leaks, the above investigations

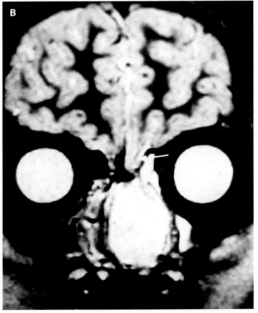

Figure 12–8 (**A**) A CT scan showing the skull base defect of a congenital meningoencephalocele (*white arrow*). (**B**) A T2-weighted MRI showing a large CSF-filled sac filling the nasal cavity with an associated stalk of brain tissue prolapsing through the skull base defect (*white arrow*). This meningoencephalocele was managed endoscopically.

are the only ones recommended. Intrathecal contrast does not improve the sensitivity of the detection of the site of a CSF leak. Intrathecal radioisotope may confirm the presence of CSF in the nasal cavity but does not add information to that obtained by a positive β2-transferrin test.[3] If the site of the leak is not able to be determined with the above investigations, the patient is taken to theater and intrathecal fluorescein is injected into the CSF space and the site of the leak sought while the patient in under general anesthetic.[5,11,12]

◆ SURGICAL TECHNIQUE

Broad-spectrum intravenous antibiotics are given with induction of anesthesia.

Intrathecal Fluorescein

Most patients undergoing elective CSF leak repair will have intrathecal fluorescein injected before surgery.[4,5,11,12] Patients who have a CSF leak during surgery will have the leak repaired at the time of the surgery without the placement of fluorescein intrathecally. All our patients preoperatively sign a separate consent form designed specifically to explain the risks of the administration of intrathecal fluorescein. The most common side effects are paresthesias and tingling in the hands and feet and convulsions. These side effects were reported when significantly higher concentrations of fluorescein were used and have not been seen in our series or other very large patient series.[4-6,11-14] In elective CSF leak closure, the lumbar drain is placed while the patient is awake. Ten milliliters of CSF is removed from the intrathecal space. A 40- to 60-kg person will have 0.2 mL 5% fluorescein mixed with 10 mL CSF administered while patients of 60 kg and heavier have 0.25 mL 5% fluorescein mixed with 10 mL CSF administered.[4,5,11,12] The fluorescein-stained CSF is re-injected through a filter into the intrathecal space at a rate of 1 mL per minute. This is done while the patient is awake so that any possible side effects can be identified. Once the fluorescein-stained CSF has been re-injected, the patient is kept in the theater recovery area for 1 to 2 hours in the head-down position to allow for the fluorescein to enter the cranial cavity and mix with the CSF around the brain. If there is a significant flow of CSF at this time, the appearance of fluorescein within the CSF is fairly rapid (within 20 minutes) but may take significantly longer in low-flow CSF leaks or where there is a relative paucity of CSF within the system. Once the patient is anesthetized, the patient is placed in the head-down position during preparation of the patient's nose with local anesthetic solution. This draping and set-up of the theater equipment usually takes ~10 to 20 minutes allowing additional time for the fluorescein to penetrate the intracranial cavity.

Intrathecal fluorescein can be invaluable for locating those difficult-to-find CSF leaks. Fluorescein can help identify the site of a small CSF leak or a leak that is intermittent or that has recently stopped leaking (usually just prior to the surgery). If a blue-light filter is used on the light source,

even the smallest quantities of fluorescein can be visualized intraoperatively and the leak can then be closed.[5,6] If at this stage the leak is still not visible, the patient should be placed in the head-down position and a forced inspiration maneuver (Valsalva-like) performed by the anesthetist. This should be repeated several times while the surgeon examines the most likely site for the CSF leak. If no leak is seen, the patient should be placed head down and ventilated for a further 30 minutes before the nasal cavity and sinuses are reexamined for fluorescein-stained CSF.[6] Again, the blue-light filter can be very useful. If the site of the leak is still not apparent, manipulation of the CSF space is attempted. The lumbar drain is attached to an arterial pressure monitor with a three-way tap. The CSF pressure is measured (normal 0 to 15 mm water). Twenty milliliters of Ringer's lactate is injected into the intrathecal space through the lumbar drain and the pressure remeasured. After 40 mL has been injected, the head-down forced inspiration maneuver is repeated with the blue-light filter to see if the leak is visible. The Ringer's lactate aliquots can be repeated but the intrathecal pressure must be measured after each aliquot to ensure that it does not go over 30 mm of water. In our series, one patient required 120 mL of Ringer's before the leak became apparent.[6]

A cornerstone of this procedure is the identification of the site of the CSF leak. The leak cannot be closed if the site cannot be identified.

Another major advantage of the fluorescein-stained CSF is the ability of the surgeon to test if the CSF leak closure is watertight once the leak has been repaired.[5] After the repair has been performed as described below, the patient is placed head down and the forced inspiration maneuver repeated. The smallest leak of CSF can be easily seen as the CSF is a bright yellow/green color.

◆ BATH-PLUG TECHNIQUE FOR CEREBROSPINAL FLUID LEAK REPAIR

This technique forms the mainstay for the closure of CSF leaks with more than 90% of our patients undergoing this technique. Once the site of the CSF leak has been identified, the dural defect is enlarged until the bony rim of the skull base can be clearly seen. As the dural defect is enlarged, a strong flow of fluorescein-stained CSF is usually apparent. It is important to remove the prolapsed dura and meninges and not to attempt repair of a dural or meningeal defect as the dura and meninges provide no support for the tissue used to repair the defect. The bone of the skull base is solid and if the repair is based around this solid support, a good result is more likely. On occasion, the bone of the skull base may be fractured and unstable. If small pieces of bone are visible, these should be removed before repair. Large pieces of bone should be left in place and the dura opened to the edge of these large pieces. If large bony fragments are present, the bath-plug technique is still suitable but the graft needs support as the suture is pulled after intracranial placement of the graft. Once the bony rim of the defect has been identified, the nasal mucosa around the defect is stripped away for

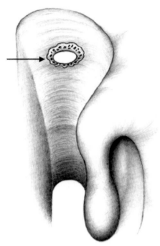

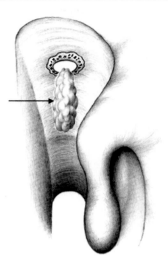

Figure 12–9 The bony margins of the defect in skull base are identified, prolapsing dura removed, and the mucosa circumferentially stripped away from edge of defect for ~5 mm (*black arrow*). (From Wormald PJ, McDonogh M. The bath-plug closure of anterior skull base cerebro-spinal fluid (CSF) leaks. Am J Rhinol 2003;17:299–305. Reprinted with permission.)

Figure 12–10 Demonstration of the fat plug (*black arrow*) relative to the size of the defect. Note that the fat plug is the same diameter as the defect. (From Wormald PJ, McDonogh M. The bath-plug closure of anterior skull base cerebro-spinal fluid (CSF) leaks. Am J Rhinol 2003;17:299–305. Reprinted with permission.)

at least 5 mm. This allows the free mucosal graft to stick to the bone and ultimately a better seal is achieved (**Fig. 12–9**).

The skull base defect is measured using a curette. For example, the defect may be two curettes wide and three long. If a 3-mm curette is used, then the defect would be 6 × 9 mm. A 6 × 9 mm fat graft is then harvested from the earlobe. If the defect is larger than 12 mm, fat is obtained either from the region of the greater trochanter of the thigh or from the abdomen. If possible, the earlobe is the preferred region for obtaining the fat graft as the fat globules are tightly knitted and easy to work with. However, if there have been multiple

piercings of the earlobe, or the defect is large, then the greater trochanter region is preferred as the fat globules in this region are again more fibrous and tightly knitted than the fat from the abdomen. The fat plug should be the same diameter as the defect (otherwise there will be difficulty introducing it through the defect) and ~1.5 to 2 cm long (**Fig. 12–10**).

A 40 Vicryl suture is knotted through the one end of the fat plug and the suture passed down the length of the fat plug (**Fig. 12–11**).

A free mucosal graft is harvested from the lateral nasal wall (usually on the opposite side to that which has the CSF leak).

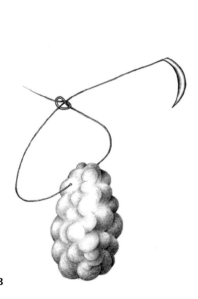

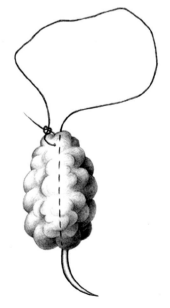

A–B

Figure 12–11 (A,B) The 40 Vicryl suture is knotted at the one end of the fat plug before been passed along the length of the fat plug. (From Wormald PJ, McDonogh M. The bath-plug closure of anterior skull base cerebro-spinal fluid (CSF) leaks. Am J Rhinol 2003;17:299–305. Reprinted with permission.)

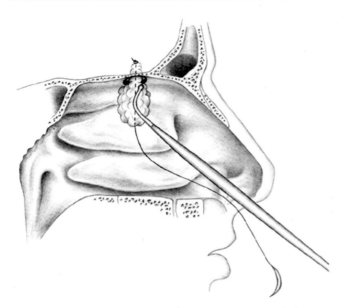

Figure 12–12 The fat plug is gently manipulated through the skull base defect into the intracranial cavity. Only a small piece of fat is introduced with each maneuver. (From Wormald PJ, McDonogh M. The bath-plug closure of anterior skull base cerebro-spinal fluid (CSF) leaks. Am J Rhinol 2003;17:299–305. Reprinted with permission.)

The mucosa is taken from the lateral nasal wall anterior to the middle turbinate and is usually ~3 × 3 cm (larger if the defect is large). The fat plug is placed below the defect and the malleable frontal sinus probe (Medtronic, Jacksonville, FL, USA) is used to gently introduce the fat plug through the defect. The malleable frontal sinus probe does not have a ball-tip on the end that aids the introduction of the fat plug. If a probe with a ball-tip is used, the fat tends to stick to the ball, and as the probe is pulled back after introducing fat intracranially, fat is pulled with the probe resulting in difficulty introducing the fat plug intracranially.[5] The important part of this technique is to introduce only a very small amount of fat through the defect with each maneuver. If a large amount of fat is introduced through the defect with one maneuver, significant pressure may be required and the probe can slip a significant distance into the intracranial cavity with the potential to injure intracranial structures.[5] If small amounts of fat are introduced with each maneuver, then greater safety is achieved as the probe does not need to enter the intracranial cavity by more than a few millimeters with each maneuver (**Fig. 12–12**).[4,5]

Consideration needs to be given to the possibility that there may be a vessel present in the region where the fat plug is introduced. This likelihood is increased with repair of meningoencephaloceles, as vessels are present that supply blood to the prolapsed brain and dura. In addition, the brain tissue that prolapses into the defect is often adherent to the edges

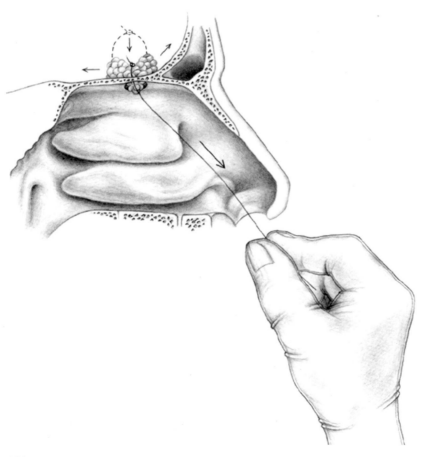

Figure 12–13 The Vicryl suture is gently pulled while the fat graft is supported. This expands the fat graft on the intracranial surface and pulls the fat into the defect giving a solid seal of the defect. (From Wormald PJ, McDonogh M. The bath-plug closure of anterior skull base cerebro-spinal fluid (CSF) leaks. Am J Rhinol 2003;17:299–305. Reprinted with permission.)

of the defect, decreasing the amount of intracranial space available for introduction of the fat plug. In these situations, the technique of placing one layer of fascia lata intracranial and the second layer as an on-lay is preferred. However, if the fat plug is manipulated gently into the intracranial cavity, the likelihood of damage of intracranial structures is very small. In our large series, no such injuries occurred.

Once the fat plug has been safely introduced through the defect, the plug is stabilized with the probe and the Vicryl suture is gently pulled. This expands the fat plug on the intracranial side of the defect and allows the CSF pressure to increase the seal of the fat in the defect (much like the water pressure of the bath sealing the bath plug in the drain) (**Fig. 12–13**).

The seal is tested by placing the patient head down and asking the anesthetist to perform a forced inspiration maneuver. No fluorescein-stained CSF should be seen. This maneuver further pushes the fat plug into the defect and a little prolapse of fat through the defect is normal. The patient is placed head up (15 degrees) and the free mucosal graft is slid up the Vicryl suture until it covers the defect. Ensure that the graft is correctly oriented with the mucosal surface facing the nasal cavity (**Fig. 12–14**).

Fibrin glue is applied and the Vicryl suture is cut. Gelfoam is placed over the free mucosal graft and fibrin glue reapplied. Several layers can be placed in this manner. No other nasal packing is used.

◆ SPECIAL SITUATIONS

Meningoencephaloceles with a Cerebrospinal Fluid Leak (See DVD Video)

The meninges and protruding brain tissue are resected up to the skull base. This is normally done with a powered microdebrider. If significant brain tissue is seen on the MRI prolapsing into the nasal cavity or sinuses, a neurosurgical consultation should be sought regarding the safety of resection of the brain tissue. After resection, the dural edges are cauterized with a suction bipolar forceps to ensure hemostasis. Exposure of the bony limits of the skull base defect is important as proper closure of the defect cannot be achieved by placing grafts against prolapsed dura, and such a repair is doomed to failure. Once the bone of the skull base defect is clearly exposed and surrounding mucosa on the nasal surface gently removed from the edges of the bony defect, the prolapsing brain tissue can be addressed. The brain tissue is shrunk using the suction bipolar until the stump of remaining brain tissue lies within the intracranial cavity. At this point, an assessment needs to be made as to whether the edges of the prolapsed brain tissue are in contact with the edges of the skull base defect and whether it is adhesive to the dura around the defect. This is often the case, and in these patients a fat plug graft is not suitable because there is insufficient space on the intracranial surface of the defect to place the fat plug. This is especially true in defects larger than 5 mm as greater amounts of brain tissue tend to prolapse into the larger defects with a greater chance of this prolapsed brain becoming adherent to the dura around the defect. The first step is to use the suction bipolar forceps to shrink the brain tissue adherent to the edges of the defect. Any blood vessels visualized are cauterized with the suction bipolar. The malleable suction Freer elevator from the Frontal Sinus Malleable Set* or from the Skull Base Set* (Medtronic ENT) is bent to the appropriate angle and the brain tissue gently mobilized from the dural edges around the defect to create sufficient space circumferentially around the bony defect. The fascia lata graft is measured to be ~10 to 20 mm larger than the defect's diameter so that there are at least 5 mm of graft to be slid into this space between brain and dura around the whole circumference of the defect. In some instances, the two-surgeon approach can be useful. The second surgeon

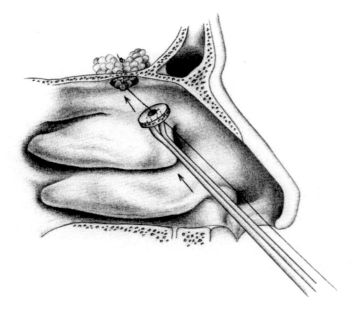

Figure 12–14 The free mucosal graft is slid up the Vicryl suture to cover the slightly protruding fat plug and skull base defect. (From Wormald PJ, McDonogh M. The bath-plug closure of anterior skull base cerebro-spinal fluid (CSF) leaks. Am J Rhinol 2003;17:299–305. Reprinted with permission.)

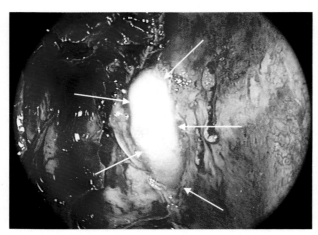

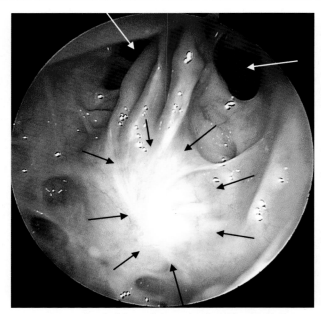

Figure 12–15 This patient presented with a right-sided spontaneous CSF leak and at surgery a 1.5-cm × 8-mm defect was found in the olfactory fossa. The brain was adherent to the dura around the defect and needed to be carefully mobilized before the fascia lata graft was placed. This photo shows the fascial graft in place as an underlay (*white arrows* mark the limits of the defect). No fluorescein can be seen and a solid seal has been achieved. This graft was covered with a free mucosal graft and fibrin glue and Gelfoam. No nasal pack was placed.

Figure 12–16 The skull base defect is outlined by the *black arrows* and the frontal sinus ostia by the *white arrows*. Note the remucosalization of the region of the defect.

can gently push the prolapsing brain tissue intracranially to allow the graft to be placed. The CSF and brain tissue then seal this graft into place and in most cases no further fluorescein-stained CSF should be visible (**Fig. 12–15**).

For large skull base defects (>2 cm) a second layer of fascia lata is placed on the nasal surface followed by fibrin glue. In smaller defects, a free mucosal graft with the mucosa harvested from the middle turbinate or floor of the nose is placed over this intracranial graft followed by fibrin glue. Defects from the posterior wall of the frontal sinus up to the anterior face of the pituitary and from lamina papyracea to lamina papyracea have been successfully closed using this two-layer facia lata approach. When large defects are closed, the fibrin glue is covered by Gelfoam and then a nasal pack is placed in the nose for 5 days. No lumbar drain is used in large defects as this is likely to result in air being sucked into the intracranial cavity rather than improving the chances of a seal. **Figure 12–16** illustrates the postoperative view of the skull base after a large defect was closed with the two-layered fascia lata technique.

Some authors have recommended the use of bone or cartilage in the repair of large skull-base defects but we have found this to be unnecessary. If cartilage or bone is introduced intracranially, it pushes the fat plug or fascia away from the dura and bony rim of the defect and does not allow for a solid seal. In patients in whom we placed bone or cartilage in an attempt to provide a solid reconstruction of the skull base, these were removed intraoperatively because the defect could not be adequately sealed and CSF continued to leak. In none of the patients who have had large defect reconstructions of their skull bases have we seen any recurrence of encephaloceles over many years of follow-up. The argument

that bone or cartilage is needed to provide stability to the skull base to prevent encephalocele development is false.

Defects in the Lateral Wall of a Very Pneumatized Sphenoid Sinus: The Transpterygopalatine Fossa Approach (See DVD Video)

In this series, there were four patients who had a defect in the lateral wall of a very pneumatized sphenoid sinus. All presented with meningoceles or meningoencephaloceles with associated CSF leaks. See **Fig. 12–17**.

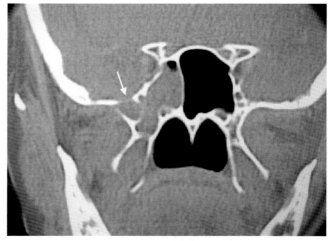

Figure 12–17 Defect in the right lateral wing of the sphenoid (*white arrow*) with CSF-filled sphenoid sinus.

In three of the four patients, multiple previous attempts at closure had been made at other institutions usually by attempting to obliterate the sphenoid with fat. These had failed, and the patients were referred to our department for closure. To close these leaks, adequate exposure of the lateral wall of the sphenoid is required. This is achieved by removal of the posterior wall of the maxillary sinus and removal of the contents of the medial region of pterygopalatine fossa with preservation of the maxillary nerve. The Vidian nerve and pterygopalatine ganglion may need to be sacrificed during this exposure. The posterior wall of the pterygopalatine fossa (which is also the anterior wall of the sphenoid) is removed and direct access through the pterygopalatine fossa is achieved. This will usually involve division of the sphenopalatine artery and other branches of the maxillary artery. Division of such a large artery is preceded by cauterization with the suction bipolar forceps* (Medtronic ENT), otherwise significant bleeding may result. The posterior wall of the pterygopalatine fossa is thick and is resected with the high-speed DCR diamond burr. Care is taken not to injure the maxillary nerve as it traverses the pterygopalatine fossa. Once direct access is achieved in this manner, the meningocele or meningoencephalocele is dealt with in the same manner as described above.

◆ POSTOPERATIVE CARE

The patient is given broad-spectrum antibiotics for 5 days postoperatively. Saline nasal spray is started immediately after the operation. The patient is instructed not to blow the nose for at least 2 to 3 weeks postoperatively. The lumbar drain is kept on free drainage at the level of the shoulder. With this arrangement, CSF should only drain if the intracranial pressure rises and so the lumbar drain serves as a safety valve for the first 24 hours. If the lumbar drain drains more than 5 to 10 mL per hour, it is raised above the shoulder to slow the drainage. After 24 hours, the lumbar drain is removed and the patient is slowly mobilized over the following 24 hours and then discharged.

◆ RESULTS

To date, 39 patients have been managed with this technique.[4,5] If these patients are divided into the four broad categories, there were 7 traumatic CSF leaks, 8 spontaneous CSF leaks, 12 meningoencephaloceles, and 12 iatrogenic CSF leaks. The average age was 40 years, and the male to female ratio was 1.2:1. **Table 12–1** summarizes the site, size, and success of the closure of the bath-plug technique.

Eight of the iatrogenic CSF leaks were referred to our department from outside institutions for closure. Thirty-six of the 39 leaks were closed at the first operation giving a primary success rate of closure of 93%. The mean follow-up time for all patients was 28 months (STD = 23) ranging from 4 to 75 months. The three patients that failed surgery were revised and all are currently successfully closed. Two of these patients had CSF leaks in the lateral wall of the sphenoid sinus and both had undergone multiple previous attempts at closure before referral to our department.[4,5] These patients were examined for evidence of raised intracranial pressure, and in one patient there was mild left papilledema. This patient probably has mild idiopathic interventricular hypertension and is currently being monitored to ensure no other problems develop. The third patient had a previous cranialization of the frontal sinus and developed a CSF leak in the posterior wall of the cranialized frontal sinus. Access was achieved by a modified endoscopic Lothrop procedure but the leak was high and lateral in the frontal sinus and difficulty was had with the placement of the fat plug. The patient started leaking within 48 hours of the repair and was taken back to theater where the fat plug was found to be partially extruded. A new fat plug was placed and closure was successful.

The results of the closure of large skull-base defects after the endoscopic removal of large sections of the skull base to provide access to the intracranial cavity for tumor removal are not included in the above results. We have found that two layers of fascia lata with one placed intracranially and the other on the nasal surface of the skull base in combination with fibrin glue, Gelfoam, and nasal packing give a reliable closure. The one leak we have had in this patient group was the first patient operated upon in whom we closed a large 3 × 3 cm defect with fat and fibrin glue alone.

◆ KEY POINTS

The CSF leak cannot be closed if it cannot be identified. There were five patients in this series in whom a fine-cut CT scan and an MRI scan could not identify the site of the leak preoperatively. Intrathecal fluorescein was placed in all elective CSF leak closures including those in whom the radiologic investigations indicated the likely site of the leak. This is an off-label usage of fluorescein so all patients had counseling regarding the potential complications of its usage and signed a separate consent form for its use.[4,5,11,12] In four patients, the blue-light filter and manipulation of the CSF space was needed before the site of the leak could be identified. Although placement of a lumbar drain and the off-label use of fluorescein are controversial, we have found these to be very useful in some patients in whom there was difficulty identifying the site of the CSF leak. In addition, the staining of the fluorescein allows the surgeon to carefully evaluate the security of the seal of the CSF leak by testing the leak by raising the intracranial pressure and looking for any evidence of fluorescein-stained CSF. Finally, the lumbar drain is kept in for 24 hours to prevent any sudden increases in CSF pressure from putting excessive pressure on the repair.

The introduction of a fat plug into the intracranial space has the potential risk of damage to intracranial vascular structures. The risk of such vessels being in the region of the CSF leak is higher in patients who have a meningoencephalocele especially if the brain is adherent to the dura around the skull base defect. We have modified our technique in these cases to use a two-layer closure (small defects, fascia and mucosa; and large defects, two layers of fascia). If there is concern regarding vessels in the region of the defect, appropriate radiologic investigations should be performed. The advent of radiologic software that is able to reconstruct the vasculature of the skull base without the need to perform an angiogram makes this a

Table 12–1 Summary of Patients Treated with the Bath-Plug Closure for Cerebrospinal Fluid Leak Repair

Patient No.	Site	Size (mm)	Follow-up (Months)	Second Closure Required	Successful
Traumatic CSF leaks					
1	Lateral wall of sphenoid	4 × 3	28	No	Yes
2	Around carotid in sphenoid with bony fragment	4 × 3	5	No	Yes
3	Posterior table of frontal sinus	3 × 3	6	No	Yes
4	Cribriform plate	6 × 4	5	No	Yes
5	Ethmoid	3 × 3	26	No	Yes
6	Sphenoid	7 × 5	26	No	Yes
7	Sphenoid	6 × 6	18	No	Yes
Iatrogenic CSF leaks					
1	Posterior ethmoid in association with skull base dehiscence from previous trauma	3 × 2	15	No	Yes
2	Posterior wall of frontal sinus. Sinus previously cranialized with mucocoele formation.	6 × 4	28	Yes	Yes
3	Posterior ethmoids.	4 × 3	32	No	Yes
4	Posterior ethmoids after resection of adenocarcinoma. Previous CSF leak at same spot with previous resection of adenocarcinoma	4 × 5	12	No	Yes
5	Posterior ethmoids	6 × 4	4	No	Yes
6	Posterior ethmoids	5 × 5	12	No	Yes
7	Adjacent to anterior ethmoidal artery	3 × 3	74	No	Yes
8	Sphenoid after intracranial meningioma removal	3 × 3	15	No	Yes
9	Post–craniofacial surgery in anterior ethmoids	3 × 3	20	No	Yes
10	Post–adenocarcinoma resection anterior ethmoid	2 × 3	12	No	Yes
11	Post–adenocarcinoma resection anterior ethmoid	3 × 3	10	No	Yes
12	Ethmoid roof (appeared to have an abnormally thin fovea ethmoidalis on both sides and had primary surgery at another institution)	16 × 12	16	No	Yes
Spontaneous CSF leaks					
1	Cribriform plate	6 × 3	11	No	Yes
2	Cribriform plate	2 × 1	12	No	Yes
3	Cribriform plate	3 × 2	38	No	Yes
4	Lateral wall of sphenoid	6 × 4	7	No	Yes
5	Cribriform plate	5 × 5	64	No	Yes
6	Roof of sphenoid	12 × 8	70	No	Yes
7	Posterior ethmoid	8 × 6	68	No	Yes
8	Sphenoid	1 × 2	8	No	Yes
Meningoencephaloceles associated with a CSF leak					
1	Sphenoid meningocele on lateral wall of very pneumatized sphenoid. Two previous attempted closures failed. Mild intracranial hypertension.	8 × 6	5	Yes	Yes
2	Cribriform plate meningoencephalocele	10 × 8	58	No	Yes
3	Meningoencephalocele found 2 years after cribriform plate trauma as a neonate.	12 × 10	8	No	Yes
4	Sphenoid meningocele in lateral wall of very pneumatized sphenoid	8 × 6	7	No	Yes
5	Frontal sinus meningoencephalocele	6 × 4	28	No	Yes
6	Cribriform plate meningocele	3 × 3	11	No	Yes
7	Cribriform plate meningoencephalocele	4 × 4	30	No	Yes
8	Sphenoid meningoencephalocele on the lateral wall of a very pneumatized sphenoid	4 × 4	26	No	Yes
9	Anterior ethmoid meningoencephalocele	13 × 8	62	No	Yes
10	Cribriform plate meningoencephalocele	14 × 8	75	No	Yes
11	Posterior cribriform plate meningoencephalocele after craniofacial surgery 2 years previously	12 × 9	30	No	Yes
12	Sphenoid meningocele on the lateral wall of a very pneumatized sphenoid sinus	8 × 8	6	Yes	Yes
Totals					
39		5.9 × 4.5	23.5	3	39

Source: From Wormald PJ, McDonogh M. "Bath-plug" technique for the endoscopic management of cerebrospinal fluid leaks. J Laryngol Otol 1997;111:1042–1046. Adapted with permission.

relatively simple investigation to perform. If doubt exists about the resection of brain tissue, neurosurgical opinion should be sought. Finally, the manipulation of the fat plug through the defect should be very gentle and the probe should not be introduced more than a few millimeters intracranially with each maneuver. This will minimize the risk of intracranial damage. In this series of patients, no such complication occurred, and from postoperative observation of the patients, there was no need to perform any postoperative radiologic investigations.

References

1. Marshall AH, Jones NS, Robertson IJA. CSF rhinorrhoea: the place of endoscopic sinus surgery. Br J Neurosurg 2001;15:8–12

2. Hughes RGM, Jones NS, Robertson JA. The endoscopic treatment of cerebrospinal fluid rhinorrhoea: the Nottingham experience. J Laryngol Otol 1997;111:125–128

3. Hegazy HM, Carrau R, Snyderman CH, Kassam A, Zweig J. Transnasal endoscopic repair of cerebrospinal fluid rhinorrhea: a meta-analysis. Laryngoscope 2000;110:1166–1172

4. Bolger WE, McLaughlin K. Cranial bone grafts in cerebrospinal fluid leak and encephalocoele repair: a preliminary report. Am J Rhinol 2003;17:153–158

5. Wormald PJ, McDonogh M. 'Bath-plug' technique for the endoscopic management of cerebrospinal fluid leaks. J Laryngol Otol 1997;111:1042–1046

6. Wormald PJ, McDonogh M. The bath-plug closure of anterior skull base cerebro-spinal fluid (CSF) leaks. Am J Rhinol 2003;17:299–305

7. Casiano RR, Jassir D. Endoscopic cerebrospinal fluid rhinorrhea repair: is a lumbar drain necessary? Otolaryngol Head Neck Surg 1999;121:745–750

8. Badia L, Loughran S, Lund V. Primary spontaneous cerebrospinal fluid rhinorrhoea and obesity. Am J Rhinol 2001;15:117–119

9. Ommaya AK, DiChiro G, Baldwin M, Pennybacker JB. Non-traumatic cerebrospinal fluid rhinorrhea. J Neurol Neurosurg Psychiatry 1968;31:214–225

10. Har-El G. What is 'spontaneous' cerebrospinal fluid rhinorrhea? Classification of cerebrospinal fluid leaks. Ann Otol Rhinol Laryngol 1999;108:323–326

11. Gacek RR. Arachnoid granulation cerebrospinal fluid otorrhea. Ann Otol Rhinol Laryngol 1990;99:854–862

12. Mattox DE, Kennedy DW. Endoscopic management of cerebrospinal fluid leaks and cephaloceles. Laryngoscope 1990;100:857–862

13. Syms CA, Syms MJ, Murphy TP, Massey SO. Cerebrospinal fluid fistulae in a canine model. Otolaryngol Head Neck Surg 1997;117:542–546

14. Mao VH, Keane WM, Atkins JP. Endoscopic repair of cerebrospinal fluid rhinorrhea. Otolaryngol Head Neck Surg 2000;122:56–60

15. Zweig JL, Carrau RL, Celin SE. Endoscopic repair of cerebrospinal fluid leaks to the sinonasal tract: predictors of success. Otolaryngol Head Neck Surg 2000;123:195–201

13

Endoscopic Resection of Pituitary Tumors

Pituitary tumors are most commonly benign pituitary adenomas, and only rarely are pituitary carcinomas or posterior pituitary neoplasias diagnosed.[1] Pituitary adenomas present most commonly in the third and fourth decades of life.[1] Their clinical presentation depends on whether the tumor is secreting (less common) or nonsecreting (more common).[1] Secreting adenomas present with the endocrine manifestations of the hormone secreted.[1,2] The most common is a prolactin-secreting tumor, followed by growth hormone, adrenocorticotropic hormone (ACTH), follicle-stimulating hormone, and luteinizing hormone.[1,2] Nonsecreting adenomas usually present due to their mass effects. Symptoms may include headache, hypopituitarism, visual loss and visual field defects (most commonly bilateral hemianopia), and cranial nerve defects.

Magnetic resonance imaging (MRI) is the radiologic investigation of choice for pathologic tumor evaluation and for defining the involvement of surrounding structures. Pituitary adenomas are divided, for clinical purposes, into microadenomas (<1.0 cm in diameter) and macroadenomas (>1.0 cm in diameter). Microadenomas are often difficult to see on MRI, but the normal anterior pituitary gland will usually be visible with a gadolinium-enhanced T1-weighted image allowing the microadenoma to be identified. In patients who have macroadenomas, the normal anterior pituitary will usually not be visualized. There are several grading systems available, but the most commonly used is based on extrasellar extension of the tumor (**Table 13–1**).[3]

In recent years, the surgical approach to the pituitary fossa has been either transseptal or transethmoid.[4,5] The transseptal

Table 13–1 Wilson Grading System for Pituitary Adenomas Based on Extrasellar Extension[3]

• *Stage 0*	No suprasellar extension
• *Stage A*	Extension into suprasellar cistern only
• *Stage B*	Extension into anterior recess of the third ventricle
• *Stage C*	Obliteration of anterior recess and deformation of floor of third ventricle
• *Stage D*	Intradural extension into anterior, middle, or posterior fossa
• *Stage E*	Extradural invasion into cavernous sinus

approach is performed through either a sublabial incision or through a hemitransfixion incision. Once the septal flaps have been raised and the anterior face of the sphenoid removed, the Cushing speculum is inserted. The microscope is swung into place and the anterior face of the pituitary fossa visualized. The sphenoid rostrum is removed and the intersinus septum identified and removed. The advantage of this technique is that the surgeon can now use an instrument in each hand to proceed with the surgery. The disadvantages of this technique are the morbidity associated with a sublabial incision and dissection and the incidence of septal perforations, adhesions, and postoperative sinusitis. In addition, the surgeon cannot visualize lateral or superior extensions of the tumor.

Recently, several surgeons have advocated a transnasal approach where the sphenoid sinus and the pituitary fossa are approached transnasally with lateralization of the middle turbinate and resection of the superior turbinate and anterior face of the sphenoid.[5–9] The Cushing speculum is introduced through the nares and into the sphenoidotomy and opened.[6,7] Opening of the speculum tends to further fracture the middle turbinate laterally as well as fracture the septum toward the opposite nasal cavity. Once the speculum is in place, the microscope is again brought in by the surgeon and the anterior face of the pituitary fossa resected with the surgeon using an instrument in each hand.[6,7] The advantages of this technique are the lack of any incisions around the face, but the disadvantage is the fracture or displacement of the septum and middle turbinate. Such a fracture of the septum is usually unstable and will often result in a septal deviation postoperatively. The middle turbinate may remain displaced and may cause obstruction of the sinus ostia, although this would be unusual.

The major reason for developing endoscopic pituitary tumor resection techniques is to minimize intranasal complications and to provide superior visualization. The endoscopic view is panoramic when compared with the microscopic view, and this helps with identification of critical anatomic landmarks within the sphenoid. In addition, angled endoscopes allow tumor that extends outside the sella to be seen, and this improves the surgeon's ability to achieve complete tumor resection.[8,9] Tumor remnants in the recesses of the sella that would not have been seen with the microscope may be visualized

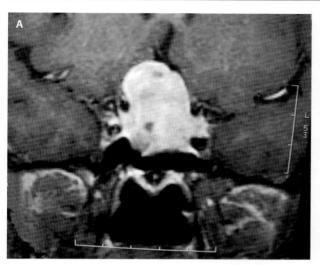

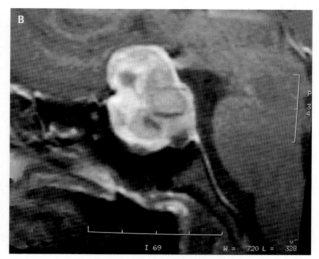

Figure 13–1 **(A)** Coronal MRI showing suprasellar extension of tumor. **(B)** Parasagittal plane MRI of the same tumor. Angled telescopes can be very helpful to visualize extensions above the sella as shown in these two MRI scans.

with an endoscope (**Fig. 13–1**). If complete tumor resection is achieved, there is less likelihood of recurrence.

◆ PREOPERATIVE ASSESSMENT

The standard radiologic evaluation prior to endoscopic resection of a pituitary tumor is a standard computed tomography (CT) scan of the sinuses and an MRI scan of the brain. These two modalities allow assessment of both the nose and sinuses and the pituitary tumor. The MRI scan requested is performed according to the image-guidance protocol for our computer-aided surgical (CAS) guidance system.

Image guidance during surgery adds to the safety of the procedure by confirming the positions of the optic nerves

and carotid arteries. In addition, during tumor resection, image guidance is used to confirm the limits of the pituitary fossa and the position of the internal carotid arteries within the cavernous sinuses, which may add to the safety of the procedure. In the preoperative evaluation of the radiology images, special attention needs to be paid to the course of the internal carotid arteries. Normally, the carotid arteries enter the base of the sphenoid sinus and turn vertically to ascend to the base of the pituitary gland where they move posteriorly and turn back on themselves forming the internal carotid siphon lateral to the pituitary gland in the cavernous sinus. They then travel anteriorly and can usually be seen on the lateral nasal wall before turning vertically and posteriorly to run lateral to the optic nerve into the anterior cranial fossa (**Fig. 13–2**).

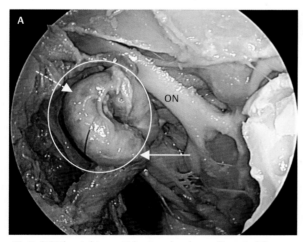

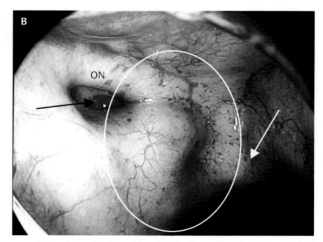

Figure 13–2 **(A)** The right carotid artery has been dissected from the surrounding bone. The *solid white arrow* indicates the beginning of the siphon where the vertical portion of the artery arches posteriorly and is then reflected anteriorly to form an anterior bend before exiting the cavernous sinus into the anterior cranial fossa behind the optic nerve (ON). The portion of this artery usually

seen in the lateral sphenoid wall is indicated by the *white oval*. The region of the carotid artery that would be directly adjacent to the pituitary gland is marked with the *solid white arrow*. **(B)** The anterior bend of the cavernous sinus is seen on the lateral nasal wall just below the optic nerve (ON). The optico-carotid recess is marked with a *black arrow* and the pituitary gland by the *white arrow*.

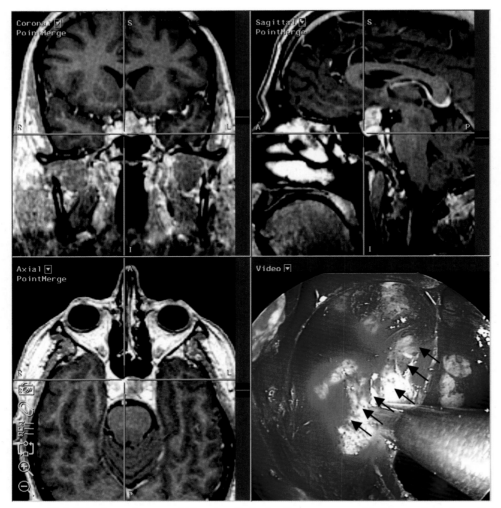

Figure 13–3 This picture from our CAS system illustrates the course of the internal carotid arteries in all three planes as they approach the midline bilaterally with a small window between them through which the pituitary tumor can be accessed. The *black arrows* indicate on the endoscopic image the medial extent of the right carotid artery. The septation on the anterior face of the pituitary is almost in the midline.

In some patients, the carotid may turn medially as it moves anteriorly after the siphon and in so doing cover the anterior face of the pituitary fossa limiting the access to the gland (**Fig. 13–3**). In such a patient, care needs to be exercised so that the carotid is not injured as the dura is opened for access to the pituitary tumor.

◆ SURGICAL TECHNIQUE

Macroadenomas

Patients are catheterized prior to surgery. This allows manipulation of fluid balance during surgery and allows the patient's postoperative urine output to be monitored. This is important in identifying and managing diabetes insipidus due to disturbance in antidiuretic hormone (ADH) regulation. This may result from the manipulation of the pituitary stalk (relatively common and usually transient) or from injury or dysfunction of the posterior pituitary gland during the procedure. Intravenous antibiotic prophylaxis is given—usually cephalosporin, gentamicin, and metronidazole. Standard preparation of the nose is performed with topical vasoconstriction and infiltration. Any significant septal deviation is dealt with via either a Killian or Freer (hemitransfixion) incision. Correction of any septal defect allows both nasal cavities to be used for access to the sphenoid during the surgery. If a significant septal deflection is not dealt with, significant trauma of that nasal cavity may occur. During surgery, instruments are often passed through the nasal cavity without endoscopic visualization. Difficulty in passing instruments in such a blinded manner can be due to septal deflection and may slow the surgery significantly.

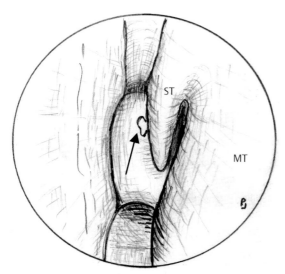

Figure 13–4 Endoscopic view of the left superior meatus and sphenoid ostium indicated with a *black arrow* and the superior turbinate (ST) and middle turbinate clearly visible.

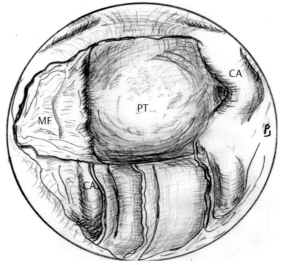

Figure 13–6 The bone of the anterior face of the pituitary fossa (PF) is widely removed. The mucosal flap (MF) has been laid aside and the bone of the pituitary fossa (PF) exposed from one cavernous sinus to the other.

The endoscope and microdebrider are passed medial to the middle turbinate, and the superior turbinate and often the sphenoid ostium are identified (**Fig. 13–4**).

The next step is to remove bilaterally the lower two-thirds of the superior turbinate and expose the natural ostium of the sphenoid sinus. A large sphenoidotomy and posterior ethmoidectomy are performed bilaterally as indicated by the shaded area in **Fig. 13–5**.

The posterior 1 cm of the septum is removed with the cutting burr and back-biting forceps and the sphenoid sinus septum visualized. The sphenoidotomy should allow passage of an instrument below the pituitary fossa and laterally onto the internal carotid artery and optic nerve eminences. The

floor of the sphenoid is lowered with a cutting burr attached to the microdebrider. A similar sphenoidotomy is performed on the other side (**Fig. 13–6**). The sphenoid sinus septum is removed flush with the pituitary fossa. If the anterior wall of the pituitary fossa is thick, the drill is used to thin this down until it is soft. Most patients with macroadenomas will have a soft anterior face of the pituitary as the pressure exerted by the expanding tumor thins the bone. However, patients who have a microadenoma may have thick bone forming the anterior face of the pituitary.

The key to endoscopic pituitary surgery is to have access to the pituitary fossa from both sides of the nose. This allows two surgeons to work off the video monitor at the same time.

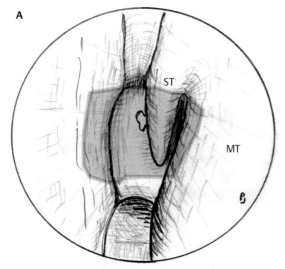

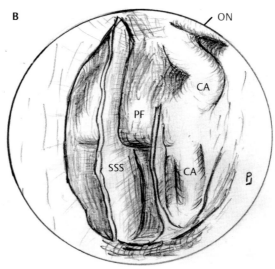

Figure 13–5 **(A)** The area to be resected, including the lower two-thirds of the superior turbinate (ST), posterior ethmoids, and large sphenoidotomy is shaded. **(B)** After resection, the carotid artery (CA), optic nerve (ON), pituitary fossa (PF), and sphenoid sinus septum (SSS) are seen.

Our team consists of a neurosurgeon (with endoscopic interest and skill) and a sinus surgeon. The roles of these surgeons are interchangeable with both surgeons able to perform all parts of the procedure. Having two surgeons allows an endoscope with camera attached and two instruments to be used at all times during the procedure. If significant bleeding occurs, a blood-free field can be maintained by one of the surgeons using a high-volume suction. The bone of the anterior face of the pituitary is fractured and removed with a Kerrison punch. Wide opening of the anterior face of the pituitary is achieved with bone removal from one cavernous sinus to the other. Care is taken with the superior bone removal as a fold of dura occurs below the optic nerves that is closely attached to the bone. If the Kerrison punch is not kept solidly in contact with the undersurface of the bone, this dural fold can be caught by the punch and a cerebrospinal fluid (CSF) leak can result.

The suction bipolar* (Medtronic Xomed) is used to cauterize the dura before a sickle knife or no. 11 scalpel blade on a no. 7 BP handle is used to create an inverted U-shaped incision into the dura (**Fig. 13–7**). We prefer the inverted U-shaped incision to the cruciate incision as the dural corners of the cruciate incision partially block the view into the sella during surgery. The inverted U-shaped incision allows an unobstructed view of the diaphragma and the lateral walls and lateral and superior recesses of the sella, where residual tumor may be missed if a clear view is not obtained.

In patients with a macroadenoma, tumor under pressure will often ooze through these dural incisions. A Deckers or Blakesley forceps is used to remove a sample of tumor for histology. Malleable suction ring curettes* (Medtronic ENT Skull Base Set) and standard pituitary ring curettes are used to first clear the tumor along the floor of the pituitary fossa until the posterior wall of the pituitary fossa is felt (**Fig. 13–8**).

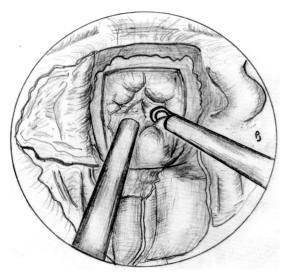

Figure 13–8 The first surgeon is using a suction ring curette to remove tumor from the lower half of the pituitary fossa while the second surgeon is holding the endoscope and a second suction to keep the surgical field clear or to retract the dura so that the first surgeon may obtain a better view of the lateral walls and diaphragma region.

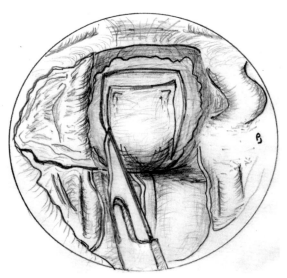

Figure 13–7 Inverted U-shaped incision performed with a no. 11 blade. This allows the dura to be flapped inferiorly and to be replaced at the end of the surgery as part of the repair of the anterior face of the pituitary.

Attention is then turned to tumor sited laterally on the cavernous sinuses. The ring curette is gently scraped along the cavernous sinus and the tumor removed using the suction on the ring curette. The curette can be felt rolling over the carotid artery. Finally, the tumor on the pituitary fossa diaphragma is removed. Care should be taken to visualize the diaphragma as it descends with the tumor removal. In patients who have a significant suprasellar tumor extension, a 30-degree endoscope can be used to visualize this suprasellar extension and to remove it under direct vision. This use of angled endoscopes is the great advantage of the endoscopic approach. It allows tumor that is traditionally not able to be visualized with the standard microscopic approach to be seen and removed under vision. In addition, the Malleable Skull Base Set* (Medtronic, Jacksonville, FL, USA) has malleable suction ring curettes that can be bent so that even a large suprasellar component can be reached from below. **Figure 13–9** shows a patient with a very large suprasellar extension. In this patient, 90% of the tumor was removed from below. Initially, we had thought that we were able to remove the entire tumor, but on postoperative MRI there remained a small piece of tumor in the region between the third and lateral ventricles. This residual tumor was removed about 6 months later through an interhemispheric approach. Intraoperative MRI may well have been able to detect this tumor fragment at the time of surgery, which may have avoided the need for a second operation.

The other significant advantage of the two-surgeon approach is the ability of one surgeon to hold the diaphragma up while the other surgeon removes tumor that may otherwise be left unresected in the angle between the diaphragma

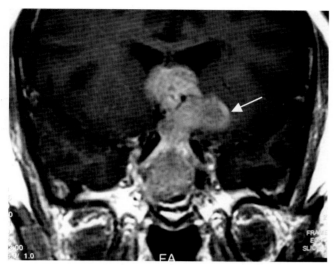

Figure 13–9 The large suprasellar extension is seen and the lateral extension of the tumor between the third and lateral ventricles marked by *arrows*. This is the area where residual tumor was seen on the follow-up MRI scan that then required a second transcranial operation for removal.

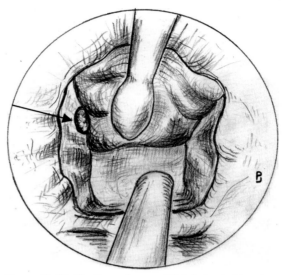

Figure 13–10 The Freer elevator (FE) is being held up by one surgeon while the second surgeon visualizes the residual tumor (RT) in the angle between the cavernous sinus and diaphragma and removes it.

and cavernous sinus (**Fig. 13–10**). In our experience, this is the most common area for residual tumor, and this area is not usually visible with the microscope as it sits above the level of the anterior bony opening made in the pituitary fossa. In addition, the diaphragma may obliterate this angle as it descends. Gently holding the diaphragma up with a Freer elevator helps to keep this angle open and allows the other surgeon to gently remove any residual tumor (**Fig. 13–10**).

To remove any microscopic or small pieces of tumor that may still be adherent to one of the walls of the sella, a small neuropattie is placed into the sella and wiped around the sella (**Fig. 13–11**). This also absorbs blood clots and allows

clear visualization of the diaphragma and lateral walls and floor of the sella. The 30-degree endoscope is usually placed within the sella cavity and rotated so that anterosuperior and anterolateral recesses can be clearly seen. In **Fig. 13–11B**, the white arrow indicates anterolateral residual tumor that was missed by a solely microscopic hypophysectomy for a growth hormone-secreting tumor. This residual tumor could be clearly seen with the angled endoscope and was removed, and the growth hormone levels have remained low to normal in the postoperative period. This case illustrates one of the most important advantages of the endoscopic approach to resection of both macro- and microadenomas.

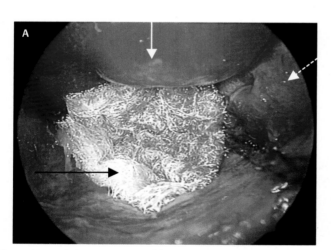

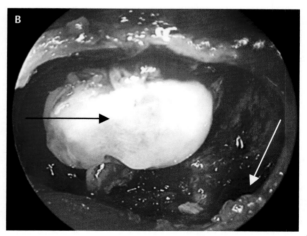

Figure 13–11 **(A)** A neuropattie (*black arrow*) is placed against the posterior wall of the sella. The diaphragma (*solid white arrow*), cavernous sinus (*broken white arrow*), and floor of the sella can all be clearly seen. **(B)** A hypophysectomy had been performed by a microscopic approach 3 weeks previously, and although the growth

hormone levels initially dropped, they rose to high levels in the third week. The patient underwent endoscopic exploration, and residual tumor was seen in the lateral anterior region (*white arrow*), and removal of this has resulted in a cure for the patient. The diaphragma can be clearly seen (*black arrow*).

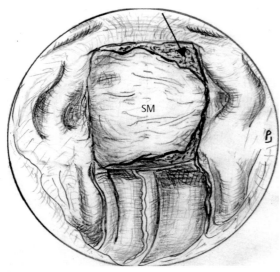

Figure 13–12 The inferiorly based dural flap is positioned over the Gelfoam paste and then the sphenoid mucosal (SM) flap is placed over the dura to cover the anterior face of the sella. Fibrin glue is applied.

Once the tumor has been completely removed, Gelfoam paste (Gelfoam powder mixed with saline to form a paste) is placed within the pituitary fossa. The preserved dural flap and sphenoid mucosa are positioned over the anterior face of the sella, and fibrin glue is applied to the surface (**Fig. 13–12**).

The middle turbinates are repositioned in their correct orientation and the operation is complete. No packing is placed within the sphenoid or the nasal cavity. If the patient has a CSF leak from the diaphragma, then the hole in the diaphragma is identified and a conically shaped fat graft is placed into the defect and gently pushed through the hole with the Malleable Probe* (Medtronic Skull Base Set) until the leak is completely sealed. This plug forms a dumbbell with some of the fat through the defect but with most of the fat still in the sella. The rest of the sella is filled with fat, and a fascia lata graft is placed over the fat with the edges of the graft tucked under the dura of the opening into the sella. The dura and sphenoid mucosa are placed over this facia and fibrin glue applied. This region is covered with Gelfoam, and the sphenoid sinus is packed with bismuth iodoform paraffin paste (BIPP)-impregnated ribbon gauze or antibiotic-soaked ribbon gauze. The gauze allows pressure to be placed on the fascia during the healing period. The ribbon gauze is trailed into the nasal cavity and is removed after 5 days in the outpatient department. No additional nasal packing is used. If the CSF leak was profuse, a lumbar drain is inserted postoperatively for 2 to 3 days to ensure the pressure is taken off the fat plug during healing.

Microadenomas

The image-guidance scan for these patients is a MRI scan. This helps with the intraoperative localization of the microadenoma and ensures that the correct portion of the gland is removed. Essentially the same approach is used for microadenomas as is used for macroadenomas up to the point where the dura is incised. After opening the dura, incisions are made over the region of the microadenoma. Using blunt dissection, this region of the gland is explored. Usually, the tumor is soft and a different consistency from the rest of the gland and in most cases can be dissected from the gland. However, some microadenomas are unable to be differentiated from normal gland, and the gland may need to be sliced in multiple places before the tumor is found. Care should be taken to avoid confusing the posterior pituitary gland with tumor as it is softer and often a paler color than the anterior pituitary gland.

◆ POSTOPERATIVE CARE

Patients are monitored in high dependency (or step-down unit) overnight with routine neurologic observations and hourly monitoring of urine output. If the urine output is greater than 250 mL per hour for more than 2 hours, an endocrinologist should be consulted and desmopressin may be given. Cortisol is usually not given in the perioperative period, but levels are monitored by the endocrinologists and augmentation prescribed if necessary. If the procedure was uncomplicated, the patient is mobilized the following day and discharged when the endocrinologists are satisfied with the patient's hormone status.

◆ RESULTS[10]

Thirty-two consecutive and unselected patients have undergone an entirely endoscopic resection of their pituitary tumors utilizing the technique described above. Of these patients, five were microadenomas. In the macroadenoma group there were six patients with extensive suprasellar and/or parasellar extensions. Postoperative imaging showed residual tumor in four patients with tumor located lateral to the carotid artery in three of these patients.[10] In the microadenoma group, all patients have normalized their hormone status. Six CSF leaks were seen during surgery and repaired. Two patients developed CSF leaks postoperatively, and one patient who had a very fibrous tumor developed a leak after revision surgery and required two returns to theater before closure of the leak was achieved. No other complications were seen. In the remaining 22 patients, complete removal of the macroadenoma was achieved and verified with postoperative MRI scanning.[10] Five patients have required continued treatment for diabetes insipidus, and eight have required ongoing hormonal replacement therapy. These results are compatible with the published results of most international centers.[11,12]

◆ KEY POINTS

The two major advantages of this technique are the minimal trauma involved in accessing the pituitary gland with bilateral sphenoidotomies and in some cases septoplasty being the only surgery necessary for the approach to the pituitary.

In addition, there is considerable advantage in the use of angled telescopes in the pituitary fossa during the resection of the tumor. This allows for tumor that may remain unseen with the traditional microscopic approaches to be resected under direct vision (**Fig. 13–11**). It also allows the descending diaphragma to be held up so that any residual tumor remaining in the angle between the diaphragma and the cavernous sinus can be visualized with a 30-degree angled telescope and removed under vision.

The technique does require two surgeons working together off the video monitor, and our team consists of a neurosurgeon and an otolaryngologist. Both surgeons have developed the skills to do all parts of the surgery, and this maintains the skill level and enthusiasm for the different aspects of the operation.

References

1. Otori N, Haruna S, Kamio M, Ohshi G, Moriyama H. Endoscopic transethmosphenoidal approach for pituitary tumors with image guidance. Am J Rhinol 2001;15:381–386
2. Sawers HA, Robb O, Walmsley D, Strachan F, Shaw J, Bevan J. An audit of the diagnostic usefulness of PRL and TSH responses to domperidone and high resolution magnetic resonance imaging of the pituitary in the evaluation of hyperprolactinaemia. Clin Endocrinol (Oxf) 1997;46:321–326
3. Wilson CB. A decade of pituitary microsurgery. The Herbert Olivecrona lecture. J Neurosurg 1984;61:814–833
4. De Divitiis E, Cappabianca P, Laws E. Microscopic and endoscopic transphenoidal surgery. Neurosurgery 2002;51:1527–1530
5. Thomas R, Monacci W, Mair E. Endoscopic image-guided transethmoid pituitary surgery. Otolaryngol Head Neck Surg 2002;127:409–416
6. Mason RB, Nieman L, Doppman J, Oldfield E. Selective excision of adenomas originating in or extending into the pituitary stalk with preservation of pituitary function. J Neurosurg 1997;87:343–351
7. Aust MR, McCaffrey T, Atkinson J. Transnasal endoscopic approach to the sella turcica. Am J Rhinol 1998;12:283–287
8. Shah S, Hal-El G. Diabetes insipidus after pituitary surgery: incidence after traditional versus endoscopic transphenoidal approaches. Am J Rhinol 2001;15:377–379
9. Cooke RS, Jones RA. Experience with the direct transnasal transphenoidal approach to the pituitary fossa. Br J Neurosurg 1994;8:193–196
10. Uren B, Vrodos N, Wormald PJ. Fully endoscopic transsphenoidal resection of pituitary tumors: technique and results. Am J Rhinol (submitted)
11. Cappabianca P, Cavallo LM, Colao A. Endoscopic endonasal transsphenoidal approach: outcome analysis of 100 consecutive procedures. Minim Invasive Neurosurg 2002;45:193–200
12. Kabil MS, Eby JB, Shanihan HK. Fully endoscopic endonasal vs. transseptal transsphenoidal pituitary surgery. Minim Invasive Neurosurg 2005;48:348–354

14

Endoscopic Orbital Decompression for Exophthalmos, Acute Orbital Hemorrhage, and Orbital Subperiosteal Abscess

Endoscopic orbital decompression plays an important role in the management of patients with Graves' orbitopathy, in patients with acute orbital hemorrhage with proptosis, and for the drainage of orbital subperiosteal abscesses.

◆ EXOPHTHALMOS IN GRAVES' DISEASE

Exophthalmos in Graves' disease is thought to result from the deposition of immune complexes in the extraocular muscles and fat, which in turn leads to edema and fibrosis.[1] The resultant increase in intraorbital pressure pushes the globe forward causing proptosis. If this proptosis becomes severe enough, the eyelids cannot close properly, and chemosis with or without exposure keratitis of the cornea may occur. In addition, the crowding of the orbital apex by the significantly enlarged extraocular muscles places pressure on the optic nerve. In a small minority of patients, stretching of the optic nerve by increasing proptosis may play a role in the development of optic neuropathy and visual loss. Visual loss is uncommon in Graves' disease, occurring in only 2% to 7% of patients.[2,3] If medical treatment (high-dose steroids with or without low-dose radiotherapy) fails, surgical decompression of the eye is indicated.[4] Whereas this has in the past been performed via external procedures, excellent reduction of proptosis is now possible with endoscopic techniques.[5,6] **Figure 14–1** shows the extraocular muscle enlargement commonly seen in patients with Graves' disease and visual loss.

Preoperative diplopia is seen in up to 30% of patients with Graves' disease. If **Fig. 14–1** is reviewed, it can be seen that the extensive muscle enlargement limits globe movement in the extremes of gaze, which in turn will cause diplopia. After decompression, significant medial and inferior prolapse of orbital tissue occurs, and diplopia can be seen in up to 30% of patients who did not have preoperative diplopia. Decompression of the lateral wall is thought to balance this intraorbital tissue displacement with resultant less likelihood

of postoperative diploplia.[7] Although orbital decompression results in significant reduction in proptosis, the patient's eyes may still have a staring appearance due to fibrosis and shortening of the levator palpebrae muscle. This results in increased scleral show, and although there may have been significant reduction of proptosis, the cosmetic appearance would still not be ideal. A release of the levator muscles can be performed, which can reduce or eliminate the scleral show.

◆ INTRAORBITAL HEMORRHAGE

Intraorbital hemorrhage is fortunately a rare occurrence and usually occurs during endoscopic sinus surgery (ESS) as a result of injury to the anterior ethmoidal artery. The damaged artery retracts into the orbit and continues to bleed within the orbital contents with increasing intraorbital pressure. This pressure results in progressive proptosis with stretching or compression of the optic nerve. This combined with impairment of arterial blood flow to the retina from increasing intraorbital pressure can result in progressive visual loss. Color vision is reduced before visual acuity is lost. If impending visual loss is suspected, the patient should be tested for loss of red color discrimination and tested for a relative afferent pupil defect. Color vision is tested by showing the patient a picture with red in it and asking the patient to name the colors in the picture. Once visual acuity is lost, the time before irreversible blindness occurs is variable but can be as short as 40 minutes if blood flow to the retina is lost. It is therefore important that if intraorbital hemorrhage occurs, the surgeon should immediately take appropriate steps to reduce intraorbital pressure and restore blood flow to the retina and optic nerve. Other than progressive proptosis, subconjuctival and periorbital hemorrhage may also be visible. If the proptosed globe is palpated, it is hard and resists direct pressure. If the optic fundus can be visualized, the retinal arterial circulation may be seen to be intermittent or pulsatile.

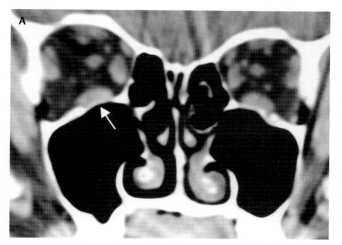
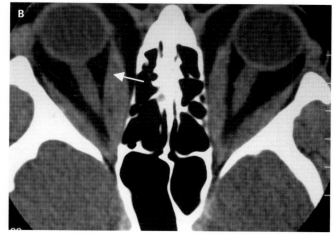

Figure 14–1 Extraocular muscle enlargement marked with *white arrow* in (**A**), a coronal soft-tissue CT scan, and in (**B**), an axial CT scan. Note the orbital apex crowding.

If an intraorbital hemorrhage is recognized intraoperatively and the patient is still on the operating table, an orbital decompression should be performed as described below. If the patient is in a recovery area or on the ward and significant proptosis and visual loss is noticed, then the following steps should be taken:

- Sit the patient up in bed
- Remove any nasal packing
- Infiltrate the lateral canthus with local anesthetic and perform a lateral canthotomy and cantholysis

These are important steps with which to buy time allowing the patient to be taken back to theater for reexploration and orbital decompression.

Surgical Technique of Lateral Canthotomy and Cantholysis

Local anesthetic (lidocaine 2% with 1:80,000 adrenaline) is placed in the lateral canthal region. A sharp scissors is used to make a horizontal incision through skin and soft tissue at the lateral junction of the eyelids onto the bone of the orbital rim (**Fig. 14–2**).

The eyelid is drawn outward with a forceps exposing the tendon attaching the inferior tarsal plate to the bone and the scissors are turned vertically and this tendon cut (**Fig. 14–3**).

Orbital fat should be seen as this tendon is cut, and the eyelid should be able to be laid on the cheek without tension

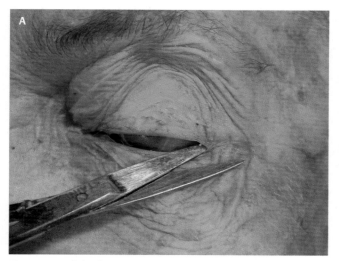
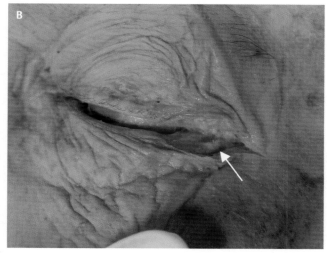

Figure 14–2 (**A**) A horizontal cut is demonstrated on a cadaver. The horizontal cut is made onto the orbital rim through the lateral canthus. (**B**) Pulling the eyelid down reveals the lateral canthal tendon (*white arrow*).

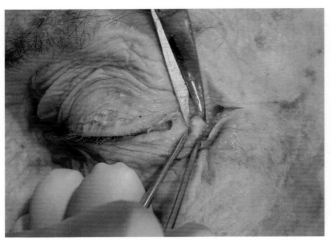

Figure 14–3 The lateral canthal tendon is held between the forceps with the scissors held vertically to cut the tendon.

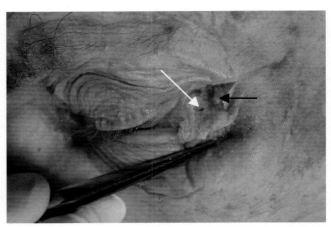

Figure 14–4 The eyelid is laid on the cheek. The cut lateral canthal tendon is marked with a *black arrow* and the orbital fat with a *white arrow*.

(**Fig. 14–4**). This reduces the intraorbital pressure and should allow reperfusion of the optic nerve and retina. However, it may be insufficient and is used only to buy time and allow the patient to return to theater for a formal decompression of the orbit.

No stitches are placed in this wound, and a dressing is placed over the wound. The wound and the lateral canthal tendon can be sutured after 24 to 48 hours. The lateral canthal tendon is sutured to the orbital periosteum. As the incision is in the crease formed by the eyelids, scarring is uncommon.

Surgical Technique for Endoscopic Orbital Decompression[5]

After standard preparation and infiltration of the nasal cavity and lateral nasal wall, an uncinectomy is performed.

The natural ostium of the maxillary sinus is identified and enlarged into the area of the posterior fontanelle with straight through-biting Blakesley forceps and the microdebrider.[5] It is essential to create the largest possible antrostomy as this gives access to the floor of the orbit and after the decompression prevents obstruction of the ostium if significant prolapse of fat occurs. If the antrostomy is small, blockage of the antrostomy and resultant sinusitis may develop.

An axillary flap is performed and the frontal recess cleared of cells with identification of the frontal ostium. A total sphenoethmoidectomy is performed with identification of the sphenoid sinus ostium.[5] This ostium is enlarged into the posterior ethmoids allowing entry into the sphenoid through the posterior ethmoids. The skull base is identified and cleared so that the entire lamina papyracea is viewable (**Fig. 14–5**).

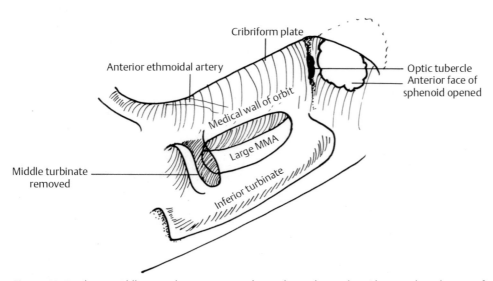

Cribriform plate

Anterior ethmoidal artery

Optic tubercle
Anterior face of
sphenoid opened

Medical wall of orbit

Large MMA

Middle turbinate removed

Inferior turbinate

Figure 14–5 A large middle meatal antrostomy and complete sphenoethmoidectomy have been performed. The middle turbinate is not shown.

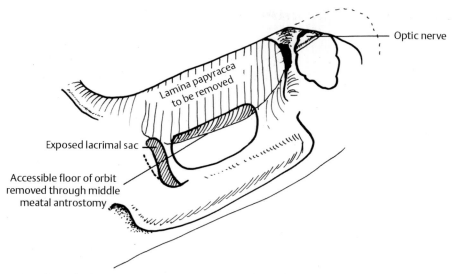

Optic nerve

Lamina papyracea to be removed

Exposed lacrimal sac

Accessible floor of orbit removed through middle meatal antrostomy

Figure 14–6 The lacrimal sac has been exposed as well as the frontal ostium, skull base, and sphenoid sinus. The bone 1 cm below the frontal ostium should be preserved to prevent prolapsed orbital fat obstructing the frontal sinus.

The hard bone of the frontal process of the maxilla is palpated with a Freer elevator and the soft lacrimal bone identified (in much the same way as is done for endoscopic dacryocystorhinostomy (DCR). This soft lacrimal bone may be left and the junction of the lacrimal bone and lamina papyracea identified. If there is doubt about the lacrimal bone, this may be flaked off and the lacrimal sac palpated to accurately identify the lacrimal sac. The blunt end of the Freer elevator is then gently pushed through the lamina papyracea and the thin bone forming the lamina papyracea flaked off.[5] Great care must be taken to preserve the orbital periosteum at this early stage as a tear of the orbital periosteum with prolapse of orbital fat can obscure the remaining lamina papyracea and make its removal more difficult. Care should also be taken not to remove the bony lamina papyracea for at least 1.5 cm below the frontal ostium. This bone is left in place to prevent prolapse of orbital fat obstructing the outflow tract of the frontal sinus. If chronic frontal sinusitis results after endoscopic orbital decompression, this can be difficult to treat. The remaining bone of the lamina papyracea is removed up to the skull base and posterior as far as the sphenoid sinus. After removal of the orbital periosteum, this is sufficient for orbital decompression for intraorbital hemorrhage or for a small reduction in proptosis cosmetic exophthalmos from Grave's disease (around 2 mm).[5-11] If a greater amount of decompression and globe retrogression is required, further decompression can be achieved by removal of the posterior half of the orbital floor.[5,11] The bone thickens at the transition from medial orbital wall to floor of the orbit. Angled curettes and Blakesley forceps are used to fracture this bone and remove it. The infraorbital nerve is identified as it runs along the floor of the orbit (roof of the maxillary sinus). The posterior floor of the orbit is removed up to the infraorbital nerve. Only the posterior half of the orbital floor can be accessed through the maxillary antrostomy. This is a technical problem as access to the anterior half of the orbital floor is usually not possible through the antrostomy with currently available instrumentation (**Fig. 14–6**).[5,11]

The average amount of globe retrogression with the removal of both the medial wall and floor of the orbit is 5 mm.[5-11] The orbital periosteum is either incised in a series of horizontal incisions or removed entirely. Retention of a medial strip of orbital periosteum may reduce the incidence of postoperative diplopia. If still greater regression of the globe is necessary, then the anterior part of the orbital floor and lateral orbital wall is approached through a subciliary incision. The conjunctiva is incised and further dissection identifies the lower-lid fat pads. The orbital rim is identified and orbital periosteum elevated. The remaining anterior floor of the orbit is removed both medial and lateral to the infraorbital nerve. This is done with Kerrison forward- and backward-biting punches. This dissection is continued onto the lateral orbital wall and the lateral orbital wall removed with a diamond drill. This lateral decompression balances to some extent the orbital fat prolapse and may result in less postoperative diplopia. It certainly increases the amount of orbital regression that can be achieved, and in our series this three-walled decompression averaged 5 to 7 mm.

Results of Orbital Decompression for Graves' Disease

The degree of regression of proptosis in the 16 orbits decompressed was 5.4 mm.[5] If only the medial wall and floor were operated on, the average globe regression was 5.75 mm. In four orbits, only the medial orbital wall was removed with an average globe regression of 1.75 mm. In six orbits, a three-wall decompression was performed with an average regression of the globe of 6.5 mm. These results are slightly different from those results we published recently as we have added three subsequent patients who underwent bilateral three-wall orbital decompression.[5] Of the 16 orbits done, one patient with complete long-standing visual loss had no improvement in vision. All other patients had normal vision preoperatively, and no patient had worsening of vision in the postoperative period.[5] Two patients who did not have preoperative diplopia developed postoperative diplopia. In both of these patients, their diplopia was transient, lasting between 1 and 3 months before fully resolving. Four patients had preoperative diplopia that continued postoperatively and required extraocular muscle surgery for correction.

◆ SUBPERIOSTEAL ABSCESS

Patients presenting with orbital complications of sinusitis commonly have a degree of cellulitis and edema (chemosis) around the eye with associated proptosis. There may also be some restriction of eye movement. Patients typically give a history of nasal obstruction, purulent rhinorrhea, and facial pressure or pain. Endoscopy reveals an inflamed and edematous nasal mucosa usually with the presence of pus in the middle meatus (**Fig. 14–7**).

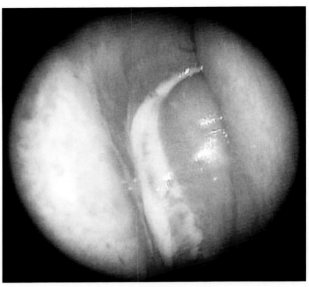

Figure 14–7 Pus can be seen in the middle meatus. The mucosa is edematous with obliteration of the space between the middle turbinate and lateral nasal wall.

Surgical Technique

If a subperiosteal abscess is suspected, a computed tomography (CT) scan of the sinuses with contrast will reveal the classic presentation of a mass located on the lamina papyracea or in relation to the floor of the frontal sinus. The rim of the mass will enhance with the contrast as seen in **Fig. 14–8**. In addition, the proptosis will be visible on the axial scans.

The surgeon should consider their endoscopy experience and skill level before deciding if a patient with a subperiosteal abscess should be managed endoscopically or through an external approach. The external approach is quick, easy, and the abscess can usually be rapidly and safely drained.

If the surgeon is skilled and experienced in ESS, endoscopic drainage of the subperiosteal abscess can be performed. The difficulty with this procedure is the significant vascularity that is associated with acute sinusitis. If a mucosal surface is touched with an instrument or endoscope, it will usually bleed, and if the surgeon is inexperienced, they may lose orientation and complications may occur. Frequent packing with decongestant-soaked neuropatties throughout the procedure helps to minimize the bleeding but will not control it entirely. In a patient with acute sinusitis, the anesthetist needs to optimize the patient's hemodynamic parameters to create the optimal surgical field (see Chapter 2). If the anesthetist is

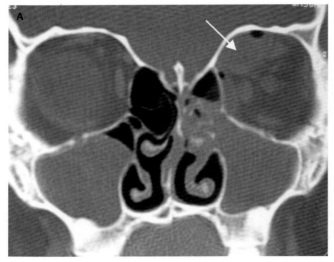

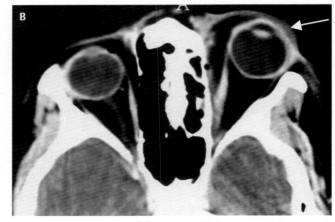

Figure 14–8 Coronal CT scans show (**A**) subperiosteal abscess (*white arrow*) associated with the roof of the orbit and (**B**) proptosis (*white arrow*) of left globe on the axial soft tissue.

inexperienced with creating optimal conditions for sinus surgery patients, as may be the case on an emergency operating surgery list, this may lead to more troublesome bleeding.

The surgical approach is to perform an uncinectomy and enlarge the maxillary ostium to a moderate degree. Uncinectomy alone without antrostomy carries the risk of postoperative closure of the maxillary sinus as the inflammation and edema predisposes to scarring and adhesion formation. Clearance of the frontal recess depends on whether the frontal sinus is thought to be the origin of the subperiosteal abscess. If the abscess is located adjacent to the ethmoidal sinuses (the most common location), then the frontal recess should be left alone and no surgery performed in this region. Clearance of the bulla ethmoidalis and posterior ethmoids is performed with identification of the lamina papyracea. The lamina papyracea over the subperiosteal abscess is widely exposed and removed. If the abscess is related to the floor of the frontal sinus, it can still be drained endoscopically. A mini-trephine is usually placed in the frontal sinus before dissection of the frontal recess. This aids in identification of the frontal sinus outflow track (the pathway along which the instruments will be passed to remove the cells of the frontal recess). The frontal recess is cleared and the frontal ostium identified. The lamina papyracea directly behind the lacrimal sac is removed, and using a curette the orbital periosteum (which is mobile) is kept intact and gently pushed laterally while the curette advances into the subperiosteal abscess. The abscess is drained.

A malleable suction Freer elevator or frontal sinus suction* (Medtronic ENT) is introduced into the cavity and any fibrin within the cavity removed. A narrow triangulated corrugated Penrose drain is slid into the abscess cavity and left in place. This ensures that pus does not reaccumulate in the abscess cavity. It is shortened the next day and removed the second day after surgery. Endoscopic drainage of subperiosteal abscesses remains highly effective but it must be emphasized that the surgeon should be experienced.

◆ KEY POINTS

Orbital decompression for exophthalmos from Graves' disease is an effective method for reduction of proptosis for cosmetic proptosis, eye complications from exposure of the cornea, and for visual loss. The amount of regression of proptosis is related to the number of walls decompressed at the time of surgery. Three-walled decompression may give a more balanced decompression with less likelihood of postoperative diplopia. However, this still has to be conclusively demonstrated.

Intraorbital hemorrhage should be managed with lateral canthotomy and cantholysis (if the patient has left the operating suite) followed by orbital decompression with removal of the medial orbital wall. Orbital decompression can be performed without canthotomy and cantholysis if the complication is noticed intraoperatively.

Endoscopic decompression of a subperiosteal abscess should only be performed by very experienced endoscopic sinus surgeons as the surgical field can be very bloody, and this can increase the degree of difficulty significantly and complications are more likely. If the surgeon is not experienced, then the abscess should be drained via an external incision.

References

1. Konishi J, Herman MM, Kriss JP. Binding of the thyroglobulin and thyroglobulin–antithyroglobulin immune complex to extraocular muscle membrane. Endocrinology 1974;95:434–466
2. Warren JD, Spector JG, Burde R. Long term follow-up and recent observations on 305 cases of orbital decompression for dysthyroid orbitopathy. Laryngoscope 1989;99:33–40
3. Garrity JA, Fatourechi V, Bergstralh EJ. Results of transantral orbital decompression in 428 patients with severe Graves' opthalmopathy. Am J Ophthalmol 1993;116:533–547
4. Asaria RHY, Koay B, Elston JS, Bates GEM. Endoscopic orbital decompression for thyroid eye disease. Eye 1998;12:990–995
5. Wee DT, Carney S, Wormald PJ. Endoscopic orbital decompression. J Laryngol Otol 2002;116:6–9
6. Lund VJ, Larkin G, Fells P, Adams G. Orbital decompression for thyroid eye disease: a comparison of external and endoscopic techniques. J Laryngol Otol 1997;111:1051–1055
7. Kennedy DW, Goodstein ML, Miller NR, Zinreich SJ. Endoscopic transnasal orbital decompression. Arch Otolaryngol Head Neck Surg 1990;116:275–282
8. Metson R, Dallow RL, Shore JW. Endoscopic orbital decompression. Laryngoscope 1994;104:950–957
9. Metson R, Shore JW, Gliklich RE, Dallow RL. Endoscopic orbital decompression under local anesthesia. Otolaryngol Head Neck Surg 1995;113:661–667
10. Neugebauer A, Nishino K, Neugebauer P, Konen W, Michel O. Effects of bilateral orbital decompression by an endoscopic endonasal approach in dysthyroid orbitopathy. Br J Ophthalmol 1996;80:58–62
11. Koay B, Bates G, Elston J. Endoscopic orbital decompression for dysthyroid eye disease. J Laryngol Otol 1997;111:946–949

15

Endoscopic Optic Nerve Decompression

The most common indication for endoscopic optic nerve decompression is traumatic optic neuropathy.[1] Currently, it is thought that ~5% of severe head injuries will have a concomitant injury to the optic nerve, optic tract, or optic cortex.[1-3] If the literature is reviewed, however, there are only a limited number of patients who have undergone this procedure.[4] Major brain injury occurs in 40% to 72% of patients with traumatic optic neuropathy,[5] and the management of this injury obviously takes precedence. This may result in the optic nerve injury only being diagnosed some time after the original injury. Some authors believe that early diagnosis and treatment of traumatic optic neuropathy may be of greater benefit to the patient[6,7] and advocate diagnosis of the optic nerve deficit by the presence of an absolute or relative afferent pupillary defect supported by disk edema and congestion of the vessels.[6] These findings, in combination with the computed tomography (CT) scan, possibly a magnetic resonance imaging (MRI) scan, and visual evoked potentials, may provide sufficient evidence to undertake optic nerve decompression.[6,7] However, the patient-management protocol suggested in this chapter is more conservative as there is still considerable debate about the value of both high-dose steroid treatment and surgical optic nerve decompression.[3-5,7] Currently, there are no properly conducted randomized controlled trials comparing high-dose steroid therapy, surgical decompression, and observation.[8] In a meta-analysis of all published cases in the literature, Cook et al concluded that treatment in the form of high-dose steroids or surgery or both was better than no treatment.[4] Tandon et al evaluated the role of steroids with and without surgery in a large study of 111 patients who were placed in two groups: one group of patients had high-dose steroids and if they failed to improve underwent an optic nerve decompression, whereas the second group had steroids alone.[1] This study showed that the patient group treated with steroids and surgery had significantly better outcome than the patient group treated with steroids alone.[1] Sofferman in a study on an animal model of traumatic optic neuropathy showed that injury to the optic nerve results in a progressive loss of myelin but with preservation of axons so that in theory the progression of the injury may be reversed with steroid or surgical decompression.[7]

Traumatic optic neuropathy is thought to result from two distinct injuries to the nerve. The primary injury results from either a direct contusive force on the optic canal and nerve, or as a result of elastic deformation of the sphenoid with a transfer of force into the intracanalicular optic nerve disrupting the axons and blood vessels.[5] This primary injury may result in compression of the nerve by bony fragments or in hemorrhage into the nerve sheath. If this injury is not treated, a secondary injury may occur. As the nerve swells in its dural sheath and bony canal, compression of the blood supply to the nerve occurs with resultant ischemia and continued axon loss.[5,7] Our department has adopted a conservative approach to traumatic neuropathy with all patients undergoing high-dose steroid treatment first before being offered surgical intervention. The exception is when bony fragments are seen to impinge on the optic nerve.

◆ MEDICAL TREATMENT FOR TRAUMATIC OPTIC NEUROPATHY

Currently megadose intravenous methylprednisolone is used following the spinal cord injury management protocol. Methylprednisolone 30 mg/kg intravenous loading dose is given followed by an infusion of 5.4 mg kg^{-1} h^{-1} thereafter.[4] The patient's visual acuity is monitored hourly, and surgical intervention is considered if the patient fulfills any of the criteria listed below:

- ◆ Fracture of optic canal on CT scan with vision less than 6/60.
- ◆ Fracture of the optic canal with vision >6/60 but the patient's vision deteriorates on steroids.

◆ Vision is less than 6/60 (or there is a deterioration of vision) after 48 hours of steroids with probable canal injury (indicated by the presence of fluid levels in the posterior ethmoids and sphenoid and/or the presence of fractures of the ethmoids, orbital apex, and sphenoid).

◆ SURGICAL TECHNIQUE FOR OPTIC NERVE DECOMPRESSION

The standard preparation of the nose is performed with decongestion and infiltration. An uncinectomy with exposure of the maxillary ostium is performed. An axillary flap is performed and the agger nasi cell removed. This improves access to the skull base. The fovea ethmoidalis is exposed in the region above the bulla ethmoidalis. If there is disruption of the cells of the frontal recess or reason to suggest that the frontal recess is obstructed, then this will be cleared, otherwise the cells in the frontal recess are left untouched. In some patients with severe sinus fractures, the entire skull base may be mobile. In the patient presented in **Fig. 15–1**, the entire posterior skull base was mobile.

In most patients, the posterior ethmoid cells will be full of blood, and when this is combined with mobility of the lamina papyracea and skull base, the surgeon can become disoriented. Therefore, this surgery should only be undertaken by very experienced endoscopic sinus surgeons. A posterior ethmoidectomy and sphenoidotomy should be performed as described in Chapter 8. In the posterior ethmoids, the posterior lamina papyracea and fovea ethmoidalis should be identified. If significant disruption of the posterior ethmoids and lamina papyracea has occurred, then a large middle meatal antrostomy provides an extra reference point and lessens the likelihood of surgeon disorientation. The natural ostium of the sphenoid sinus should be identified and the anterior face of the sphenoid widely opened. It is important for the surgeon to be fully aware of the anatomy of the lateral wall

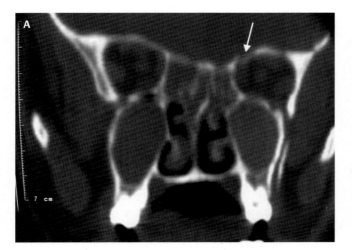
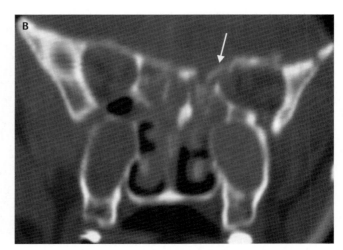
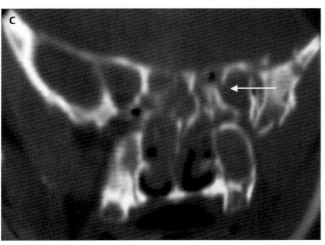
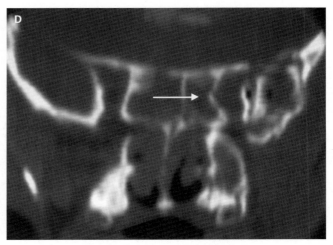

Figure 15–1 (A–D) Coronal sequential CT scans from (**A**) the posterior ethmoids to (**D**) the sphenoid sinus. The *white arrows* indicate fractures. Note the blood in the ethmoids and sphenoids.

In addition, the *white arrow* in (**B**) indicates the loose segment of skull base. The scans are of relatively poor quality due to patient movement from confusion from an associated head injury.

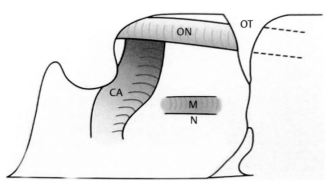

Figure 15–2 A diagram of the structures on the lateral wall of the sphenoid. The optic nerve (ON), internal carotid artery (CA), maxillary nerve (MN), and the optic tubercle (OT) can be seen.

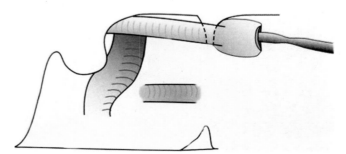

Figure 15–3 The Hajek Koeffler punch is used to widely open the anterior face of the sphenoid up to the skull base and laterally adjacent to the lamina papyracea.

of the sphenoid (**Fig. 15–2**). If available, the computer-aided surgery (CAS) navigation system may help in patients where there has been significant anatomic disruption.

The anterior face of the sphenoid needs to be taken as high as possible so that the roof of the sphenoid and the posterior ethmoids is continuous.[3,9,10] The sphenoid should be inspected and the optic nerve, carotid artery, and pituitary fossa identified.[9,10] If there has been significant disruption of the orbital apex or the lateral wall of the sphenoid, then identification of these basic structures can be difficult (**Fig. 15–3**). In these cases, image guidance may help.

The thick bone overlying the junction of the orbital apex and sphenoid sinus is known as the optic tubercle. This bone is normally too thick to flake off, and an irrigated diamond burr (the dacryocystorhinostomy (DCR) diamond burr with the 25-degree angle from Medtronic ENT) is used to thin this bone down until it is almost transparent (**Fig. 15–4**).[9,10]

A blunt Freer elevator is pushed through the lamina papyracea ~1.5 cm anterior to the junction of the posterior ethmoids air cell(s) and the sphenoid. Care should be taken to keep the orbital periosteum intact while this is done, otherwise prolapse of orbital fat can severely obstruct the dissection of the optic nerve. The bone of the posterior orbital apex is flaked off the underlying orbital periosteum (**Fig. 15–5**).[9,10]

Once the bone over the orbital apex is removed, the bone of the optic canal is approached. This bone is usually quite

thin and can, in a large proportion of patients, be simply flaked off the underlying nerve. In some cases, however, the bone over the nerve can be too thick and will need to be thinned with a diamond burr prior to removal. Once the bone is thin enough to be flaked off the underlying nerve, suitably designed instruments should be used. Any instrument that has a thick working end is unsuitable. If the back of the instrument indents the nerve as the edge of the instrument is used to engage the edge of the optic canal bone, it should not be used. Suitable instruments include the Beale elevator and the House curette both from the ear tray (**Fig. 15–6**).[9]

Once all the bone has been cleared off the optic canal and the underlying optic nerve sheath is clearly visible, the sheath should be incised.[9,10] The location of the ophthalmic artery should be kept in mind. The ophthalmic nerve artery usually runs in the posteroinferior quadrant of the nerve. In a small proportion of patients, however, this artery can migrate around the lower edge of the nerve and potentially into the surgical field[8]; though if the nerve is incised in the upper medial quadrant, the risk to this artery should be minimal.[9,11] A sharp sickle knife* (DCR mini-sickle knife [Medtronic ENT] is the most suitable) is used to incise the sheath of the optic nerve. Usually, the pressure from the swollen optic nerve will cause the sheath to split as it is incised. The underlying pressure will often cause the nerve

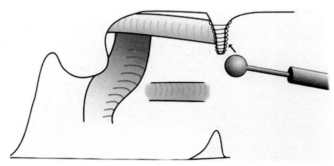

Figure 15–4 A curved irrigated diamond burr is used to thin down the optic tubercle until it is almost transparent.

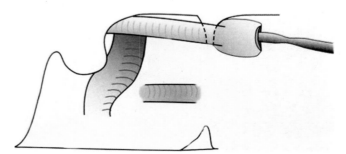

Figure 15–5 The blunt Freer elevator is used to flake off the bone 1.5 to 2 cm anterior to the optic tubercle. Care is taken to keep the orbital periosteum intact.

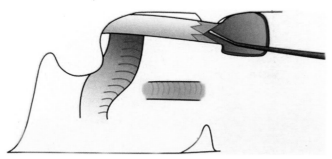

Figure 15–6 A Beale elevator is used to flake the bone off the optic nerve in the sphenoid.

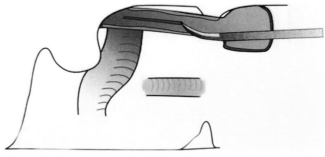

Figure 15–7 A sharp sickle knife is used to incise the sheath of the optic nerve in its superior medial quadrant.

to protrude through the incision (**Fig. 15–7**). This incision is continued onto the orbital periosteum of the posterior orbital apex with resultant protrusion of orbital fat. The orbital fat covering this area of the medial rectus muscle is thin, and care should be taken to avoid injuring this muscle. Potentially, such an incision can create a cerebrospinal fluid (CSF) leak but to date none has been seen after this incision. This may be due to the fact that the nerve has swollen and any potential CSF space has been obliterated. No packs are placed on the nerve or in the sinuses.

◆ RESULTS OF OPTIC NERVE DECOMPRESSION FOR TRAUMATIC OPTIC NEUROPATHY

Blunt Injury

Four patients presented with traumatic optic neuropathy after blunt trauma (usually a motor vehicle accident). Visible trauma to the frontal bone was seen with fractures

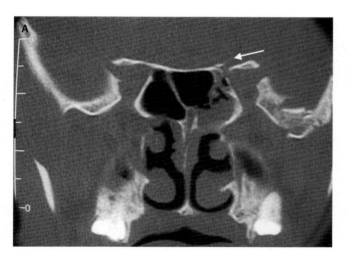

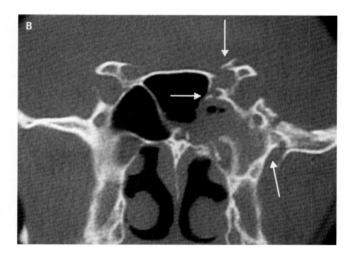

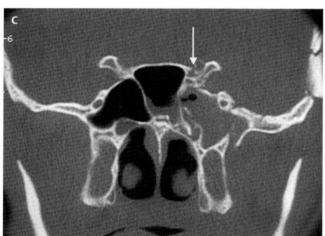

Figure 15–8 (A–C) Coronal sequential CT scans through the sphenoid sinus of one of the patients who presented with significant fractures through the optic nerve canal, around the carotid artery, and in the lateral aspects of the sphenoid (*white arrows*).

183

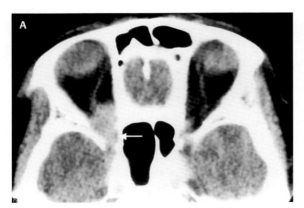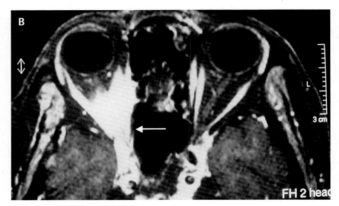

Figure 15–9 (**A**) CT scan and (**B**) MRI scan of the patient with a pseudotumor of the orbital apex.

involving the posterior ethmoids and sphenoid. Blood was seen in posterior ethmoids and sphenoid in all patients. Two patients had an obvious fracture through the bony optic canal (**Fig. 15–8**).

All patients were operated on after failed medical therapy (high-dose intravenous steroids) for the optic neuropathy, and all underwent surgery within 5 days of the original injury. Two patients with hematomas around the orbital apex (**Fig. 15–1**) improved from light perception preoperatively to 6/9 vision. The third patient improved from light perception to 6/60 vision, and the fourth patient improved from no light perception to 6/60 vision. Three of these patients were left with limited visual field defects.

Sharp Injury

Two patients suffered optic neuropathy after a penetrating knife-wound and both had no light perception after the initial injury. One patient underwent surgery 8 days after the injury and the second patient 12 days after the injury. Preoperative medical therapy was significantly delayed due to patients presenting to a rural hospital before referral to our hospital. Preoperative CT and MRI suggested the optic nerve was intact, and in one case an obvious injury to the optic canal was seen. At surgery in one patient, a bony fragment was seen to significantly indent the nerve. This was removed and the optic nerve decompressed and the sheath was slit, but the patient showed no postoperative improvement in vision. The other patient also showed no improvement after surgery. It is not known if the mechanism of injury after such a localized insult is different or whether the delayed presentation may have also contributed to the lack of improvement after surgery.

◆ PSEUDOTUMOR OF THE ORBITAL APEX AND TUMORS OF THE ORBITAL CANAL

Two patients presented with compressive lesions of the orbital apex or optic canal with progressive visual loss. One patient had a pseudotumor of the orbital apex that extended significantly into the bony optic nerve canal. This patient presented with progressive visual loss and underwent decompression of the posterior orbit and optic canal. Postoperatively she regained normal vision, which over a period of months slowly deteriorated. The surgery was revised and the annulus of Zinn was divided. This again improved her vision to 6/18 without further deterioration (**Fig. 15–9**).

The second patient presented with an 8-month progressive visual loss and at presentation could only see hand movements. He had a fairly extensive compressive lesion of his orbital apex and optic canal. After decompression, his vision remained stable but did not improve (**Fig. 15–10**). Patients with long-term visual loss may not respond as well as patients who present with more rapid visual loss due to optic nerve decompression.

◆ KEY POINTS

Optic nerve decompression is a highly complex procedure and should only be undertaken by endoscopic sinus surgeons with significant experience and skill. Potentially, injury to the skull base with a resultant CSF leak may occur, and an associated injury to the internal carotid artery may also be present (**Fig. 15–8**).[12] Injudicious manipulation of bony fragments may have catastrophic consequences for the patient. Patients should be given a trial of medical therapy before surgery is contemplated unless there is an obvious bony fragment impinging on the optic nerve.[4] Results from the small case series presented in this chapter and from larger studies in the literature[1–4,10] suggest that patients should be operated on if medical therapy fails to improve the vision within 24 to 48 hours. Significant delays again would seem to lessen the potential for success of the surgery.[5,7] Great care should be taken in exposing the optic nerve especially when flaking the bone from the nerve. Injudicious use of inappropriate instruments has the potential to worsen the vision, and this should be kept in mind during the procedure.[12] In the hands of an experienced endoscopic sinus surgeon, this procedure is a relatively safe operation with low morbidity and has the potential

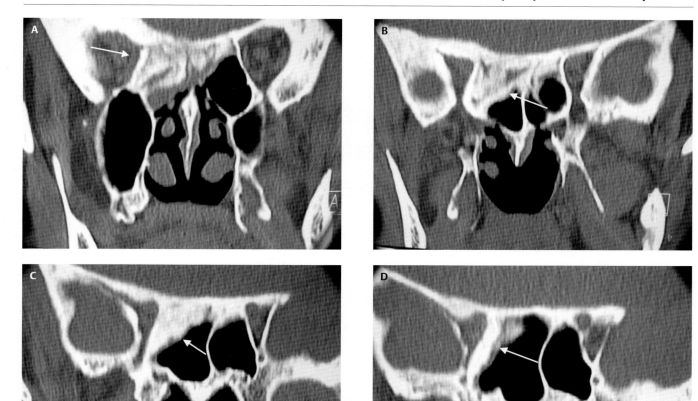

Figure 15–10 (A–D) Coronal sequential CT scans from (**A**) the posterior ethmoids to (**D**) the sphenoid sinus. The compressive lesion on the orbital apex and optic canal is indicated by the *white arrows*.

to improve and in some cases restore lost vision especially after blunt trauma.

References

1. Tandon DA, Thakar A, Mahapatra A, Ghosh P. Trans-ethmoid optic nerve decompression. Clin Otolaryngol Allied Sci 1994;19:98–104
2. Kountantakis SE, Maillard A, El-Harazi S, Longhini L, Urso R. Endoscopic optic nerve decompression for traumatic blindness. Otolaryngol Head Neck Surg 2000;123:34–37
3. Kuppersmith RB, Alford E, Patrinely J, Lee A, Parke R, Holds J. Combined transconjuctival/intranasal endoscopic approach to the optic canal in traumatic optic neuropathy. Laryngoscope 1997;107:311–315
4. Cook MW, Levin L, Joseph M, Pinczower E. Traumatic optic neuropathy. A meta-analysis. Arch Otolaryngol Head Neck Surg 1996;122:389–392
5. Steinsapir KD, Goldberg R. Traumatic optic neuropathy. Surv Ophthalmol 1994;38:487–518
6. Lubben B, Stoll W, Grenzebach U. Optic nerve decompression in the comatose and conscious patients after trauma. Laryngoscope 2001;111:320–328
7. Sofferman RA. The recovery potential of the optic nerve. Laryngoscope 1995;105:1–38
8. Steinsapir KD, Seiff S, Goldberg R. Traumatic optic neuropathy: where do we stand? Ophthal Plast Reconstr Surg 2002;18:232–234
9. Luxenberger W, Stammberger H, Jebeles J, Walch C. Endoscopic optic nerve decompression: the Graz experience. Laryngoscope 1998;108:873–882
10. Chow JM, Stankiewicz J. Powered instrumentation in orbital and optic nerve decompression. Otolaryngol Clin North Am 1997;30:467–476
11. Chou PI, Sadun A, Lee H. Vasculature and morpheometry of the optic canal and intracanalicular optic nerve. J Neuroophthalmol 1995;15:186–190
12. Metson R, Fletcher SD. Endoscopic orbital and optic nerve decompression. Otolaryngol Clin North Am 2006;39:551–561

16

Endoscopic Resection of Tumors Involving the Maxillary Sinus, Pterygopalatine Fossa, and Infratemporal Fossa

As endoscopic sinus surgery (ESS) has progressed over the past 10 years, new techniques have been introduced to aid with the resection of tumors in regions that have traditionally been difficult to access.[1] In general, the approaches described in this chapter are more suitable for benign tumors, but as techniques and adjuvant therapy develop, these techniques will be increasingly applied to the resection of malignant tumors.

To assess the endoscopic resectability of a tumor, both computed tomography (CT) and magnetic resonance imaging (MRI) scans are required.[2–4] Using both these modalities, the surgeon can determine if sinuses that are opacified on the CT scan contain retained secretions or tumor.[2,3] By being able to accurately define the extent of the tumor, resection can then be carefully planned. Endoscopic resection of the medial maxilla is useful to access the anterior posterior and lateral walls of the maxillary sinus.[3,5,6]

◆ SURGICAL TECHNIQUES FOR ACCESS TO THE MAXILLARY SINUS, PTERYGOPALATINE FOSSA, AND INFRATEMPORAL FOSSA

Canine Fossa Trephination for Access to the Maxillary Sinus

Tumors that involve the medial wall, anterior floor, or anterior or anterolateral wall of the maxillary sinus cannot be accessed through a maxillary antrostomy irrespective of how large this is made. It is necessary in these patients to provide an alternative route of access. Although this can be achieved through an inferior meatal puncture, placement of a 4-mm microdebrider blade through the inferior meatal antrostomy tends to destabilize the inferior turbinate as the blade is moved within the maxillary sinus. This is because the nasal vestibule provides a fulcrum around which the blade is rotated, causing significant dis-

ruption of the second fulcrum, which is the inferior meatal port. In addition, this route of access does not give access to the anterior and medial compartments of the maxillary sinus. The best port is provided by the canine fossa trephine, as described in Chapter 5. Because there is only a single fulcrum around which the blade rotates, good access is provided to the anteromedial, anterolateral, and floor of the sinus (**Fig. 16–1**).

Canine fossa trephination, however, is not suitable for tumors originating from or with extensive attachment to the anterior wall of the maxillary sinus as the trephine will be placed through tumor attachment.

Endoscopic Medial Maxillectomy for Access to the Anterior Wall of the Maxillary Sinus and Infratemporal Fossa[5,6]

The nasal cavity is prepared by placing cocaine- and adrenaline-soaked neuropatties in the nasal cavity. The lateral nasal wall and septum are infiltrated with 2% lidocaine and 1:80,000 adrenaline. A pterygopalatine fossa block is placed via the greater palatine canal using 2 mL of lidocaine and adrenaline (see Chapter 2). This helps to reduce bleeding during the dissection of the medial wall of the maxilla and the pterygopalatine fossa.

The first step in endoscopic medial maxillectomy is to remove the uncinate process and perform a large middle meatal antrostomy. The maxillary antrum is enlarged posteriorly up to the posterior wall of the maxillary sinus. This provides visualization of the medial orbital wall and allows removal of the residual medial maxilla without endangering the orbit. Most large tumors of the maxillary sinus and/or pterygopalatine fossa will involve the posterior ethmoids and sphenoid. In these patients, an axillary flap is performed and the frontal recess dissected with exposure of the frontal ostium. The bulla ethmoidalis is removed and a posterior ethmoidectomy and sphenoidotomy is performed. The skull base is clearly identified. Any tumor extension into the

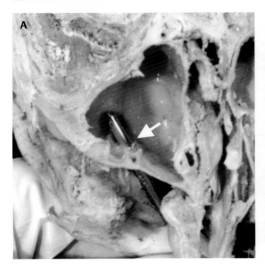
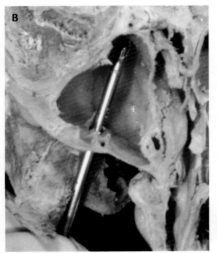
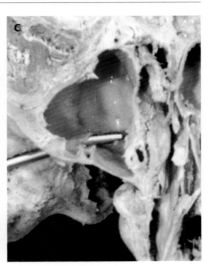

Figure 16–1 (A–C) An axially cut right maxillary sinus of a cadaver illustrating the access that can be achieved within the maxillary sinus (lateral, floor, and medial) through a canine fossa trephine.

The *white arrow* indicates the trephination port in the anterior face of the maxillary sinus

anterior and posterior ethmoids can be assessed, and if necessary biopsies or frozen sections of the mucosa from these regions can be sent for examination. This helps ensure complete tumor clearance.

To perform the medial maxillectomy, the inferior turbinate is medialized. A Tilley packing forceps is used to crush the turbinate just distal to the junction of the anterior end of the turbinate and the lateral nasal wall.[5] If there is a large intranasal component of a soft nonvascular tumor, the tumor is debulked (**Fig. 16–2**). If the tumor is very vascular or firm, then it can be pushed superiorly or partially debulked. Because of the posterior location of angiofibroma, debulking is usually not necessary.

Turbinectomy scissors are used to cut along the crushed region of the inferior turbinate up to the point where the turbinate inserts into the lateral nasal wall. A scalpel is used to make mucosal incisions from just below the orbit, through the cut inferior turbinate onto the floor of the nasal cavity.[5] This incision is continued along the floor of the nose to the posterior region of the inferior turbinate. Here the mucosal incision is turned vertically toward the posterior region of the maxillary sinus antrostomy. A sharp chisel is used to cut the bone under the mucosal incisions following the mucosal incision. The posterior vertical cut needs to enter the maxillary sinus adjacent to the posterior wall of the maxillary sinus and into the large antrostomy (**Fig. 16–3**).[5]

Once the bone forming the medial maxillary wall is mobilized, the nasolacrimal duct will tether the bone anteriorly and the duct will be visualized. The duct should be transected with a scalpel. At the end of the operation, the dacryocystorhinostomy (DCR) spear knife* (Medtronic ENT) is used to open the lower half of the sac creating anterior and posterior flaps, which are then rolled out.[5–7] This prevents postoperative stenosis of the sac.[5,6] The edges of the resected portion of the maxilla are trimmed with the

microdebrider. If a 70-degree telescope is used, the entire maxillary sinus should be able to be visualized.[5] This includes the anterior wall and floor of the maxillary sinus (**Fig. 16–4**). The tumor can now be removed from the maxillary sinus under direct visualization. If additional access is required and the tumor does not attach to the anterior

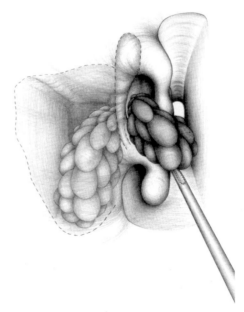

Figure 16–2 Inverting papilloma originating in the maxillary sinus is partially debulked with a microdebrider to establish the region of origin of the tumor. (From Wormald PJ, Ooi E, van Hasselt A, Nair S. Endoscopic removal of sinonasal inverted papilloma including endoscopic medial maxillectomy. Laryngoscope 2003;113:867–873. Reprinted with permission.)

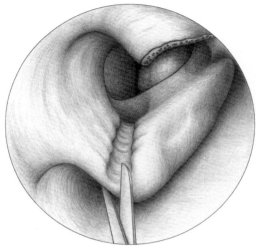

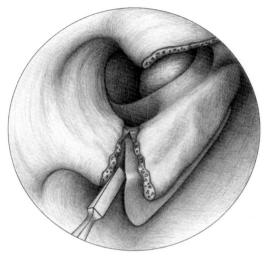

A

B

Figure 16–3 (**A**) The inferior turbinate is crushed and cut up to the insertion of the turbinate on the medial wall of the maxilla. (**B**) Mucosal incisions are followed by bony cuts made with an osteotome. (From Robinson S, Patel N, Wormald PJ. Endoscopic management of tumours within the infratemporal fossa: a 2-surgeon transnasal endoscopic approach. Laryngoscope 2005;115(10):1818–1822. Reprinted with permission.)

wall of the maxillary sinus, a canine fossa puncture can be performed. This allows instruments or an endoscope to be introduced through the anterior wall of the maxillary sinus, which can be useful to access areas within the sinus that may be otherwise difficult to access. Malleable suction dissectors* (both curette and Freer elevator) (Medtronic ENT) are also very useful as these instruments can be bent to the required angle for dissection in difficult areas such as the anterior wall or anterolateral region of the maxillary sinus.

If the anterior face of the maxillary sinus cannot be well seen or if better access to the anterior face is required for a tumor that attaches extensively to the anterior face of the maxillary sinus, further resection of the anteromedial wall and frontal process of the maxilla can be performed (**Fig. 16–5**). In such cases, a canine fossa trephine is not thought to be suitable due to the small risk of seeding the tumor into the soft tissues of the cheek. Although seeding is unlikely to occur, this risk is thought to be greater if the entry point into the maxillary sinus is through tumor rather than through normal mucosa.

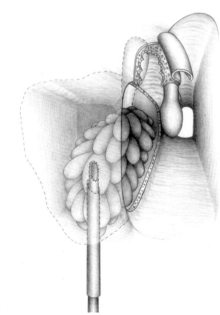

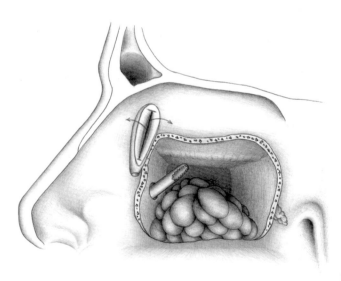

A

B

Figure 16–4 (**A**) View after endoscopic medial maxillectomy as viewed with a 0-degree endoscope. (**B**) The view of the maxillary sinus with a 70-degree endoscope. Note the microdebrider blade that has been placed through the canine fossa trephine. (From Wormald PJ, Ooi E, van Hasselt A, Nair S. Endoscopic removal of sinonasal inverted papilloma including endoscopic medial maxillectomy. Laryngoscope 2003;113:867–873. Reprinted with permission.)

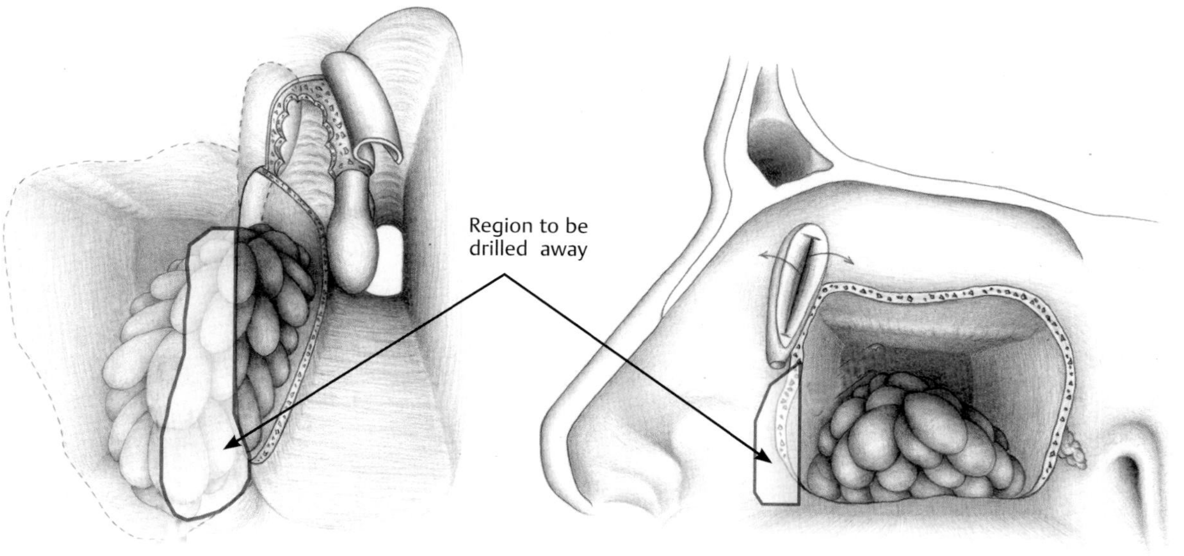

Figure 16–5 (A, B) Region of the frontal process of the maxilla that should be drilled away if direct access to the anterior wall of the maxillary sinus is needed. (From Wormald PJ, Ooi E, van

Hasselt A, Nair S. Endoscopic removal of sinonasal inverted papilloma including endoscopic medial maxillectomy. Laryngoscope 2003;113:867–873. Reprinted with permission.)

If access is still difficult and the anterior wall of the maxillary sinus is not fully accessible, a transseptal route provides a better angle of approach to this region. This access is achieved by performing a hemitransfixion incision in the opposite nasal vestibule and then removing a small horizontal area of cartilage and/or bone opposite the region of the anterior maxillary sinus. The instrument can then be passed through the hemitransfixion incision, through the cartilage window, and then through the horizontal mucosal incision in the opposite nasal cavity, giving greater access to the anterior wall of the maxillary sinus. This approach significantly improves the angle of approach and usually allows complete access to the entire anterior maxillary wall (**Fig. 16–6**). This region is best approached using either a 60-degree microdebrider blade or a 70-degree diamond burr (Medtronic ENT).

Access to the Pterygopalatine Fossa

Access to the pterygopalatine fossa is achieved by removing the posterior wall of the maxillary sinus. In most cases, a medial maxillectomy is unnecessary as most of the pterygopalatine fossa can be accessed through a large middle meatal antrostomy. If necessary, this antrostomy can be taken through the inferior turbinate to the floor of the nose by partial inferior turbinate resection. The mucosa from the posterior wall of the maxillary sinus is elevated and preserved (**Fig. 16–7A**). This exposes the bone, and removal of this bone is necessary to expose the pterygopalatine fossa. To remove this bone, it is necessary to expose the sphenopalatine artery (**Fig. 16–7B**) as described in Chapter 10. The artery is cauterized with suction bipolar forceps. A Hajek Koeffler punch or 45-degree through-biting Blakesley forceps is used to remove the bone anterior to the sphenopalatine artery

(**Fig. 16–7C**). The punch is introduced into the sphenopalatine foramen and the bone anterior to the foramen removed until the posterior wall of the maxillary sinus is reached. Further removal of this bone can be done with either with the punch or with a 45-degree through-biting Blakesley.

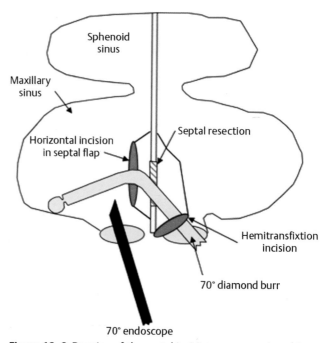

Figure 16–6 Drawing of the septal incisions necessary to achieve good access to the entire anterior wall of the maxillary sinus for tumors either originating from this region or with a significant anterior wall attachment.

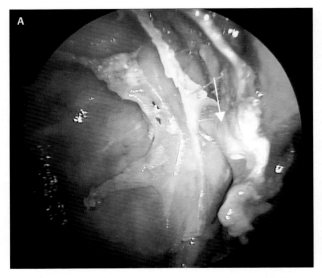

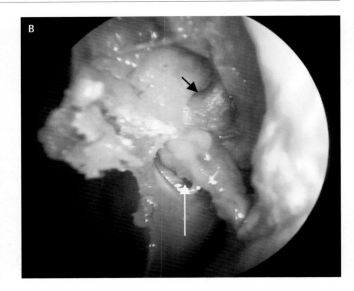

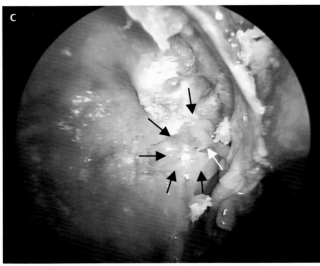

Figure 16–7 (**A**) The sphenopalatine artery is identified (*white arrow*). The maxillary sinus mucosa is still intact over the posterior wall of the sinus. (**B**) Further dissection posterior to the sphenopalatine artery shows the posterior nasal branch (*black arrow*) exiting the posterior aspect of the sphenopalatine foramen. (**C**) The bone directly anterior to the sphenopalatine artery (*white arrow*) has been removed. The bony edges are marked with *black arrows*. For complete exposure of the pterygopalatine and infratemporal fossae, this bone needs to be completely removed.

Bone is removed until the contents of the pterygopalatine fossa are exposed.

Access to the Infratemporal Fossa

To access the infratemporal fossa, all of the bone of the posterior and lateral wall of the maxillary sinus needs to be removed. Most of the bone can be removed through the same nostril as the tumor using either the Hajek Koeffler punch or through-biting Blakesley (**Fig. 16–8**). For complete access, the bone should be removed from the roof to the floor of the maxillary sinus.

Bone removal can continue until the anterior wall of the maxillary sinus is reached by inserting the punch or Blakesley forceps through the opposite nostril via a septal port. The septal port for the infratemporal fossa is very similar to that used to access the front wall of the maxillary sinus. This angle

of approach allows the instruments to be advanced up to the anterior maxillary sinus wall as described in **Fig. 16–6**.

◆ ENDOSCOPIC ANATOMY

Endoscopic Anatomy of the Greater Palatine Canal and the Pterygopalatine Fossa

The greater palatine canal and the pterygopalatine fossa are continuous (**Fig. 16–9**). The pterygopalatine fossa is similar to an inverted cone, and the bottom of this cone forms the greater palatine canal. The pterygopalatine fossa contains the distal branches of the maxillary artery, namely the sphenopalatine artery and the greater palatine artery. In addition, the Vidian nerve enters the posterior aspect of the fossa before moving laterally to end in the pterygopalatine ganglion suspended from the maxillary nerve. The pterygopalatine

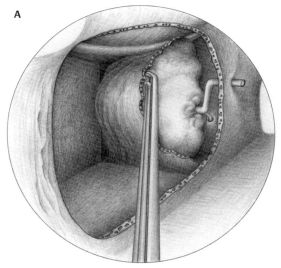

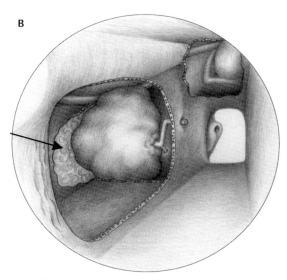

Figure 16–8 (**A**) In this drawing, the Hajek Koeffler punch is used to remove the posterior wall of the maxillary sinus through the same nasal cavity as the tumor. (**B**) The bone removal has continued onto the lateral wall of the maxillary sinus (*black arrow*).

(From Robinson S, Patel N, Wormald PJ. Endoscopic management of tumours within the infratemporal fossa: a 2-surgeon transnasal endoscopic approach. Laryngoscope 2005;115(10):1818–1822. Reprinted with permission.)

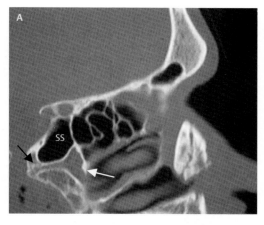

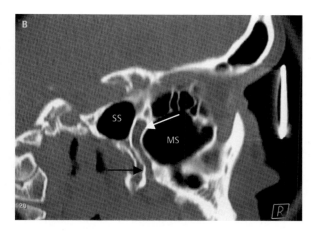

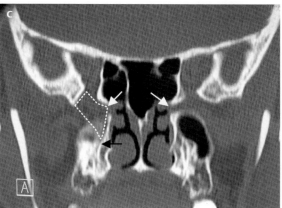

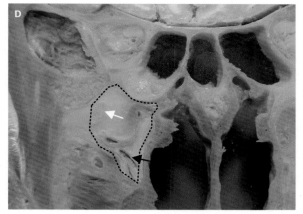

Figure 16–9 (**A**) Parasagittal CT scan showing the cone-shaped pterygopalatine fossa (*white arrow*). The Vidian canal can be seen entering the posterior wall of the pterygopalatine fossa (*black arrow*). (**B**) In this CT scan, the pterygopalatine fossa (*white arrow*) is seen to sit between the maxillary sinus (MS) and the sphenoid sinus (SS). The pterygopalatine fossa is continuous with the greater palatine canal (*black arrow*). Note it narrowing as it becomes the

pterygomaxillary fissure before it expands into the infratemporal fossa. (**C**) Coronal CT scan in which the cone-shaped fossa is outlined by a *broken white line,* and the sphenopalatine foramina are indicated with *white arrows.* (**D**) In this cadaver dissection, the fossa is outlined with a *black broken line.* The *white arrow* indicates the maxillary nerve in the infraorbital fissure and the *black arrow* the descending palatine artery.

fossa narrows gradually as it opens laterally into the region of the infraorbital fissure and then widens again as it becomes the infratemporal fossa (**Fig. 16–9**).

The roof of the pterygopalatine fossa is formed by the infraorbital fissure, foramen rotundum, and the maxillary nerve coursing from the foramen rotundum from medial to lateral across the roof of the fossa just below the orbital apex. The medial wall is formed by the palatine bone, sphenopalatine foramen, and sphenopalatine artery, the floor is formed by the greater palatine canal, and the lateral wall is formed by the pterygomaxillary fissure. In **Fig. 16–10**, the relationships between the foramina that enter the posterior wall of the pterygopalatine fossa, namely the palatovaginal canal, the Vidian canal, and the foramen rotundum, are demonstrated. In addition, the infraorbital fissure and pterygomaxillary fissure are seen. The sphenopalatine foramen is not seen, as the medial wall is not depicted.

If the anatomy of this region is viewed endoscopically and each layer removed so that the underlying layer can be appreciated, a good understanding of the anatomy can be achieved (**Fig. 16–11**). The first fact to be appreciated is that

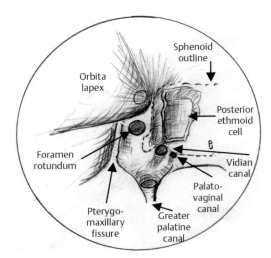

Figure 16–10 This drawing depicts the relationships of the structures entering the posterior region, roof, and floor of the right pterygopalatine fossa. The medial wall with the sphenopalatine foramen is not depicted.

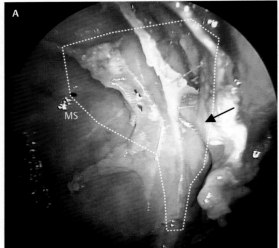

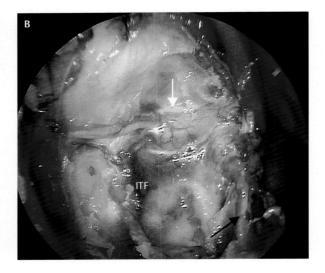

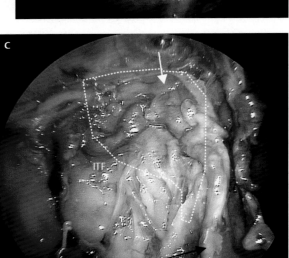

Figure 16–11 In (**A**), the mucosa overlying the posterior wall of the maxillary sinus is still intact. The *broken white line* outlines the dimension of the pterygopalatine fossa. In (**B**), the bone of the posterior wall of the maxillary sinus has been removed but the periosteum is still intact. However, in (**C**) the maxillary nerve (*white arrow*) and artery in the greater palatine canal (the descending palatine artery) (*black arrow*) can be clearly seen.

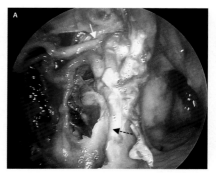
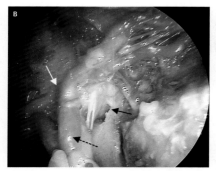
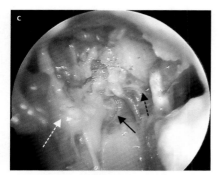

Figure 16–12 (**A**) An orientation picture demonstrating the maxillary nerve (*white arrow*) entering the foramen rotundum along the roof of the fossa. In (**B**), the maxillary nerve is seen posteriorly (*white arrow*) with the Vidian nerve seen exiting the Vidian canal (*solid black arrow*) passing forward and laterally into the fossa. The descending palatine artery is marked with a *broken black arrow*. (**C**) The sphenopalatine artery and postnasal artery have been removed to show the Vidian nerve forming the pterygopalatine ganglion (*broken white arrow*) in the fossa. The palatovaginal canal is marked with a *broken black arrow*.

the pterygopalatine fossa forms a relatively small part of the total area behind the posterior wall of the maxillary sinus. Second, the first structures to be encountered when entering the fossa are the blood vessels. The neural structures all lie deep to this plexus of arteries.

Further dissection in the roof to the fossa allows the maxillary nerve to be seen just below the orbit in the roof of the fossa. If this nerve is followed posteromedially, the foramen rotundum can be seen (**Fig. 16–12**). If we now remove the major blood vessels from the fossa, we can identify the Vidian nerve entering the fossa posteriorly. In **Fig. 16–12C**, the sphenopalatine artery and the postnasal artery have been removed to display the Vidian nerve

exiting the Vidian canal and forming the pterygopalatine ganglion.

Infraorbital Fissure

The other relationship that is important to understand is how the pterygopalatine fossa and infratemporal fossa relate to the infraorbital fissure. It is through this fissure that tumors can extend from the infratemporal fossa and pterygopalatine fossa up toward the orbital apex and then posteriorly toward the cavernous sinus and carotid artery. **Figure 16–13** shows the infraorbital fissure with the maxillary

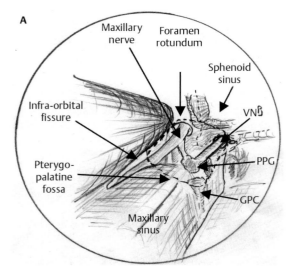
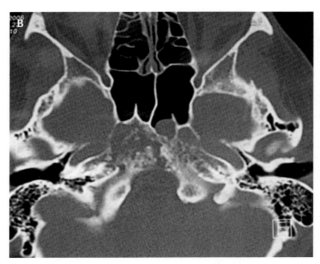

Figure 16–13 This drawing illustrates the important relationships between the right maxillary nerve and the infraorbital fissure and the pterygopalatine fossa as viewed from an anterosuperior aspect. The maxillary nerve exits the foramen rotundum and crosses the roof of the pterygopalatine fossa (*broken line* outlining the dimensions of the fossa) and occupies the gap created by the infraorbital fissure. Note that the medial aspect of the fissure connects to the pterygopalatine fossa, and the lateral (more anterior) part of the fissure connects to the infratemporal fossa. This relationship is important as it helps one to understand how tumors spread from one fossa to another and on occasions into orbital apex. OA, orbital apex; VN, Vidian nerve; PPG, pterygopalatine ganglion; GPC, greater palatine canal.

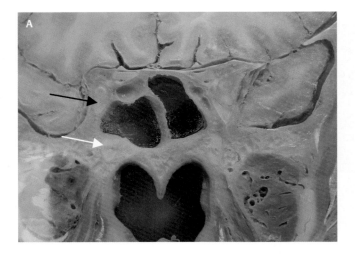
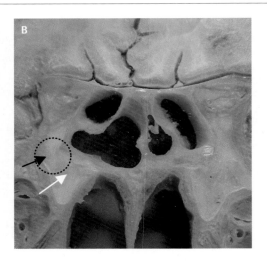
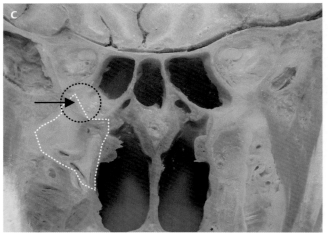
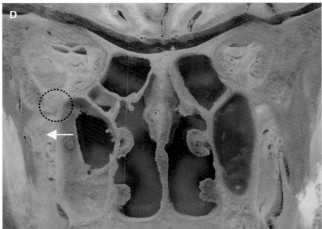

Figure 16–14 (**A**) The *solid black arrow* indicates the maxillary nerve as it exits the cavernous sinus in the lateral wall of the sphenoid. The *white arrow* indicates the Vidian nerve in the Vidian canal. (**B**) The *black arrow* again illustrates the infraorbital nerve and the *white arrow* the Vidian nerve, both now in the pterygopalatine fossa. (**B–D**) The infraorbital fissure is indicated

by the *dotted circle*. In (**C**), the pterygopalatine fossa is indicated by the *white dotted outline*. Note that in (**C**), the medial end of the infraorbital fissure is in the pterygopalatine fossa, and in (**D**) the lateral end of this fissure is in the roof of the infratemporal fossa (*white arrow*).

nerve running through it. Note how the medial part of the fissure communicates with the pterygopalatine fossa, and the lateral part of the fissure communicates with the infratemporal fossa.

As the orbital apex and sphenoid are approached, the inferior portion of the lamina papyracea thickens as it forms the medial wall of the infraorbital fissure. The lateral wall of the fissure is formed by the medial wall of the middle cranial fossa. **Figure 16–14** starts in the sphenoid, and as the cuts move anteriorly the foramen rotundum can be seen and then the pterygopalatine fossa. The maxillary nerve can consistently be seen in the infraorbital fissure, and it is around this structure that tumor can insinuate to reach the orbital apex and then expand into the space between the lateral sphenoid wall and middle cranial fossa. Significant expansion can occur so that the tumor may reach the cavernous sinus and even the carotid artery.

To understand how the medial aspect of the infraorbital fissure can be surgically accessed, **Fig. 16–15** demonstrates the anatomy as it would be seen if this region were to be approached endoscopically. Note that the posterior wall of the maxillary sinus has been removed and a complete sphenoethmoidectomy has been performed on the right side. The orbital apex (O), ethmoidal skull base (SB), sphenoid sinus, and the optic nerve (ON) can be seen. Note the lateral wall and floor of the sphenoid sinus are marked with white arrows. It is this corner formed by the floor and lateral walls of the sphenoid that needs to be drilled away to access the orbital apex lateral to the lateral wall of the sphenoid. In **Fig. 16–15B**, the space between the lateral wall of the sphenoid and the medial wall of the middle cranial fossa is outlined by a black dotted line. The broken black arrow indicates the direction that the tumor will take once it has occupied this space and expands the space and heads posteriorly toward the cavernous sinus and carotid

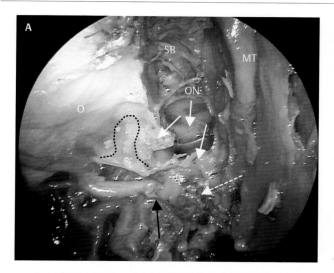

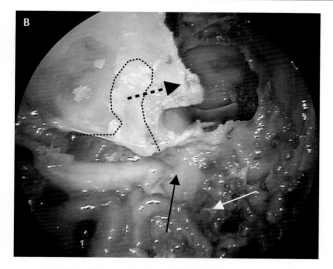

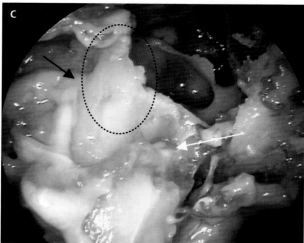

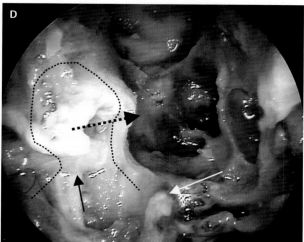

Figure 16–15 (**A**) Illustrates the right orbital apex (O), ethmoid skull base (SB), optic nerve (ON), middle turbinate (MT), maxillary nerve (*black arrow*), Vidian nerve (*broken white arrow*), and the floor and lateral wall of the sphenoid (*solid white arrows*). The entrance into the space between the lateral wall of the sphenoid and medial wall of the temporal lobe is outlined with a *dotted black line*. (**B**) A magnified view with the space above the infraorbital fissure outlined with a *dotted black line* and a *broken black arrow* indicating the direction of tumor extension

once tumor enters this space. In (**B–D**), the maxillary nerve and foramen rotundum are indicated with a *black arrow* and the Vidian nerve and canal by a *white arrow*. In (**C**), the area of bone to be removed to enter the space between the lateral wall of the sphenoid and medial temporal lobe is outlined with a *dotted black line*. In (**D**), the maxillary nerve is further exposed after removal of this bone and the space between the sphenoid and temporal walls seen. The direction of tumor spread within this space is indicated by the *broken black arrow*.

artery. To expose the maxillary nerve in the lateral wall of the sphenoid and thereby access this space between the middle cranial fossa and sphenoid, the bone of the lateral sphenoid wall and floor needs to be drilled away. This area of bone is indicated in **Fig. 16–15C** by the dotted oval. Once this bone has been removed, the space between the lateral sphenoid wall and medial wall of the temporal lobe becomes more easily visible (outlined by the black dotted line in **Fig. 16–15D**).

Region of the Middle Cranial Fossa

To access the region of the middle cranial fossa and foramen ovale, further removal of the lateral wall of the sphe-

noid is necessary. To achieve this, both the Vidian nerve in the floor of the sphenoid sinus and the maxillary nerve in the lateral wall of the sphenoid are exposed and the bone around these nerves removed with a diamond burr. The Vidian canal leads directly to the second genu of the internal carotid artery as it turns vertically and runs up the lateral wall of the sphenoid toward the pituitary fossa. In **Fig. 16–16A**, the line drawing illustrates the relationship between the Vidian canal and the maxillary nerve as the bone is removed between these structures. This bone removal exposes the space between the middle cranial fossa plate and the lateral wall of the sphenoid both below and above the maxillary nerve. The space above the maxillary nerve is just below the orbital apex, and tumors expanding

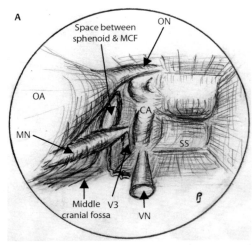

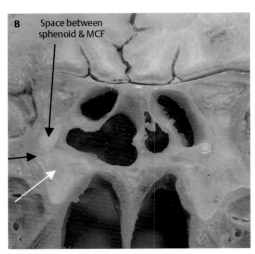

Figure 16–16 (A, B) The relationship between the orbital apex (OA), optic nerve (ON), middle cranial fossa (MCF), maxillary nerve (MN), and the space that is present between these structures is demonstrated. As one moves posteriorly within this space, the cavernous sinus and mandibular nerve (V3) are approached. In

addition, the relationship between the Vidian nerve (VN) and the carotid artery (CA) in the sphenoid sinus (SS) floor is demonstrated. In (**B**), the space between the middle cranial fossa and the lateral wall of the sphenoid is seen. The *black arrow* indicates the maxillary nerve (V2) and the *white arrow* the Vidian nerve.

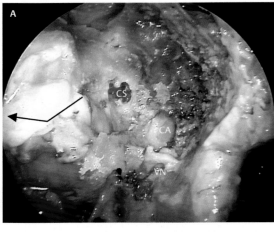

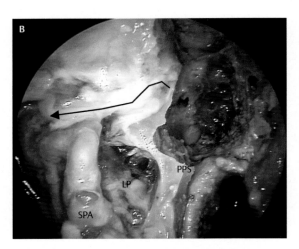

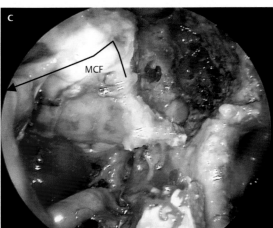

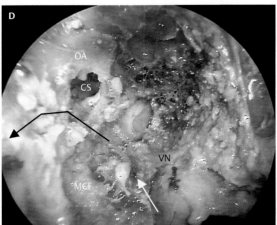

Figure 16–17 In (**A**), the bone below and lateral to the Vidian nerve (VN) is removed. The maxillary nerve running in the lateral wall of the sphenoid is exposed (*black arrow*). The cavernous sinus (CS) and carotid artery (CA) have also been exposed. Note how the Vidian nerve approaches the carotid artery in an anteroposterior direction. In (**B**), the endoscope has been drawn back to give a less magnified view. The maxillary nerve running through the pterygopalatine fossa is indicated with the *black arrow*. The superior

head of the lateral pterygoid (LP) is pushed inferiorly exposing the space between the middle cranial fossa and the lateral wall of the sphenoid. The pterygoid process of the sphenoid (PPS) that separates this space from the nasal cavity is seen. (**C, D**) Further removal of this bone exposes the middle cranial fossa (MCF). As the posterior wall of the sphenoid is approached, the foramen ovale (*white arrow*) is seen with the mandibular branch of the trigeminal nerve exiting the foramen.

into this region will cause compression of the orbital apex. The relationship of the orbital apex, lateral wall of the sphenoid, and medial wall of the middle cranial fossa is demonstrated in **Fig. 16–16B**.

To further illustrate this series of complex anatomic relationships, the following dissections have been done to illustrate how the progressive removal of the bone of the inferior and lateral wall of the sphenoid will expose the space between the lateral wall of the sphenoid and the middle cranial fossa (**Fig. 16–17**). It is important to understand that as this space progresses posteriorly, the cavernous sinus and then the carotid artery are encountered. As removal of the floor of the sphenoid continues laterally, the pterygoid process of the sphenoid is removed up to the maxillary nerve. This exposes the upper head of the lateral pterygoid muscle, which lies up against the middle cranial fossa. As the bone removal continues posteriorly, the foramen ovale and the mandibular branch of the trigeminal nerve are seen, which are lateral and anterior to the carotid artery. The Vidian nerve is medial and marks the position of the carotid at the junction of the floor and posterior wall of the sphenoid. Directly above the foramen ovale in the lateral wall is the cavernous sinus (CS), and above the cavernous sinus is the orbital apex (OA). The relationship between the medial pterygoid muscle, pterygoid process of the sphenoid, space between the lateral sphenoid wall and middle cranial fossa, maxillary and mandibular branches of the trigeminal nerve, Vidian nerve and carotid artery are demonstrated in **Fig. 16–17**.

The final dissection of the lateral wall of the sphenoid exposes the cavernous sinus anterior to the carotid artery. If the remaining bone of the lateral wall of the sphenoid is removed, the cavernous sinus and mandibular branch of the trigeminal nerve (V3) will be exposed above the foramen ovale (white arrow in **Fig. 16–18A**). Further bone removal laterally will remove the bone overlying the medial middle temporal fossa and expose the underlying dura as

seen in **Fig. 16–18B** (white arrow). Although dura covers the cavernous sinus as it is approached from the sphenoid sinus, this covering is very thin and tenuous with multiple small veins joining or leaving the cavernous sinus so that such a dissection can be quite bloody and the bleeding difficult to control. The relationship of the Vidian nerve (VN), carotid artery (CA), cavernous sinus (CS), V2, V3, foramen ovale, and middle cranial fossa (MCF) can be appreciated in **Fig. 16–18**.

Infratemporal Fossa

Once the bone overlying the posterior wall of the maxillary sinus has been removed, the pterygopalatine fossa and infratemporal fossa are seen (**Fig. 16–19**). The maxillary nerve (MN) can be seen at the junction of the infratemporal fossa and orbit. These fossae are covered by periosteum and the contents are exposed by removing the periosteum. Both fossae contain fat, blood vessels, and nerves. The fat and blood vessels usually lie antermedial to the neural structures. Once the fat has been removed, the underlying maxillary artery and muscles of the infratemporal fossa can be seen. The two heads of the lateral pterygoid muscle (LTM) can be seen originating directly behind the greater palatine canal with the maxillary artery (broken black arrow) entering the infratemporal fossa between the two heads of the lateral pterygoid muscle. As one moves further laterally, the temporalis muscle (TM) and the deep portion of the masseter muscle (MM) come into view (**Fig. 16–19C**). Inferior to the masseter is the gingivobuccal sulcus filled with fat (white arrow). Behind the masseter lies the ramus of the mandible, which forms the lateral border of the infratemporal fossa.

It is important to understand the muscles of the infratemporal fossa as they form the boundaries of the fossa, and when tumors expand the fossa, they will push these

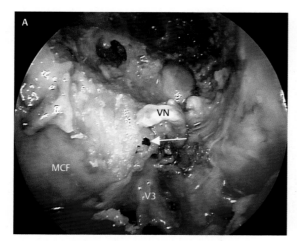 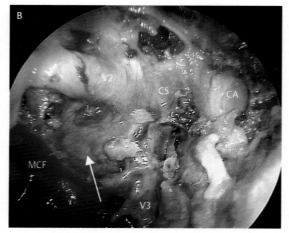

Figure 16–18 In (**A**), the foramen ovale (*white arrow*) and the mandibular branch of the trigeminal nerve (V3) are seen anterior and lateral to the Vidian nerve (VN). In (**B**), the residual bone of

the lateral sphenoid wall has been removed and the middle cranial fossa (MCF) dura exposed (*white arrow*). The dura overlying the cavernous sinus (CS) has been exposed.

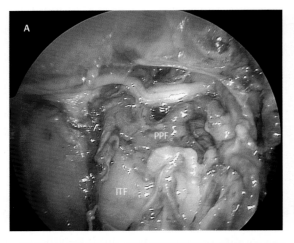

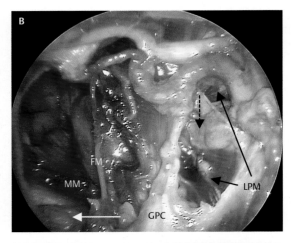

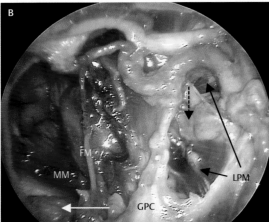

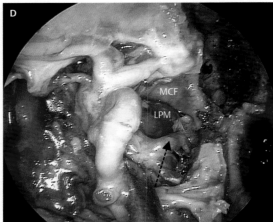

Figure 16–19 In (**A**), the pterygopalatine (PPF) and infratemporal (ITF) fossae can be seen. In (**B, C**), the fat has been removed exposing the greater palatine canal (GPC) and descending palatine artery, the maxillary nerve (MN), the two heads of the lateral pterygoid muscle (LPM), temporalis muscle (TM), and masseter muscle (MM). The maxillary artery is indicated by the *broken black*

arrow and the gingivobuccal fat pad by the *white arrow*. In (**D**), the maxillary artery (*black arrow*) has been pulled laterally exposing the upper head of the lateral pterygoid muscle (LPM), which has also been pulled down to expose the middle cranial fossa (MCP). The maxillary artery (*black arrow*) enters the pterygopalatine fossa between the two heads of the lateral pterygoid muscle.

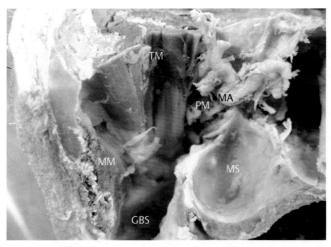

Figure 16–20 The muscles of the infratemporal fossa, the temporalis muscle (TM), masseter muscle (MM), and lateral pterygoid muscle (PM) can be seen. The maxillary sinus (MS) and maxillary artery (MA) form the medial limits of the infratemporal fossa.

muscles away. In **Fig. 16–20**, the more anterolateral muscles, the temporalis and masseter muscles, are clearly seen. Behind the maxillary artery and descending palatine artery, the pterygoid muscles can just be made out. The potential space of the gingivobuccal sulcus can also be clearly seen in this dissection.

◆ TUMORS INVOLVING THE MAXILLARY SINUS, PTERYGOPALATINE, AND INFRATEMPORAL FOSSAE

Antrochoanal Polyps

Antrochoanal polyps commonly form from the posterior wall of the maxillary sinus. These tumors need to have the site of origin resected to prevent recurrence. The first step is to perform a large middle meatal antrostomy and to expose the site of origin of the tumor. If the entire site can be easily accessed through the middle meatal antrostomy, then the tumor and the site of origin are resected with a margin of normal mucosa. If the site of origin is not easily accessible through a middle meatal antrostomy, a canine fossa trephination should be performed and the microdebrider or Freer elevator placed through the trephine site and the origin of the polyp resected with the margin of normal tissue.

Inverting Papillomas

The other very common benign tumor involving the maxillary sinus is inverting papilloma (IP). Small IP tumors of the maxillary sinus that do not arise from the anterior wall of the maxillary sinus can be resected by creating a large middle meatal antrostomy and a canine fossa trephine (described in Chapter 5). The endoscope can be placed into the maxillary antrostomy while the dissecting instrument is placed through the canine fossa puncture. This can be reversed with the endoscope being placed through the canine fossa puncture and instrument through the maxillary antrostomy. Using this technique, almost the entire maxillary sinus can be accessed. The only area where access may not be adequate

is the anterior face of the maxillary sinus. Tumors located on the anterior face may need to undergo endoscopic medial maxillectomy for complete resection. All other small or localized tumors can be resected using this two-site approach.

Endoscopic Resection of Large or Anterior Wall Maxillary Sinus Tumors

If a tumor cannot be accessed with the canine fossa trephination or it originates from a large area or from the anterior wall of the maxillary sinus, endoscopic medial maxillectomy should be performed. If additional access is required, the frontal process of the maxilla can be drilled away. This can be combined with a transseptal access to improve the angulation to the anterior wall as described earlier in this chapter. All walls of the maxillary sinus should be able to be accessed, and the tumor and underlying mucosa should be removed. In **Fig. 16–21**, the patient has a large inverting papilloma extending laterally beyond the limits of the maxillary sinus.

This inverting papilloma was based on the inferior turbinate. Resection of the medial maxilla removed a large part of the tumor origin. In addition, the tumor took origin from the adjacent floor and posterior wall of the maxillary sinus. This could

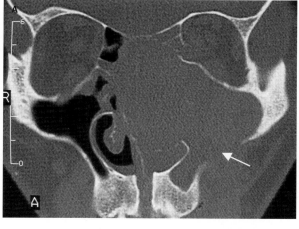
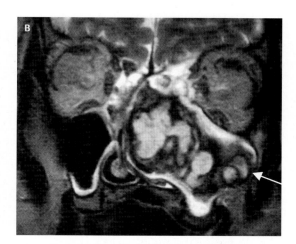
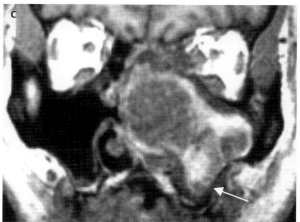
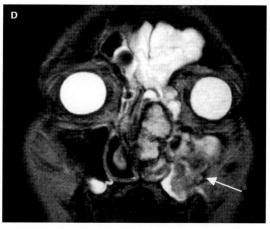

Figure 16–21 A large inverting papilloma eroding the lateral wall of the maxillary sinus (*white arrow*). (**A**) The CT and the MRI (T2 weighting in [**B, D**] and T1 in [**C**]) show the tumor's extent.

MRI (scan [**D**], T2 weighting) shows an obstructed frontal sinus with mucus lighting up in the frontal sinus.

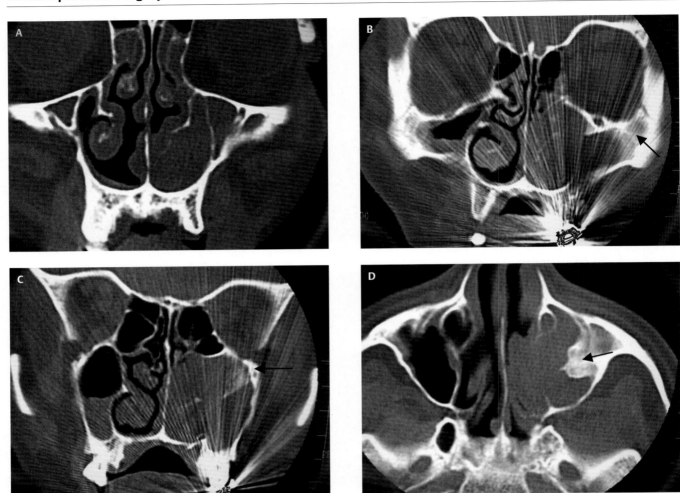

Figure 16–22 (A–D) Inverting papilloma originating around the neo-osteogenesis seen on the lateral wall of the maxillary sinus (*black arrow*).

be easily accessed after endoscopic medial maxillectomy. The bone in the region of origin of the tumor was able to be drilled with a diamond burr to ensure no tumor had infiltrated into crevices within the floor of the maxillary sinus.

The following patient presented with an inverting papilloma that took origin around a region of new bone formation on the lateral and anterior wall of the maxillary sinus. This anterior and lateral area was able to be accessed (after an endoscopic medial maxillectomy) with a 70-degree diamond burr and the origin of the tumor completely cleared with drilling of the underlying bone (**Fig. 16–22**). It is common for inverting papilloma to originate from a region of new bone formation, and therefore it is important to drill away this new bone as mucosa may invaginate into the new bone, and failure to remove this may result in tumor recurrence.[8]

Results of the Endoscopic Resection

Patients with inverting papilloma were classified according to the classification of Krouse[4] presented in **Table 16–1**. The published series of patients who have undergone endoscopic resection of inverting papillomas, including those

patients with large and extensive lesions that have had an endoscopic medial maxillectomy as part of the tumor resection, are presented in **Table 16–2**. As can be seen from these results and from recent publications by Krouse[9] and a review article by Melroy and Senior,[10] the results obtained by endoscopic removal of inverting papillomas are better than those achieved in the past using an open approach.

Table 16–1 Krouse Staging System for Inverted Papilloma

Stage	Extent of Tumor
I	Tumor confined to nasal cavity. No malignancy.
II	Tumor involving the ostiomeatal complex and ethmoids and/or medial wall of maxillary sinus. No malignancy.
III	Tumor involving the inferior, superior, lateral, or anterior wall of maxillary sinus, sphenoid, and/or frontal sinus. No malignancy,
IV	All extranasal/extrasinus tumors. All tumors associated with malignancy.

Source: Data from Krouse JH. Development of a staging system for inverted papilloma. Laryngoscope 2000;110:965–968.

Table 16–2 Presentation, Origin, Stage, Procedure, and Outcome for Endoscopic Removal of Inverting Papilloma Including Patients Who Underwent Medial Maxillectomy for Removal of the Inverting Papilloma

Case No.	Age and Sex	Symptoms	Origin	Stage	Endoscopic Procedure	Current Status and Follow-up
1. †	51 M	Left nasal obstruction, rhinorrhea	Left maxillary antrum, lamina papyracea, sphenoid sinus	IV	Medial axillectomy, canine fossa puncture, ethmoidectomy, sphenoidotomy, and clearance of the frontal recess	Had recurrence of tumor after 4 months in left infratemporal fossa —surgically cleared and now disease free after 3 years
2.	54 M	Left nasal obstruction, epistaxis	Left maxillary sinus and inferior turbinate	II	Medial maxillectomy, canine fossa puncture, and DCR	Disease free
3.	71 M	Right nasal obstruction, rhinorrhea	Right uncinate process	II	Middle meatal antrostomy (MMA)	Disease free
4.	41 M	Left nasal obstruction (previous lateral rhinotomy for IP)	Left lamina papyracea, frontal sinus	III	MMA, ethmoidectomy, sphenoidotomy, and endoscopic Lothrop procedure	Disease free
5.	74 M	Left nasal obstruction	Left nasal septum	I	Middle meatal antrostomy, ethmoidectomy	Disease free
6.	72 M	Asymptomatic	Left middle turbinate	I	Resection of middle turbinate, ethmoidectomy, sphenoidotomy	Disease free
7.	46 M	Left nasal obstruction	Left maxillary sinus	II	MMA, ethmoidectomy, and sphenoidotomy	Disease free
8.	53 M	Right frontal sinusitis (previous lateral rhinotomy for IP)	Right maxillary sinus floor	III	Medial maxillectomy and canine fossa puncture	Disease free
9.	60 F	Right nasal obstruction, rhinorrhea	Right maxillary sinus floor	III	MMA and canine fossa puncture	Disease free
10.	78 F	Right epistaxis and nasal obstruction	Right maxillary sinus floor	III	Medial maxillectomy, ethmoidectomy, DCR, and canine fossa puncture	Disease free
11.	53 M	Left nasal obstruction (previous Caldwell Luc)	Left maxillary sinus floor	III	MMA, ethmoidectomy, and frontal recess clearance	Disease free
12.	44 M	Right nasal obstruction	Left middle meatus	I	MMA, ethmoidectomy, middle turbinectomy	Disease free
13.	67 M	Left nasal obstruction	Sphenoid and posterior ethmoids	III	MMA, ethmoidectomy, superior turbinectomy, and extended sphenoidotomy	Disease free
14.	58 F	Right nasal obstruction and blood-stained discharge	Posterior septum	I	Sphenoethmoidectomy, septal, middle, and superior turbinate resection	Disease free
15.	71 M	Right nasal obstruction	Right middle meatus and medial wall maxillary sinus	II	Ethmoidectomy, frontal recess clearance, middle turbinectomy, medial maxillectomy, and canine fossa puncture	Disease free
16.	50 F	Left nasal obstruction, epistaxis, and discharge	Left superior rim of maxillary sinus ostium	II	Anterior ethmoidectomy, MMA, and canine fossa puncture	Disease free
17.	56 M	Right nasal obstruction	Middle meatus on posterior rim of maxillary ostium	II	Ethmoidectomy and MMA	Disease free

Source: Used with permission from Wormald PJ, Ooi E, van Hasselt A, Nair S. Endoscopic removal of sinonasal inverted papilloma including endoscopic medial maxillectomy. Laryngoscope 2003;113:867–873. † Recurrence found associated with squamous cell carcinoma deposits.

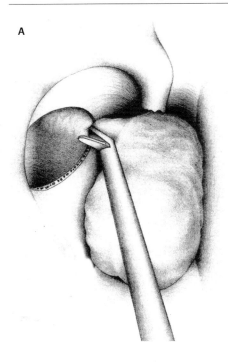

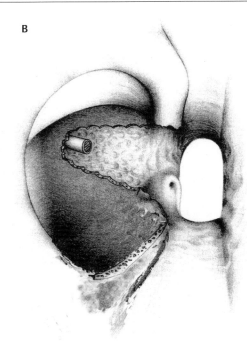

Figure 16–23 **(A)** The nasal component of the tumor has been mobilized and the large middle meatal antrostomy performed. A 45-degree through-biting Blakesley is used to remove the posterior wall of the maxillary sinus. **(B)** The tumor has been removed and the pterygopalatine fossa exposed. The maxillary artery is seen in the tumor bed. (From Wormald PJ, van Hasselt CA. Endoscopic removal of juvenile angiofibromas. Otol Head Neck Surg 2003;129(6):684–691. Reprinted with permission.)

The recurrence rates of inverting papilloma with open procedures average at 18% while those performed endoscopically average 12%.[10]

Endoscopic Removal of Juvenile Nasopharyngeal Angiofibromas

Small Juvenile Nasopharyngeal Angiofibromas

There is currently widespread acceptance that small juvenile nasopharyngeal angiofibromas (JNAs) occupying the nasal cavity alone or with minimal extension into the pterygopalatine fossa or adjacent sinuses can be managed endoscopically.[6,10] The first step is to embolize the tumor within 24 hours of the surgery to reduce its vascularity. If the embolization is done prior to 24 hours, the tumor may open up significant collateral blood supply and regain a degree of its vascularity. The second step is to perform a large middle meatal antrostomy with removal of the posterior fontanelle and a sphenoethmoidectomy to provide access over the top of the tumor into the sphenoid sinus. Thereafter, the intranasal component of the tumor is mobilized with a malleable suction Freer* (Medtronic ENT). Often it is stuck to the septum and posterior bony choana, but there is always a surgical plane directly on the tumor surface. If there is sufficient room in the nose, the tumor does not need to be debulked, but if the nasal component is very large, this may need to be resected before any extension of the tumor is dealt with. After mobilization of the nasal component, the tumor is divided at its entry into the sphenopalatine foramen using a Coblation wand. The concomitant tissue removal and hemostasis achieved with the Coblation wand

reduces bleeding from the cut surface of the tumor. The nasal component is then delivered via the nasopharynx through the mouth. Next, the extension of tumor into the pterygopalatine fossa needs to be exposed. The posterior wall of the maxillary sinus is removed, starting at the pterygopalatine foramen and moving laterally until the tumor in the pterygopalatine fossa and the attached maxillary artery are exposed (**Fig. 16–23**). Large tumor extensions into the pterygopalatine fossa need to be dealt with as described in the next section.

Endoscopic Removal of Large Juvenile Nasopharyngeal Angiofibromas[11]

The most common benign tumor involving the pterygopalatine fossa (and infratemporal fossa) is the juvenile angiofibroma (JNA). These tumors normally originate in the region of the sphenopalatine foramen and expand into the pterygopalatine fossa. Large tumors that extend into the infratemporal fossa will usually have a large intranasal component that may extend into nearby sinuses, especially the sphenoid sinus. Other benign tumors seen in this region are rare but may include inverting papillomas extending from the nasal cavity or tumors originating from the nerve sheath (schwannomas), cartilage, or muscle. The reason why there has been debate about the most appropriate method for removing these tumors is the significant vascularity that is associated with these tumors. Massive bleeding can occur during tumor resection, and if the surgeon is not prepared or is unable to manage such hemorrhage, complications can result. There are two significant steps that are now possible to allow these large JNAs to be

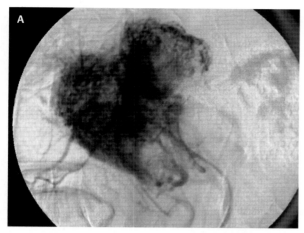
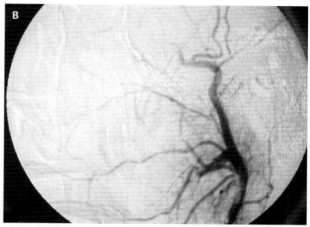

Figure 16–24 (**A**) The significant vascular blush of the tumor. (**B**) This blush has been removed by embolization of the maxillary artery feeding the tumor.

tackled endoscopically. The first step is to preoperatively embolize the tumor, thereby significantly reducing the vascularity and improving visualization during resection (**Fig. 16–24**).[6,11]

The second step is the two-surgeon approach, which allows the second surgeon to place a high-volume suction in the operative field when bleeding is problematic and alternatively to place traction on the tumor facilitating the dissection.[6,11]

Before surgery is performed, a large JNA needs careful assessment to decide if it is endoscopically resectable. Large JNAs tend to expand into potential spaces and to follow pathways of least resistance. In the pterygopalatine fossa and infratemporal fossa, several areas need to be critically evaluated before the surgeon decides if the tumor is endoscopically resectable.[11] In the pterygopalatine fossa, the infraorbital fissure needs to be closely evaluated. There is a potential space between the lateral wall of the sphenoid and the middle cranial fossa as seen in the previous anatomic review of this region. The tumor can infiltrate around the infraorbital nerve and enter the potential space above the nerve and expand this space. Further growth will cause the tumor to push posteriorly toward the cavernous sinus and second genu of the carotid artery. Such a case is illustrated in **Fig. 16–25** where the tumor abuts the cavernous sinus and carotid and compresses the orbital apex within this potential space above the infraorbital fissure.

In this case (**Fig. 16–25**), the maxillary nerve would be completely surrounded by tumor, and it would be unlikely that the tumor could be separated from the nerve, and indeed the nerve needed to be sacrificed during the dissection. In most cases where the tumor does not expand through the infraorbital fissure, the nerve is pushed upward by the tumor and can usually be dissected free from the tumor. The nerve should be identified both distally and proximally early in the dissection and preserved. The suction dissection instruments are used to separate the nerve from the tumor. Fibrous tissue that will not dissect away is divided with endoscopic soft tissue scissors from the Medtronic Skull Base Set*

(Medtronic ENT). These scissors come in 3-, 5-, and 7-mm blade lengths with a left-curved, right-curved, and straight blade in each of these sizes.

The other region that is often involved in the spread of large JNAs is the Vidian canal.[11] The tumor grows in this region in close proximity to the mouth of the Vidian canal. This funnel-shaped opening allows the tumor to grow down the canal and expand the canal. This region and particularly the Vidian canal should always be assessed on both CT and MRI imaging. It is vitally important to understand the anatomy and relationships of the Vidian canal and to be able to assess tumor spread in this region. As was demonstrated earlier in this chapter, the Vidian canal runs in the floor of the sphenoid in an anteroposterior direction toward the carotid artery as it moves from its lacerum segment into its cavernous segment. Tumor may expand this canal and erode the floor of the sphenoid and in some cases (**Fig. 16–26**) abut the carotid artery. It is our belief that failure to fully evaluate the Vidian canal at the time of removal of the JNA is one of the biggest causes of tumor recurrence. Small pieces of tumor lying within the canal can easily be missed and may grow progressively over time after tumor removal.

Endoscopic Two-Surgeon Technique for Tumors of the Pterygopalatine Fossa and Infratemporal Fossa

Although excellent access is provided by an endoscopic medial maxillectomy, the key to successful endoscopic removal of large JNAs is having two surgeons operating at the same time.[6,11,12] This is achieved by providing access to the tumor bed for the second surgeon through the septum. At the beginning of the procedure, a Freer (hemitransfixion) incision is made on the opposite side to that of the tumor. Using standard septoplasty techniques, the mucosa is elevated off the cartilage of the septum. The cartilage of the septum is preserved but most of the posterior bony septum is resected. At the point where access is required, a horizontal incision is made in the opposite septal mucosa

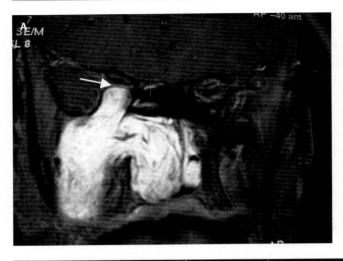

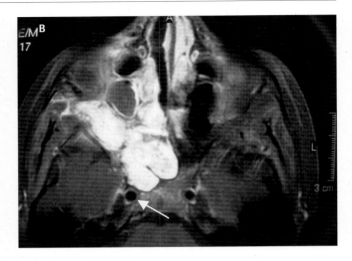

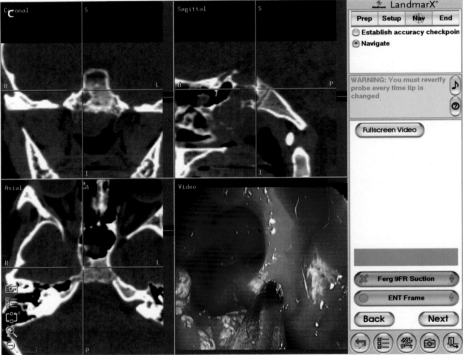

Figure 16–25 (**A**) In coronal MRI scan, the tumor extends around the infraorbital nerve into the space between the lateral wall of the sphenoid sinus and the temporal lobe and significantly compresses the orbital apex (*white arrow*). (**B**) In axial MRI scan, the tumor can be seen extending posteriorly into this space and abutting the cavernous sinus and carotid artery (*white arrow*). (**C**) In the intraoperative image-guidance picture, the suction probe is placed in this space between the lateral wall of the sphenoid and temporal lobe after tumor resection as can be seen by the crosshairs on the adjacent CT scans.

to allow instruments placed through the opposite nostril and into the Freer incision to cross the septum and access the tumor region on the opposite side of the nose (**Fig. 16–27**).

During removal of the tumor, the second surgeon can provide significant traction on the tumor. This traction is vital to help the primary surgeon keep the dissection progressing around the posterior region of the tumor. This rotation of the tumor will also allow the feeding vessel (usually the maxillary artery) to be identified and clipped or cauterized before it is divided. If significant bleeding occurs, then a large-volume suction can be placed in the field and allow the suction bipolar cautery to be used to cauterize these vessels. Once the tumor is removed, the tumor bed can be closely

inspected to ensure no tumor remnant remains, especially in the region of the Vidian canal. If remnants are seen, they are carefully removed. Once hemostasis is achieved with the suction bipolar forceps, the preserved mucosa from the posterior wall of the maxillary sinus is replaced. Surgicel or Gelfoam powder can be placed in the cavity if required, and the horizontal incision in the septal mucosa is sutured. This stitch is continued anteriorly as a through-and-through plication suture of the septum until it is brought out at the base of the Freer incision and used as a continuous suture to close this incision.

The final step is to ensure that the lacrimal sac is adequately exposed to prevent postoperative stenosis and epiphora. Without intraoperative management of the lacrimal sac, the

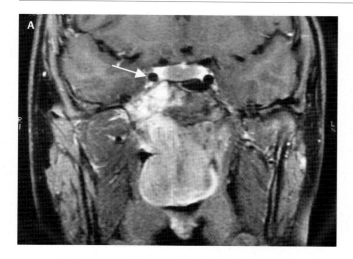

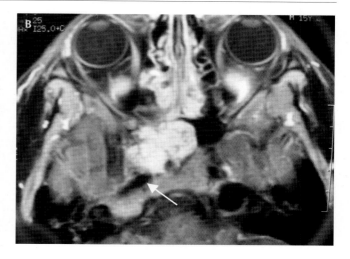

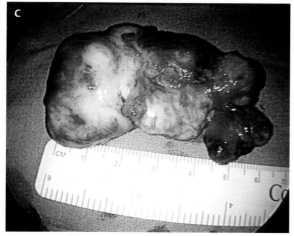

Figure 16–26 (A) In coronal MRI scan, the tumor fills the nasopharynx, and expands the Vidian canal posteriorly until it abuts the internal carotid artery (*white arrow*). **(B)** This abutment of the carotid artery (*white arrow*) is seen in this axial MRI. **(C)** After endoscopic removal of the tumor, it is placed on a ruler for evaluation of its size.

incidence of postoperative epiphora has been described to be as high as 30%.[7]

Results of Endoscopic Removal

In a series of 14 consecutive patients with angiofibroma managed endoscopically, eight patients had extensive disease requiring endoscopic medial maxillectomy.[6,11] The classification of Radkowski et al[13] was used to classify the patients, and the distribution of the patients in each category is presented in **Table 16–3**. Only patients classified as either IIC or IIIA required endoscopic medial maxillectomy for an entirely endoscopic removal of their tumor.

All patients described in this series have had regular postoperative MRI scans. In two patients, there is residual tissue enhancement with contrast in the region of the Vidian canal. Both of these patients have had repeated MRI scans over several years without any enlargement of this enhancing area and are monitored every 6 months for any change. Whether this enhancement reflects disease recurrence or increased tissue vascularity is unclear, but revision surgery will only be offered if this tissue shows

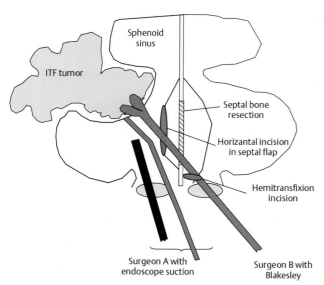

Figure 16–27 Diagram illustrating the access points for the two-surgeon technique.

Table 16-3   Radkowski et al Classification of Juvenile Angiofibromas

Stage	Description	n = 14
IA	Limited to nose and nasopharyngeal area	1
IB	Extension into one or more sinuses	0
IIA	Minimal extension into pterygopalatine fossa	2
IIB	Occupation of the pterygopalatine fossa without orbital erosion	3
IIC	Infratemporal fossa extension without cheek or pterygoid plate involvement	3
IIIA	Erosion of the skull base (middle cranial fossa or pterygoids)	5
IIIB	Erosion of skull base with intracranial extension with or without cavernous sinus involvement	0

Source: Data from Radkowski D, McGill T, Healy GB, et al. Angiofibroma: changes in staging and treatment. Arch Otolaryngol Head Neck Surg 1996;122:122–129.

growth on repeated MRI scans. The rest of the patients are currently disease free with an average follow-up time of 4.1 years. The patient numbers have increased from the recently published series[6,11] to include all patients operated on over the past 5 years.

Schwannomas Involving the Pterygopalatine and Infratemporal Fossae

Medial maxillectomy also provides access to other tumors that may involve the pterygopalatine and infratemporal fossae. In **Fig. 16-28**, a schwannoma of the maxillary nerve involves the entire pterygopalatine fossa and extends significantly into the infratemporal fossa. Medial maxillectomy allows access to the entire posterior wall of the maxillary sinus and after its removal to the tumor.

Figure 16-29 illustrates the tumor seen in **Fig. 16-28** after endoscopic medial maxillectomy and tumor removal. It was confirmed histologically to be a schwannoma.

Malignant Tumors Involving the Pterygopalatine and Infratemporal Fossae

Currently, the role of endoscopic resection for the management of malignant tumors is unclear.[14,15] Recently, there have been some studies published utilizing endoscopic resection for malignant tumors, but the authors have stressed that long-term follow-up is not available for these patients and that radical resection with open approaches remains the gold standard.[14,15] In our practice, patients are offered standard

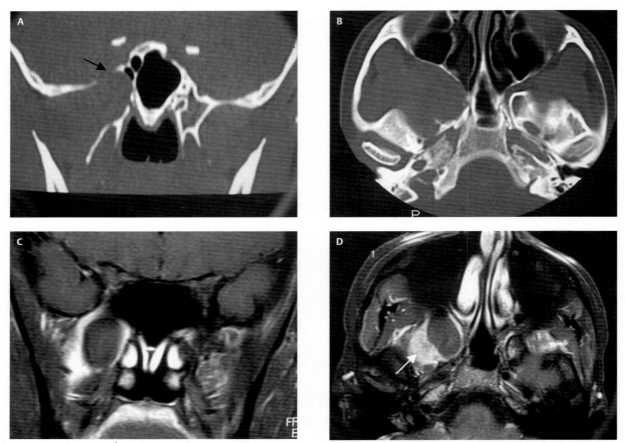

Figure 16–28. The CT marked (**A**) corresponds with the MRI marked (**C**) as do the CT and MRI marked (**B, D**). The erosion of the middle cranial fossa is marked with a *black arrow* in (**A**). The extension of the tumor into the infratemporal fossa is marked in (**D**) with a *white arrow*.

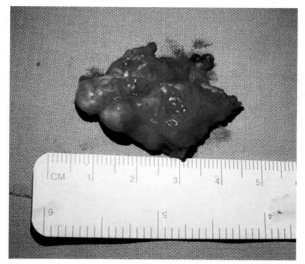

Figure 16–29 Resected schwannoma from the patient shown in **Fig. 16–28**.

external approaches and radical resection including cranio-facial resection if the tumor involves the dura. If, however, the patient declines this treatment, then endoscopic tumor removal with postoperative radiotherapy with or without chemotherapy is offered. Most malignancies in the nose and sinuses have a pushing front and do not infiltrate through the orbital periosteum or dura. These tumors are usually soft, and there is usually a surgical plane between the tumor and the natural boundaries of the nose and sinuses. The exception is squamous cell carcinoma, and we do not usually offer endoscopic resection to these patients. In some instances where there is localized infiltration of the tumor into the dura or orbital periosteum, this can be endoscopically resected, and in the case of the dura repaired. However, in most patients where such a breach of the dura or orbital periosteum is obvious on preoperative MRI scanning, external radical resection is strongly advocated.

The principle of tumor removal is to first debulk the tumor to create space in the nose in which to operate. This is easily done with a Blakesley forceps (to allow tumor to be sent for histology) and a microdebrider blade. No attempt

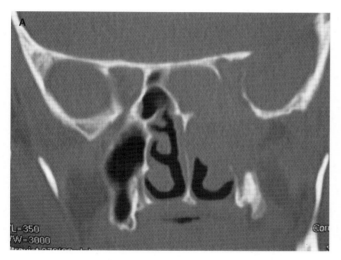

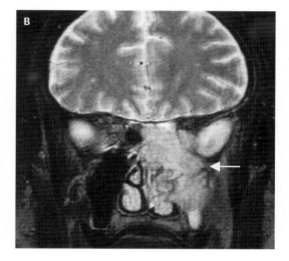

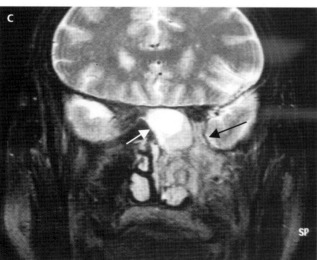

Figure 16–30 CT scan (**A**) shows erosion of the lateral wall of the sphenoid, erosion of the upper pterygoid plates, and widening of the infraorbital fissure. MRI scan (**B**) shows extension of the tumor into the infratemporal fossa (*white arrow*) and (**C**) extension of tumor through the infraorbital fissure into the potential space between the lateral wall of the sphenoid and the temporal lobe (*black arrow*). The sphenoid is filled with mucus (*white arrow*).

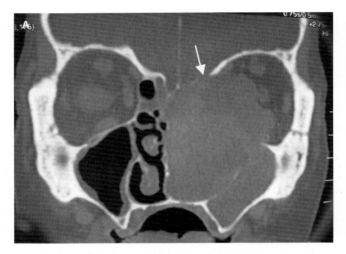

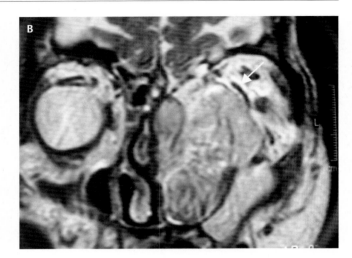

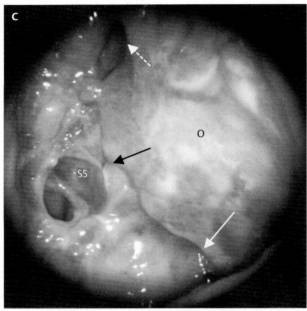

Figure 16–31 (**A**) In the CT scan, the skull base has been eroded (*white arrow*) and there is significant compression of the orbit. (**B**) In the MRI scan, the compression rather than invasion of the orbit is illustrated by the medial rectus (*white arrow*) being pushed up against the optic nerve. (**C**) In the postoperative picture, the sphenoid sinus (SS) and orbit (O) can be clearly seen with the posterior ethmoid artery (*black arrow*) and maxillary sinus (*white arrow*) and frontal ostium visible (*broken white arrow*).

is made to remove tumor from surrounding structures. Once there is space to operate, then a surgical plane is established between the tumor and the lamina papyracea or, if absent, the orbital periosteum. In the region of the skull base, this plane is established between the skull base or, if absent, the dura. To start the dissection, the junction of the tumor and lateral nasal wall is found anteriorly, and a malleable suction Freer is used to elevate the mucosa anterior to the tumor establishing the plane between mucosa and bone. This allows the surgical plane to be established around the margins of the tumor. If this plane is followed either onto the exposed orbital periosteum or dura, tumor can be dissected off the periosteum or dura without its disruption. In this way, it is usually possible to remove all macroscopic tumor leaving the underlying periosteum and dura intact. In the following case example, the patient presented with a sinonasal undifferentiated carcinoma

(SNUC) (**Fig. 16–30**). The surgical plan was to attempt endoscopic tumor removal but if necessary to combine endoscopic resection with a craniotomy. At the time of surgery, complete macroscopic resection was achieved endoscopically, and we believed that there would be no additional benefit in performing a craniotomy. The patient underwent postoperative radiotherapy and to date is still disease free (12 months follow-up).

In the following case example, a patient presents with a chondrosarcoma with significant proptosis, diplopia, and nasal obstruction (**Fig. 16–31**). He was elderly (85 years old) and generally in poor health, and the Combined Oncology Head and Neck Clinic felt that he would not be suitable for craniofacial resection and so he was offered endoscopic resection and radiotherapy. The tumor was debulked and after space was created, a good surgical plane was able to be established anterior to the tumor origin. The tumor was then dissected off the dura and the orbital periosteum. An endoscopic medial maxillectomy was performed to improve lateral access. Complete macroscopic tumor removal was achieved and the patient offered postoperative radiotherapy.

◆ POSTOPERATIVE CARE

Broad-spectrum antibiotics are continued for 5 days after surgery. Douching of the nose with saline is started immediately postoperatively. Crusting will usually continue for a few months and may worsen during and immediately after radiotherapy. In most patients, crusting is not problematic in the long-term although some patients (who have had radiotherapy) can continue to have significant crusting if mucociliary drainage is not reestablished after some months. There is no easy solution for this other than continued regular saline douching and crust removal under endoscopic control.

◆ CONCLUSION

Knowledge of the anatomy of the pterygopalatine and infratemporal fossae, infraorbital fissure, and adjacent parasphenoid region including the Vidian canal is essential if tumors in these areas are to be endoscopically addressed. This chapter presents a detailed overview of this anatomy and the various endoscopic surgical techniques used to address this region.

References

1. Hyams VJ. Papillomas of the nasal cavity and paranasal sinuses. A clinicopathological study of 315 cases. Ann Otol Rhinol Laryngol 1971;80:192–206
2. Keles N, Deger K. Endonasal endoscopic surgical treatment of paranasal sinus inverted papilloma—first experiences. Rhinology 2001;39:156–159
3. Sukenik MA, Casiano R. Endoscopic medial maxillectomy for inverted papillomas of the paranasal sinuses: value of the intraoperative endoscopic examination. Laryngoscope 2000;110:39–42
4. Krouse JH. Development of a staging system for inverted papilloma. Laryngoscope 2000;110:965–968
5. Wormald PJ, Ooi E, van Hasselt A, Nair S. Endoscopic removal of sinonasal inverted papilloma including endoscopic medial maxillectomy. Laryngoscope 2003;113:867–873
6. Wormald PJ, van Hasselt CA. Endoscopic removal of juvenile angiofibromas. Otolaryngol Head Neck Surg 2003;129(6):684–691
7. Vrabec DP. The inverted Schneiderian papilloma: a 25-year study. Laryngoscope 1994;104:582–605
8. Chiu AG, Jackman AH, Antunes MB, . Radiographic and histologic analysis of the bone underlying inverted papillomas. Laryngoscope 2006;116:1617–1620
9. Krouse JH. Endoscopic treatment of inverting papilloma: safety and efficacy. Am J Otolaryngol 2001;22:87–99
10. Melroy CT, Senior BA. Benign sinonasal neoplasms. Otolaryngol Clin North Am 2006;39:601–617
11. Douglas R, Wormald PJ. Endoscopic surgery for juvenile nasopharyngeal angiofibroma: where are the limits? Curr Opin Otolaryngol Head Neck Surg 2006;14:1–5
12. Robinson S, Patel N, Wormald PJ. Endoscopic management of tumours within the infratemporal fossa: a 2-surgeon transnasal endoscopic approach. Laryngoscope 2005;115(10):1818–1822
13. Radkowski D, McGill T, Healy GB. Angiofibroma. Changes in staging and treatment. Arch Otolaryngol Head Neck Surg 1996;122:122–129
14. Batra PS, Citardi MJ. Endoscopic management of sinonasal malignancy. Otolaryngol Clin North Am 2006;39:619–637
15. Stamm AC, Pignatari SS, Velutini E. Transnasal endoscopic surgical approaches to the clivus. Otolaryngol Clin North Am 2006;39:639–656

17

Endoscopic Resection of the Eustachian Tube and Postnasal Space

The most common tumor of the postnasal space is nasopharyngeal carcinoma. Fortunately, these tumors are radiosensitive and there is seldom a need for surgical excision. In rare cases, nasopharyngeal carcinoma that has recurred despite repeated radiotherapy may need surgical excision. In these cases, recurrent tumor is best managed by external procedures such as the maxillary swing technique, transmaxillary approach, facial translocation, transcervico-mandibulo-palatal, infratemporal fossa, and lateral infratemporal middle fossa.[1-7] These recurrent carcinomas are usually not suitable for endoscopic excision as the tumor has infiltrated the surrounding structures. There is significant fibrosis if the patient has previously undergone radiotherapy obliterating surgical planes. These tumors are removed by traditional techniques with appropriate vascular control. However, there are a small number of rare benign and malignant tumors that occur in the postnasal space and eustachian tube that are nonresponsive to radiotherapy and are best treated by primary surgical excision. Examples of these are the minor salivary gland tumors (benign and malignant), malignant melanomas, and juvenile angiofibromas. These tumors usually have an identifiable plane and a pushing front that will allow identification of the surgical plane and can be excised endoscopically even if there is limited extension into the parapharyngeal space. Endoscopic resection is appealing as it allows a complete resection of the tumor with minimal morbidity in contrast with the external approaches that have significant associated morbidity. To perform endoscopic resections in this region, a detailed knowledge of the anatomy is necessary.

◆ ANATOMY

The surgical approach to this region is via the medial pterygoid plate. The relationship of the medial pterygoid plate, medial pterygoid muscle, tensor palatini, levator palatini, and Eustachian tube (ET) needs to be understood. If the postnasal space is viewed endoscopically, the medial pterygoid plate, ET, and fossa of Rosenmueller can be clearly seen (**Fig. 17-1**).

To access the ET, the medial pterygoid plate needs to be removed and the underlying medial pterygoid muscle exposed (**Fig. 17-2**). Note how the tensor palatine muscle forms a natural surgical plane as it attaches to the anterior aspect of the ET. Inferiorly, the ET lies on the levator palatini muscle as it moves laterally to its attachment to the skull base. The lateral pterygoid muscle attaches to the lateral aspect of the lateral pterygoid plate and is usually not seen in the dissection unless there is significant infratemporal fossa extension of the tumor. Just anterior to where the ET attaches to the skull base, the mandibular branch (V3) of the trigeminal nerve is seen. Directly posterior to V3, in the apex of the fossa of Rosenmueller, the internal carotid artery can be seen (**Fig. 17-2**).

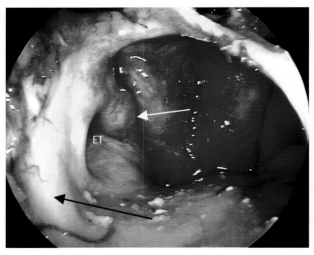

Figure 17-1 The right medial pterygoid plate can be seen as a mucosal prominence (*black arrow*) directly anterior to the ET. The fossa of Rosenmueller can be seen behind the ET (*white arrow*).

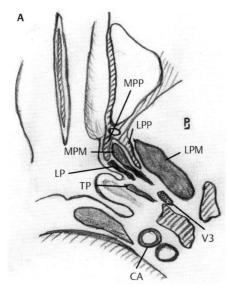

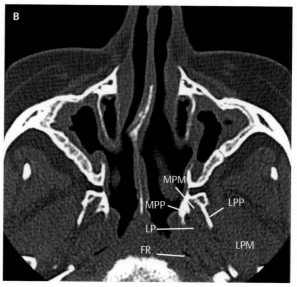

Figure 17–2 In diagram (**A**) and axial CT scan (**B**), the medial pterygoid plate (MPP) and lateral pterygoid plate (LPP) are identified. The medial pterygoid muscle (MPM) is seen between these two plates. The lateral pterygoid muscle (LPM) is seen lateral to the LPP. The levator palatini (LP) attaches to the medial aspect of the Eustachian tube (ET) while the tensor palatine lies below the ET. The fossa of Rosenmueller (FR) forms most of the posterior boundary of the ET. Note the relationship of the mandibular nerve (V3) and the carotid artery (CA) to the apex of the fossa of Rosenmueller and V3.

◆ SURGICAL TECHNIQUE

The nose is prepared in the standard fashion. A pterygopalatine fossa block is placed through the mouth and greater palatine canal into the pterygopalatine fossa. The first step for this surgery is to remove the posterior half of the inferior turbinate. A large middle meatal antrostomy is done with exposure of the posterior wall of the maxillary sinus.

The middle meatal antrostomy is taken down to the floor of the nose, and the mucosa over the medial pterygoid plate is elevated (**Fig. 17–3**).

To access this region, a two-surgeon approach is advocated. The use of both nostrils allows greater angulation and clearance of blood if significant bleeding occurs, so that surgery can continue. The access to this region is slightly different from that used for the infratemporal

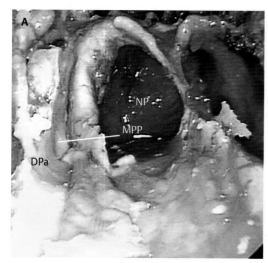

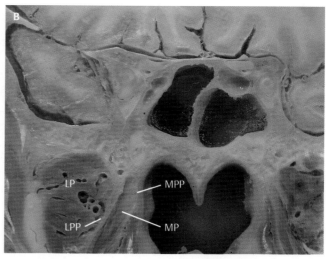

Figure 17–3 In (**A**), the mucosa overlying the medial pterygoid plate has been elevated. The descending palatine artery (DPa) has been exposed. In (**B**), the medial and lateral pterygoid plates (MPP and LPP) are marked. The medial pterygoid muscle (MP) and lateral pterygoid muscle (LP) and their relationships to the plates are seen.

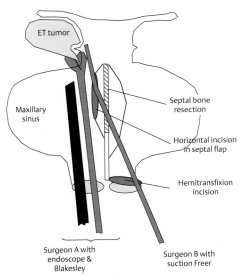

Figure 17–4 The resection of septal bone is more posterior as is the horizontal incision in the elevated septal mucosal flap. The two-surgeon technique allows greatly flexibility in instrument placement and better angulation to the region of the tumor.

fossa in that the septal resection of bone requires complete resection of all posterior septal bone. In addition, the horizontal incision in the mucosal flap of the septum is further posterior allowing easy access to the region of the ET. This allows the ET and tumor to be placed on traction when dissection is being performed in the lateral regions of the postnasal space, which increases the safety by pulling the ET and tumor medially, lessening the risk to the carotid artery (**Fig. 17–4**).

The next step is to remove the bone of the medial pterygoid plate using a skull base curved diamond burr (Medtronic ENT). As the bone is removed, the descending palatine artery is exposed. This needs to be cauterized using the suction bipolar then divided (**Fig. 17–5**). This gives the surgeon access to the medial pterygoid muscle and the lateral pterygoid plate. The medial pterygoid muscle is surrounded by a dense venous plexus, and sharp dissection of this muscle can result in significant venous bleeding. We prefer to use the Coblation wand to remove this muscle as this can be done without significant bleeding.

There is a natural surgical plane anterior to the ET. This is formed by the cartilaginous anterior aspect of the ET and

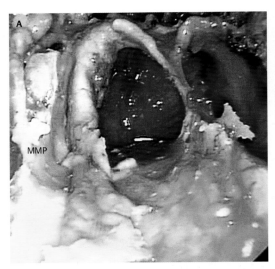

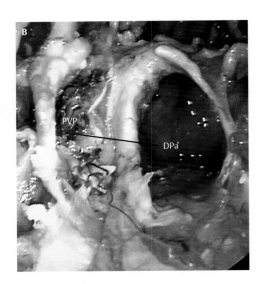

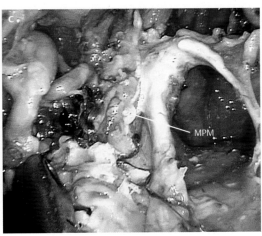

Figure 17–5 In (**A**), the medial pterygoid plate is exposed. In (**B**), this plate has been removed exposing the rich venous pterygoid venous plexus (PVP) (*colored blue* in this injected cadaver specimen). In (**C**), this venous plexus has been removed with the descending palatine artery to expose the underlying medial pterygoid muscle.

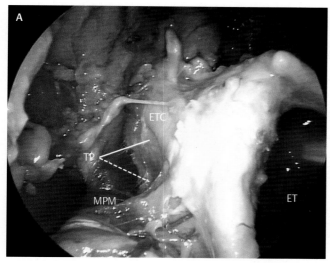

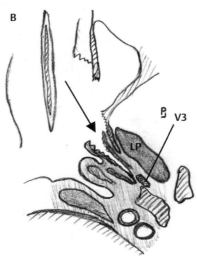

Figure 17–6 In (**A**), the right eustachian tube (ET) orifice defines the medial extent of the dissection. The medial pterygoid muscle (MPM) is being swept laterally with the dissector exposing the anterior cartilage of the ET (ETC). Attached to this cartilage is the tensor palatini (TP) fibrous aponeurosis (*solid white line*) with its

muscle fibers seen below (*broken white line*). In the axial diagram (**B**), the resection of the inferior turbinate, posterior medial maxilla, medial pterygoid plate, and medial pterygoid muscle can be appreciated. The *solid black arrow* indicates the surgical plane anterior to the ET but medial to V3.

the attached fibrous aponeurosis of the tensor palatini. If the aponeurosis is followed inferiorly, the tensor palatini muscle fibers can be seen (**Fig. 17–6**). The surgical removal of the medial pterygoid plate and partial removal of the medial pterygoid muscle with establishment of the anterior surgical plane can be also appreciated on the axial diagram also presented in **Fig. 17–5**.

The next step is to release the ET inferiorly and posteriorly (**Fig. 17–7**). These horizontal and posterior incisions are made with the Coblation wand to minimize bleeding. The horizontal incision cuts through the tensor and levator palatini muscles and further dissection enters the parapharyngeal space. The dissection is continued laterally directly under the ET thereby mobilizing the ET from the parapharyngeal space. If the fossa of Rosenmueller is to be included in the resection, the posterior incision is made onto the parapharyngeal muscle. The surgical plane is anterior to the muscle. If the plane is deep to these muscles, the carotid artery and jugular vein are at increased risk in the most lateral extent of the fossa (**Fig. 17–6**).

The ET complex is relatively immobile until the fibrous attachment of the ET to the skull base is cut. As this tissue is tough, these incisions need to be done with sharp instruments such as the angled scissors from the Skull Base Set* (Medtronic ENT). Although a scalpel was used in the cadaver dissection depicted in **Fig. 17–8**, it is not advisable to use this instrument to perform this step as the internal carotid artery is at risk during this maneuver. It is also better to use the natural curve of the scissors angled anteriorly (away from the carotid). In addition, the second surgeon should place the ET under traction, thereby allowing each cut made with the scissors to be more effective and less likely to damage the internal carotid (**Fig. 17–8**).

Once the ET has been removed, the surrounding anatomic structures can be clearly identified. In **Fig. 17–9**, the lateral pterygoid plate, foramen lacerum in the roof of the fossa of Rosenmueller, and posterior pharyngeal muscles can be seen. Above and lateral to the attachment of the ET to the skull base is the mandibular branch (V3) of the trigeminal nerve. If the lateral pterygoid plate is drilled away, then the underlying lateral pterygoid muscle is seen; and if the pharyngeal muscles are separated, then the internal carotid artery can

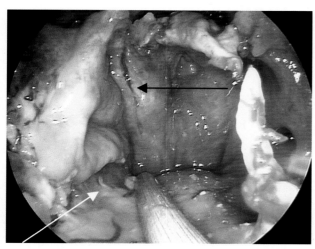

Figure 17–7 The horizontal incision (*white arrow*) exposes the underlying tensor and levator palatini muscle fibers. The vertical incision (*black arrow*) and surgical plane should be anterior to the prevertebral muscles.

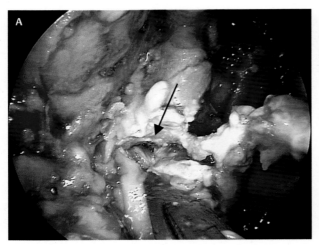

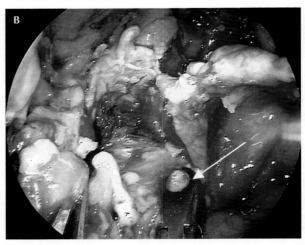

Figure 17–8 In (**A**), the superior attachment of the ET to the skull base has been cut (*black arrow*). (**B**) Traction is now placed on the ET with a Blakesley forceps, allowing the residual fibrous attachments to be clearly seen and safely divided.

be seen before it enters the petrous temporal bone (**Fig. 17–9B**). The internal carotid artery is usually posterior and in some patients more lateral than V3.

◆ POSTOPERATIVE CARE

Hemostasis is achieved with the suction bipolar forceps. A dressing of fibrillar Surgicel is applied to the surgical bed. The bed is allowed to granulate and heals with time. Broad-spectrum antibiotics are given for 5 days. To decrease postoperative crusting, the patient performs regular nasal douches using the squeeze-bottle nasal wash method. Nasal toilet is performed at 2 weeks postoperatively and as necessary thereafter. A repeat magnetic resonance imaging (MRI) scan

is performed to ensure that there is no tumor recurrence at 6 and 12 months and yearly thereafter.

◆ CASE EXAMPLES

We have had three patients in recent years in whom we have performed this surgery. The first patient had a malignant melanoma of the mucosa within the ET, and the second patient had a low-grade mucoepidermoid carcinoma originating within the ET lumen and protruding through the wall of the ET into the parapharyngeal space. A component of this tumor prolapsed into the nasopharynx and caused nasal obstruction. The third patient had a recurrent juvenile angiofibroma lateral and inferior to the ET.

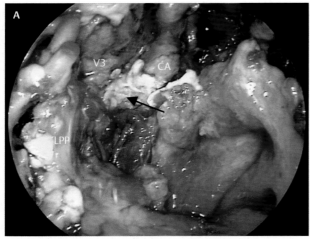

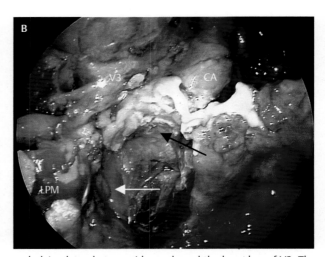

Figure 17–9 In (**A**), the lateral pterygoid plate (LPP), V3, and foramen lacerum (*black arrow*) can be seen. The internal carotid artery (CA) is seen running directly above the foramen lacerum. In (**B**), the lateral pterygoid plate has been removed exposing the

underlying lateral pterygoid muscle and the branches of V3. The pharyngeal muscles have been teased away to expose the internal carotid artery (*white arrow* and CA). The foramen lacerum (*black arrow*) is seen in the apex of the fossa of Rosenmueller.

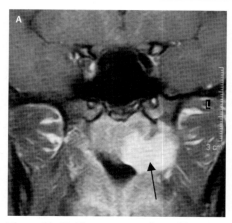
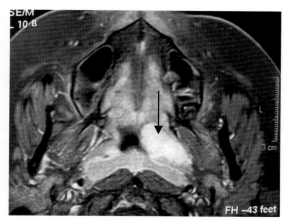

Figure 17–10 The tumor is indicated by a *black arrow* in (**A**), the coronal T1 MRI scan, and in (**B**), the axial scan.

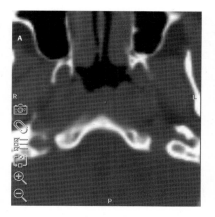
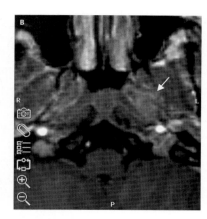
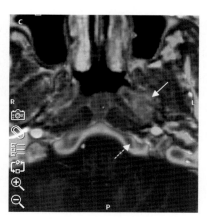

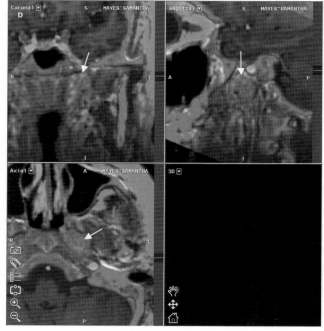

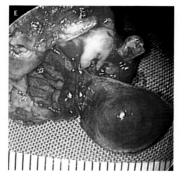

Figure 17–11 (**A**) In the axial CT scan, the tumor is not clearly seen but the bony landmarks are visible. (**B**) In the MRI scan, the tumor is clearly seen (*white arrow*) but the bony landmarks are absent. (**C**) In the merged (CT and MRI) scan, both the bony landmarks (*broken white arrow*) and tumor (*white arrow*) are clearly seen. (**D, E**) The intraoperative image guidance–merged scan with the tumor (*white arrow*) and bony landmarks seen in all three planes. In addition, the resected ET and tumor can be seen.

The patient with the mucoepidermoid carcinoma presented with nasal obstruction and the following MRI demonstrated a postnasal space mass (**Fig. 17–10**). The patient was taken to theater, and the tumor prolapsing out of the ET orifice was removed and sent for histology and the diagnosis confirmed.

The surgeon who performed the biopsy confirmed tumor remained within the ET orifice, and the patient was sent to the tumor board where it was decided that endoscopic excision was the best option for the patient. Computer-aided surgery (CAS) is an important part of the surgical plan. In these cases, both computed tomography (CT) and MRI should be loaded and a "merge" performed. This tool allows the surgeon to move between CT and MRI and to adjust the image to have any percentage blend of CT and MRI. In this case, the tumor could not be visualized on CT scanning but could be visualized on MRI scanning. "Merge" allowed the blend between CT and MRI to be adjusted so that the bony landmarks (pterygoid plates) and the tumor were clearly visible (**Fig. 17–11**). In addition, if contrast is used, the internal carotid arteries can also be clearly seen.

This tumor, the melanoma, and the angiofibroma were removed using the technique described. Biopsies of tissue remaining in the surgical bed after excision revealed no residual tumor. No additional treatment modalities were given to these patients and they have remained free of locoregional recurrence of disease. The melanoma patient has, however, developed distant metastasis.

◆ **KEY POINTS**

If endoscopic surgery is to be contemplated in this area, it is vitally important that the surgeon be familiar with the endoscopic anatomy of this region. The surgeon needs to create a mental three-dimensional image of the anatomy and be able to place the dissection at all times within the three-dimensional picture. The new CAS guidance systems help significantly, and the ability to merge the CT and MRI scans allows both bony and soft tissues to be accurately identified. Using the two-surgeon approach also adds significantly to the safety of the procedure as the second surgeon can keep the surgical field clear of blood and provide traction on the tumor at vital stages of the dissection. The biggest risk of this surgery is injury to the internal carotid artery, and both the anesthetist and surgeon should have a surgical plan ready to put into action should this complication occur (see Chapter 10).

References

1. Fee WE, Gilmer PA, Goffinet DR. Surgical management of recurrent nasopharyngeal carcinoma after radiation failure at the primary site. Laryngoscope 1988;98:1220–1226
2. Hsu MM, Ko JY, Sheen TS, Chang YL. Salvage surgery for recurrent nasopharyngeal carcinoma. Arch Otolaryngol Head Neck Surg 1997;123:305–309
3. Wei WI, Lam KH, Sham JS. New approach to the nasopharynx: the maxillary swing approach. Head Neck 1991;13:200–207
4. Hao SP, Tsang NM, Chang CN. Salvage surgery for recurrent nasopharyngeal carcinoma. Arch Otolaryngol Head Neck Surg 2002;128:63–67
5. Morton RP, Liavaag PG, McLean M. Transcervico-mandibulo-palatal approach for surgical salvage of recurrent nasopharyngeal cancer. Head Neck 1996;18:352–358
6. Fisch U. The infratemporal fossa approach for nasopharyngeal tumors. Laryngoscope 1983;93:36–44
7. Schramm VL, Imola MJ. Management of nasopharyngeal salivary gland malignancy. Laryngoscope 2001;111:1533–1544
8. Yoshizaki T, Wakisaka N, Murono S. Endoscopic nasopharyngectomy for patients with recurrent nasopharyngeal carcinoma at the primary site. Laryngoscope 2005;115:1517–1519
9. Roh JL, Park CI. Transseptal laser resection of recurrent carcinoma confined to the nasopharynx. Laryngoscope 2006;116:839–841

18

Endoscopic Resection of Clival and Posterior Cranial Fossa Tumors

Tumors of the clivus and posterior cranial fossa are very difficult to access via traditional neurosurgical approaches. In the past, skull base teams would approach the petroclival region by either a lateral or anterior route. The lateral route was via an extended middle cranial fossa approach,[1] whereas the anterior route could be transmaxillary, transoral, or trancervical.[2,3] All of these approaches involve significant resection of normal structures with inevitable associated morbidity.[1-4] Even after such a resection, the final surgical access was usually limited. The operating microscope did not allow a view around the corner, and if the tumor extended beyond the exposed area, resection under direct vision was not possible.

The advantage of the endoscopic transsphenoidal approach is that it allows access to the entire clivus down to the atlas of the cervical spine. It also allows early identification of the vital vascular structures with clear visualization of both carotid arteries and the cavernous sinuses and associated neurologic structures.[4] The most common tumor presenting the clival region is a chordoma. Although complete resection of the tumor and the surrounding bone is optimal, this is often not possible due to the location and surrounding vital structures.[2,5] It is accepted that as complete a resection as is possible should be performed.[5] In most cases, clival chordomas are slow growing and if surgery can be combined with radiotherapy (especially proton beam radiotherapy), this gives the patient the best possible chance of prolonged survival.[2,5] Because curative surgery is often not possible, the morbidity associated with tumor debulking should be as limited as possible. These factors make an endoscopic approach to these tumors attractive as it provides the best possible chance of complete surgical removal with the least surgical morbidity.[4,5] To remove the clival tumor and any associated intracranial extension, a clear understanding of the anatomy of this region is essential.

◆ ANATOMY

The Clivus

The clivus extends from the floor of the sella turcica to the foramen magnum. The thickness of the clivus depends upon the pneumatization of the sphenoid and can vary significantly (**Fig. 18–1**). When this bone is thick, it may hold significant venous channels. This makes removal of the bone a slow process as significant bleeding can occur as the cancellous bone is opened. This is generally quickly controlled by packing the area with Gelfoam paste. Further drilling will provoke more bleeding, which requires repacking, and this process can make bone removal tedious. There is no quick and easy solution to the control of the bleeding in this area, however. The lateral borders of the dissection of the clivus are the vertical portions of the carotid arteries, and these must be exposed at the beginning of the dissection to avoid inadvertent damage (**Fig. 18–1**). The inferior limit of the dissection is usually the floor of the sphenoid, but if access is required to the basi-occiput, foramen magnum, or even lower to the first cervical vertebra, then the entire sphenoid floor can be removed.

Complete removal of the clivus exposes the dura of the posterior fossa. Bone behind the inferior portion of the vertical part of the carotid arteries can be removed so that the arteries stand proud of the lateral margins. The limit to which this bone can be removed is determined by the 45-degree angle that the carotid arteries make as they run in their canals through the petrous temporal bone. This region where the petrous portion of the carotid artery turns vertically in the floor of the sphenoid is where bone should be removed to access the petrous apex. In some patients, a large cholesterol granuloma may thin down the bone separating the granuloma from the sphenoid allowing the granuloma to be drained through the sphenoid.

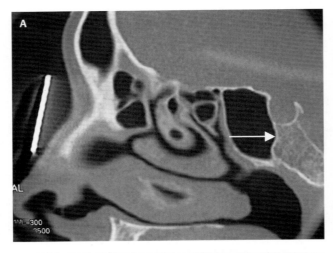

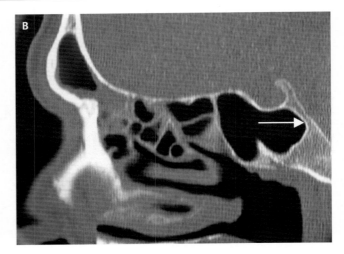

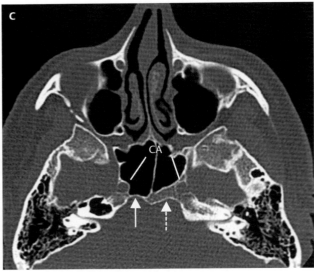

Figure 18–1 In parasagittal CT scan (**A**), the sphenoid is poorly pneumatized and the clivus is thick (*white arrow*). In (**B**), the sphenoid is better pneumatized with a resultant thinner clivus separating the sphenoid from the posterior cranial fossa (*white arrow*). In the axial CT scan (**C**), the right side of the clivus is very thin (*solid white arrow*), whereas the left side is significantly thicker (*broken white arrow*). The vertical portions of the internal carotid arteries (CA) indicate the lateral extent of the clivus.

Posterior Cranial Fossa

Once the dura of the posterior cranial fossa has been removed, the contents of the posterior cranial fossa can be seen. The first and most notable structure seen is the basilar artery, which is usually covered with arachnoid (**Fig. 18–2**). In patients, this is left undisturbed, but in the cadaver, it is removed to allow proper visualization of the surrounding structures. In most patients, the segments of the brain stem that can be easily visualized are the upper part of the medulla, the pons, and the lower edge of the midbrain. The vessels that are seen are the basilar artery, the posterior cerebral arteries, the superior cerebellar and the anterior inferior cerebellar arteries. Depending upon the state of the brain, a variable number of the cranial nerves can be seen. Dehydration of the brain by the administration of mannitol may enlarge the space around the brain stem and allow easier visualization of the nerves (**Fig. 18–2**).

If the pituitary is removed and the optic chiasm visualized, a better perspective of the cranial nerves in the posterior fossa can be achieved. In **Fig. 18–3**, if the telescope is turned laterally, cranial nerve VI can be seen just below the carotid artery and again in the cavernous sinus behind the carotid artery. Cranial nerve III can be seen exiting the brain stem just inferior to the posterior cerebral artery.

If the 30-degree endoscope is advanced further into the posterior cranial fossa, the rest of the cranial nerves can be seen (**Fig. 18–4**). The trigeminal nerve (V) exits the lateral aspect of the pons with the thin cranial nerve IV below it. Cranial nerve V enters Meckel's cave before passing into the cavernous sinus. Below cranial nerve V, cranial nerves VII, VIII, and the nervus intermedius can seen entering the internal auditory meatus. Although in this cadaver there seems to be space between the brain stem and the skull base, this is not always the case in patients and therefore caution should be exercised when contemplating removing tumors from the lateral regions of the posterior cranial fossa. Inferior to

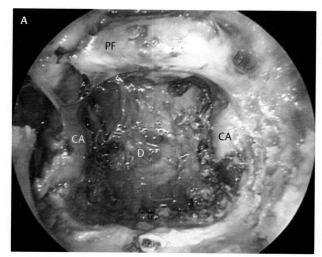

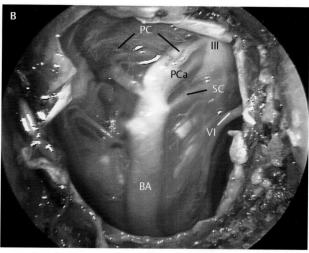

Figure 18–2 In (**A**), the posterior cranial fossa dura has been exposed from the vertical portion of the carotid artery (CA) to carotid artery (CA) and from the pituitary fossa (PF) to the floor of the sphenoid. In (**B**), the dura has been removed exposing the basilar artery (BA), posterior cerebral artery (PCa), and the posterior communicating (PC) artery of the circle of Willis. In addition, the superior cerebellar (SC) artery, third (III) and sixth (VI) cranial nerves can be seen.

cranial nerves VII and VIII, cranial nerves IX and X can be seen entering the jugular foramen.

If the endoscope is turned inferiorly, the vertebral arteries can be seen joining to form the basilar artery. Shortly thereafter, the posterior inferior cerebellar artery (PICA) is given off. The nerve roots of cranial nerve XII can be seen (**Fig. 18–5**).

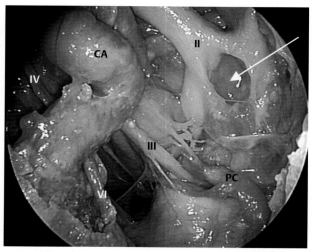

Figure 18–3 This view is obtained after removal of the pituitary gland, and the residual stalk (*white arrow*) can be seen behind the optic chiasm (right optic nerve marked as II). The third cranial nerve (III) can be seen between the posterior cerebral artery (PC) and the superior cerebellar artery. The carotid artery (CA) siphon is seen with the sixth cranial nerve (VI) below and lateral (in the cavernous sinus) to the artery.

Cavernous Sinus

The cavernous sinus lies between two layers of dura and is filled with venous sinusoids. Its medial border is the pituitary fossa and lateral border the middle cranial fossa. Anteroinferiorly, it is related to the infraorbital fissure and posteriorly to Meckel's cave. In most patients, the two cavernous sinuses are connected by the intercavernous venous connections. These are venous sinuses connecting one cavernous sinus to the other and running over the anterior face of the pituitary fossa. Fortunately, in patients with pituitary macroadenomas, the pressure of the tumor on the anterior face of the pituitary fossa will usually result in their obliteration. However, in microadenomas, these sinusoids may be present and cause significant venous bleeding when opened during entry into the pituitary fossa.

The cavernous sinus contains cranial nerves III, IV, V, and VI. **Figure 18–6** is a diagrammatic representation of the contents of the cavernous sinus adjacent to the pituitary gland.

The contents of the cavernous sinus are seldom seen during surgery as it is only possible to open the cavernous sinus if tumor has infiltrated it and obliterated the venous sinusoids. However, in such cases it is important to know the anatomy of the cavernous sinus so that these important structures are not damaged during resection of such tumors. In **Fig. 18–7**, the carotid artery is swung medially to expose the contents of the cavernous sinus. Note how cranial nerve III is a large nerve in the roof of the sinus with the smaller less easily visible cranial nerve IV directly below it. Cranial nerve VI is seen to enter the sinus lower down and from the posterior inferior aspect then to traverse from inferior to superior abutting the carotid artery. If this nerve is moved medially, the V1 and V2 branches of cranial nerve V can be seen. V3 is in the same surgical plane but lies more inferior to the dissection presented in **Fig. 18–7**.

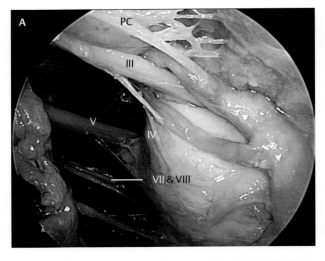

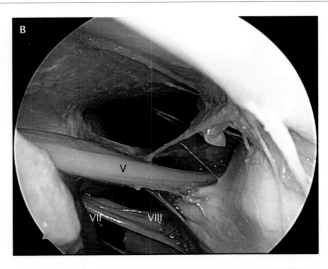

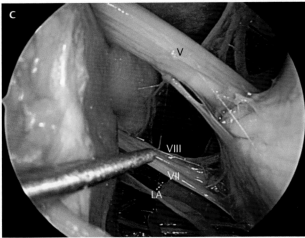

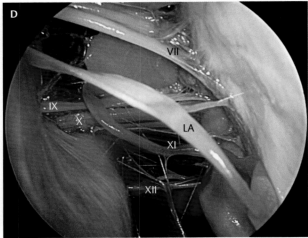

Figure 18–4 In (**A**), the posterior communicating artery (PC) of the circle of Willis is seen. Below this, cranial nerves III, V, VII, and VIII can be seen leaving the brain stem and entering the foramina of the skull base. In (**B, C**) is a closer view of the cranial nerve V with cranial nerve IV seen below it. A clear view of cranial nerves VII and VIII with the nervus intermedius lying between them is obtained. In (**D**), cranial nerves IX and X can be seen entering the jugular foramen. Below this, the roots of cranial nerve XI can be seen. The labyrinthine artery (LA) is seen anterior to these cranial nerves.

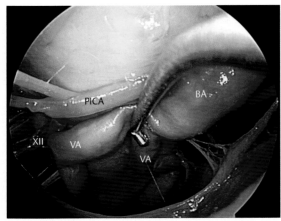

Figure 18–5 The two vertebral arteries (VA) are seen joining at the tip of the metal probe to form the basilar artery (BA). Just above the junction of the vertebral arteries, the posterior inferior cerebellar artery (PICA) is given off. The nerve roots of cranial nerve XII can be seen.

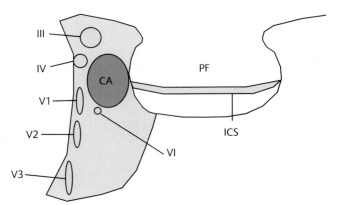

Figure 18–6 This diagrammatic representation of the right cavernous sinus shows the carotid artery (CA) within the cavernous sinus. Cranial nerve VI is the most medial nerve, and cranial nerves III, IV, and V tend to run against the lateral wall of the cavernous sinus. The intercavernous venous sinus (ICS) that connects one sinus to the other is illustrated.

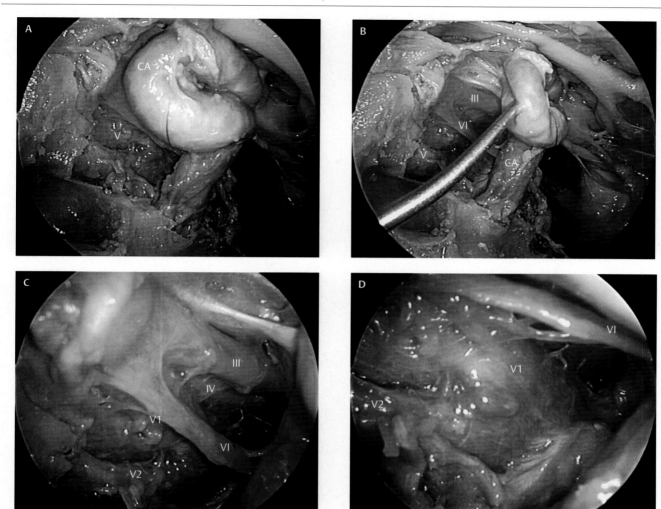

Figure 18–7 In (**A**), the medial dural wall of the cavernous sinus has been removed exposing the siphon of the internal carotid artery (CA) clearly. The cranial nerve V can be seen inferolaterally within the cavernous sinus. In (**B**), the carotid is moved medially to expose the contents of the cavernous sinus. Cranial nerves III, V, and VI can be clearly seen. (**C**) In the magnified view, cranial nerves III and IV and branches V1 and V2 can be clearly seen. V1 lies directly under cranial nerve VI. In (**D**), cranial nerve VI has been elevated and the V1 and V2 branches of cranial nerve V can be clearly seen.

◆ SURGICAL TECHNIQUE

The surgical approach to this region is very similar to the approach to pituitary tumors (see Chapter 13). The superior turbinate is removed and bilateral large sphenoidotomies are created. The posterior centimeter of the septum is removed so that two surgeons can simultaneously assess the sphenoid and the clivus. The floor of the sphenoid is resected with a straight 3.2 round cutting burr (Medtronic ENT). It is important to resect most of the floor as failure to do so will result in the anterior sill of the floor of the sphenoid driving the instruments upward toward the pituitary (**Fig. 18–8**). The parasagittal computed tomography (CT) scan illustrates this point showing that lack of resection of the floor of the sphenoid drives instruments superiorly, making access to the posterior floor of the sphenoid and adjacent clivus difficult.

The next step is to identify the vertical portions of both carotid arteries thereby delineating the lateral limits of the dissection. Usually this is done with a 25-degree skull base diamond burr (Medtronic ENT), which allows the walls of the carotids to be exposed with minimal risk of injury. The drill can contact the adventitia of the wall of the carotid without cutting this tissue, allowing the vessel to be exposed. If the lesion extends inferolaterally to the carotid canals, it can be followed as long as it is kept in mind that the petrous temporal portion of the carotid runs at ~45 degrees to the vertical portion of the carotids. In a patient with a chordoma, such an extension can be removed with a curved diamond burr. Sometimes the 70-degree reverse cut diamond burr (Medtronic ENT) is required to reach behind and below the carotid canals and into the petrous apex (**Fig. 18–9**).

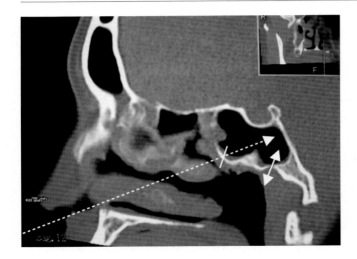

Figure 18–8 The white solid line illustrates the removal of only the anterior face, and limited removal of the floor will still result in a straight instrument being driven onto the undersurface of the pituitary fossa (*broken white arrow*). Further removal of the floor of the sphenoid up to the region of the *double-headed white arrow* will allow access to the junction of the posterior sphenoid floor and adjacent clivus. Further removal of the soft tissue in the roof of the nasopharynx will give access to the lower region of the clivus toward the foramen magnum and atlas.

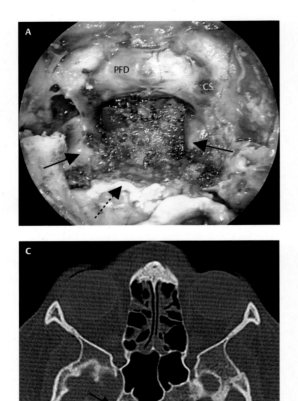

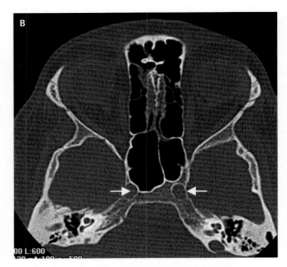

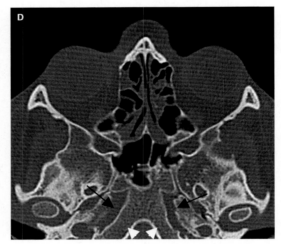

Figure 18–9 In (**A**), the vertical portions of the carotid arteries have been exposed (*solid black arrows*). Superiorly, the dura overlying the pituitary fossa (PFD) has been exposed, and the cavernous sinus (CS) on both sides can be clearly seen. Note the intercavernous venous sinus connecting the two sinuses. Inferiorly, the floor of the sphenoid has been drilled away until almost adjacent to the clival dura (*broken black arrow*). In axial CT (**B**), the vertical portions of the carotid arteries are seen (*white arrows*) with the clivus between the carotids. In axial CTs (**C, D**), the petrous portions of the carotid arteries and foramen lacerum are marked with *black arrows* and the posterolateral portions of the clivus behind the arteries are marked with *white arrows*. Note how the petrous portion of the carotid runs at a 45-degree angle to the vertical portions of the arteries.

If the tumor breaches the clival dura and protrudes intracranially, then this portion of the tumor may be separated from the clival component by sharp dissection using the endoscopic skull base scissors* (Medtronic ENT). The residual tumor protruding from the clivus into the posterior cranial fossa is now accessible without the surgeons' having to work around the often bulky clival component. The dural opening should be visualized and can be further enlarged with the scissors to allow an endoscopic view of the intracranial tumor component. Clival chordomas are usually soft and amenable to debulking with gentle suction. Care must be taken to ensure that the tumor is not entangled with any of the vascular structures of the brain stem. Traction on a tumor wrapped around a brain-stem perforator may cause catastrophic bleeding and hemorrhage into the brain stem and intraoperative death. In this situation, it is vitally important for the otolaryngologist and neurosurgeon to work closely as a team. The malleable skull base blunt hook and probe* (Medtronic ENT Skull Base Set) are used to mobilize the tumor while gentle traction is applied and the tumor is gently delivered through the dural defect into the sphenoid. Angled endoscopes and malleable suctions* (Medtronic ENT Skull Base Set) are used to visualize the intracranial

cavity to ensure no residual tumor remains. If residual tumor is seen, a suction regulator is placed in the suction line to reduce the amount of suction. The malleable skull base suction* (Medtronic ENT) is then placed through the dural defect onto the residual tumor. The suction control port of this instrument is very wide so that if a vessel or nerve is inadvertently sucked into the end of the instrument, removal of the finger from the suction port will remove all suction at the tip and the vascular structure or nerve will be released uninjured.

◆ CASE EXAMPLES

A middle-aged woman presented with a large clival chordoma that protruded into the sphenoid sinus, abutting both internal carotid arteries and extending intracranially where it abutted the basilar artery (**Fig. 18–10**).

This patient was managed with a two-surgeon approach with bilateral large sphenoidotomies, removal of the posterior 1 cm of the septum, and removal of the floor of the sphenoid. Once access had been achieved, both vertical portions of the carotids were exposed with a rough diamond

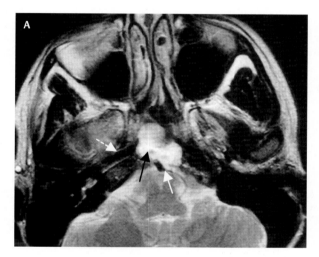

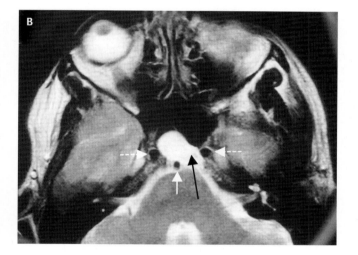

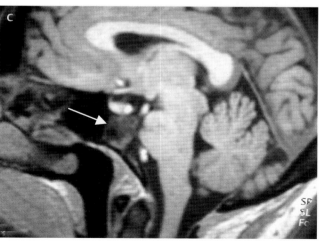

Figure 18–10 (A, B) On the axial MRI scans, the chordoma (*black arrow*) can be seen between the carotid arteries (*broken white arrows*) and abutting the basilar artery (*solid white arrow*). (**C**) In the parasagittal MRI scan, the lesion can be seen in the clivus below the pituitary and abutting the pons.

223

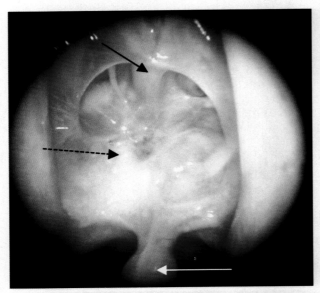

Figure 18–11 This endoscopic image of the sphenoid indicates the residual septum (*white arrow*), intersinus septum of the sphenoid (*black arrow*), and the region of the reconstruction of the posterior fossa wall (*broken black arrow*).

burr. The remaining bony clivus was removed with exposure of the clival dura with a central deficit through which the chordoma entered the posterior cranial fossa. Utilizing the two-surgeon approach, the intracranial portion of the tumor was slowly mobilized under direct vision. A 30-degree endoscope was used to visualize the inferior intracranial extension of the tumor. The malleable blunt tip and curved probes were used to gently dissect the arachnoid from the tumor and the tumor was delivered into the sphenoid and removed. Reconstruction of the skull base was achieved initially with fat alone but the patient developed a cerebrospinal fluid (CSF) leak ~1 month after surgery and the repair was then augmented with fascia lata. This repair remains intact after 4 years' follow-up (**Fig. 18–11**). To date, there is no evidence of a recurrent disease on magnetic resonance imaging (MRI) scanning.

The second case example is a middle-aged man who presented with a partial sixth cranial nerve palsy. MRI scans showed a lesion extending from internal carotid to internal carotid and extending inferior and lateral to the vertical portions of the carotids. The intracranial extension indents the anterior surface of the pons and displaces the basilar artery laterally (**Fig. 18–12**).

The other area that should always be assessed is the possible inferior bony extension of these tumors. If the CT scans of this case are reviewed, the inferolateral extension behind the petrous temporal portions of the internal carotids can be seen (**Fig. 18–13**). There is significant bony erosion of this part of the clivus down toward the foramen magnum. In this patient, more bony erosion is seen on the right side (white arrow) in the petrous apex.

This patient was approached with a two-surgeon standard pituitary exposure with wide sphenoidotomies, septal resection, and floor of sphenoid resection. Once the tumor

was fully on view, the vertical portion of the internal carotid arteries was exposed from the base of the sphenoid to the floor of the pituitary fossa using a rough diamond burr. The dura of the entire floor of the pituitary was then exposed. This delineates the superior and lateral margins of the dissection. Next, the floor of the sphenoid was drilled away and the tumor followed laterally behind the vertical portions of the internal carotids and posteriorly until the posterior cranial fossa dura was exposed. Once dura was exposed inferiorly (at the base of the clivus), laterally (behind the carotids), and superiorly (at the pituitary-clivus junction) the tumor was felt to be fully mobile. The tumor was placed under slight traction, and a gush of CSF was seen as the intracranial component was displaced in the posterior fossa dural defect. Using the skull base endoscopic scissors* (Medtronic ENT), the sphenoid/clival component of the tumor was divided from the intracranial extension at the level of the posterior fossa dura. Once the sphenoid component was removed, enough space was created so that the two surgeons could work comfortably on the remaining intracranial tumor. The dural defect was enlarged with the endoscopic skull base scissors and a view of the posterior cranial fossa obtained. Using the malleable right-angled hook and blunt tip probe (Skull Base Set, Medtronic ENT), the intracranial component was gently mobilized and delivered through the dural defect. The endoscope was switched to a 30-degree endoscope and the posterior cranial fossa reexplored. Residual tumor was seen superiorly on the anterior face of the pons. A suction regulator was placed in the suction line limiting the amount of suction, and the malleable frontal sinus suction was bent so it could be placed through the dural defect superiorly, and the residual tumor indenting the pons was gently removed. Complete macroscopic tumor resection was achieved. The skull base defect was repaired with two layers of fascia lata. One layer was placed intracranially and the other on the dura from the sphenoid. Fibrin glue and a nasal pack were put in place. Unfortunately, the patient developed a CSF leak after the pack was removed. On reexploration, the dural repair was solid with a very thin stream of CSF seen coming from the junction between the pituitary dura and the repair. This region was opened and repaired with a bath-plug type fat plug and fibrin glue.

To date, we have endoscopically removed six clival chordomas. In five of the six, complete macroscopic tumor resection was possible, and in this group there has been no recurrence of tumor since resection with a mean follow-up of 3.5 years. One patient had proton beam irradiation after surgical resection. In the sixth patient, the residual tumor is growing very slowly, and this is been monitored with sequential MRI scans. Further surgery will be offered if the tumor grows significantly or produces symptoms.

◆ KEY POINTS

Endoscopic resection of clival and posterior cranial fossa tumors presents a challenge to the skull base team. Successful management of these patients requires a detailed knowledge of the anatomy and a high level of endoscopic skill. The endoscopic skull base team, normally consisting of a rhinologist

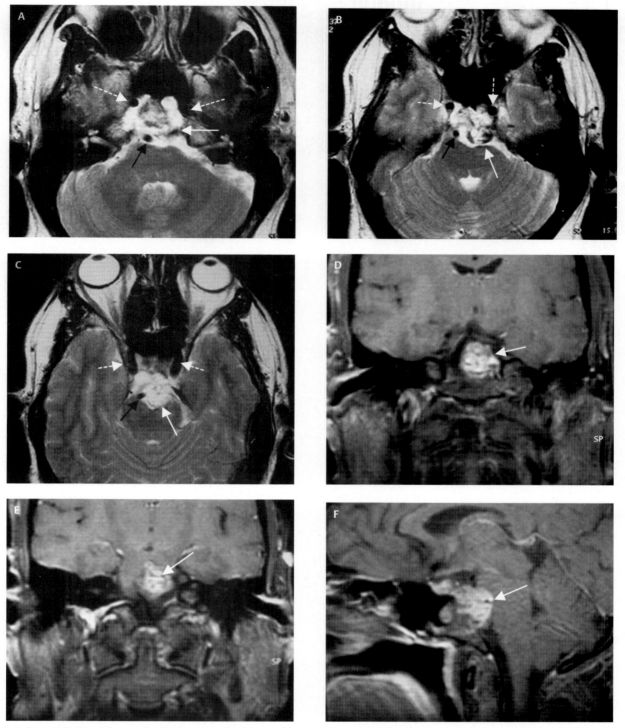

Figure 18–12 In MRI T2 axial scans (**A–C**), the tumor (*white arrow*) is seen between the two vertical portions of the carotids (*broken white arrows*). It is also evident how the tumor indents the pons and displaces the basilar artery (*black arrow*) laterally. In the coronal T1 scans (**D, E**), the tumor can be seen indenting the pons (*white arrow*). (**F**) This indentation can be fully appreciated on the parasagittal MRI T1 image. Note the significant posterior indentation of the tumor into the pons (*white arrow*).

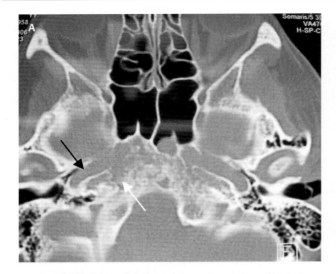

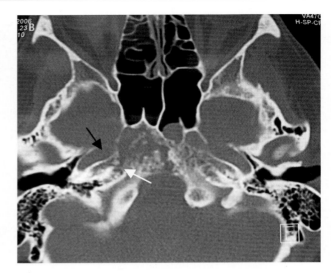

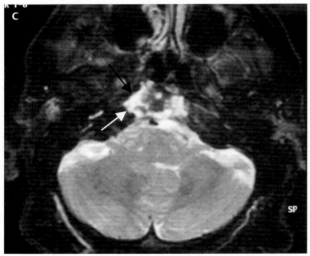

Figure 18–13 Axial CT scans (**A, B**) and T1 MRI (**C**) illustrate the horizontal portions of the internal carotid (*black arrow*) and the bony erosion immediately posterior to the carotid in the base of the clivus (*white arrow*).

and a neurosurgeon, need to build their endoscopic expertise on less challenging cases such as with pituitary tumor resection, and, once they have had sufficient expertise, to then progress to clival and posterior cranial fossa tumors.

References

1. Brackmann DE, Arriaga MA. Surgery of the posterior cranial fossa. In: Cummings CW, ed. Otolaryngology Head and Neck Surgery. 4th ed. St. Louis: Mosby; 2005

2. Lanzino G, Dumont AS, Lopez MBS, Laws E. Skull base chordomas: overview of disease, management options, and outcome. Neurosurg Focus 2001;10:E12

3. Demonte F, Diaz E, Callender D, Suk I. Transmandibular, circumglossal, retropharyngeal approach for chordomas of the clivus and upper cervical spine. Technical note. Neurosurg Focus 2001;10:E10

4. Solares CA, Fakhri S, Batra P, Lee J, Lanza DC. Transnasal endoscopic resection of lesions of the clivus: a preliminary report. Laryngoscope 2005;115:1917–1922

5. Frank G, Sciarretta V, Calbucci F, Farneti G, Mazzatenta D, Pasquini E. The endoscopic transnasal transphenoidal approach for the treatment of cranial base chordomas and chondrosarcomas. Neurosurgery 2006;59(1 Suppl 1):ONS50–ONS57

19

Endoscopic Resection of Anterior Cranial Fossa Tumors

Endoscopic techniques for transnasal resection of benign anterior cranial fossa tumors were developed for tumors involving both the nasal cavity, sinuses, and the anterior cranial fossa. However, experience with these tumors has led to the refinement of these techniques to address benign tumors of the anterior cranial fossa that do not have a nasal or sinus component. Although most of this experience has been with meningiomas, these techniques can also be used to address malignant nasal tumors that extend intracranially. The first step toward a wholly endoscopic resection of malignant sinonasal tumors was the experience gained with endoscopic management of the sinonasal component of the tumor during a standard craniofacial resection. We found that the endoscopic resection of the sinonasal component could be as effectively dealt with endoscopically as it can with external traditional approaches. In the case of large tumors involving both nasal cavities, the endoscopic approach was more effective as it dealt with both sides, as opposed to most of the external approaches that limited access to one side of the nose. A significant number of these malignant tumors attach to the skull base and associated orbit. During craniofacial resection, the skull base involved with tumor is completely excised. [1-3] The associated orbital involvement would, in most circumstances, be removed as a separate excision.

We found that endoscopically resecting the sinonasal component afforded better visualization of the tumor, allowing the nonattached tumor to be extensively debulked and the regions of tumor attachment to be accurately identified. This in turn allowed a complete resection of the sinonasal and if present the orbital component. As the experience with benign anterior skull base tumor resection developed, these techniques could in turn be applied to the resection of selected malignant tumors involving the skull base and intracranial cavity. Tumors thought to be suitable were tumors with a localized intracranial extension. Because of the infiltrative nature of squamous cell carcinomas, these were thought not to be suitable, whereas adenocarcinoma and esthesioneurob-lastoma could be addressed wholly endoscopically. Although the gold standard for these malignancies remains craniofacial resection,[1] there is increasing evidence that for selected patients, the wholly endoscopic resection yields comparable results.[2-5] Recently published series have reported similar morbidity and mortality rates and very similar local recurrence rates.[2,3,5] In addition, there are significant benefits for the patients undergoing wholly endoscopic resection as unevolved structures are not removed, and this approach avoids skin incisions with improved cosmetic results.[2-5] In addition, those patients who are medically or otherwise unsuitable for a standard craniofacial resection or who choose not to undergo this procedure can be offered the endoscopic approach as an alternative. Endoscopic resection of the anterior skull base requires a detailed knowledge of the anatomy of this region.

◆ ANATOMY OF THE ANTERIOR SKULL BASE

The anterior skull base consists of the orbital plates of the frontal bone with cribriform plate (part of the ethmoid bone) separating them. These plates attach to the planum sphenoidale (lesser wing of the sphenoid bone) posteriorly (**Fig. 19–1**). The cribriform plate gives rise to the crista galli onto which the falx cerebri attaches.

If the anterior skull base is approached endoscopically from front to back, the frontal bone (posterior wall of the frontal sinus), foveae ethmoidalis, and intervening cribriform plates can be seen. Posteriorly, the foveae ethmoidalis and cribriform plates attach to the planum sphenoidale. The important vascular structures within the anterior skull base are the anterior and posterior ethmoid arteries. Note how there is a space or cell between the frontal sinus ostium and the anterior ethmoidal artery (**Fig. 19–2**). This is always the case as the artery usually runs in the base of the second

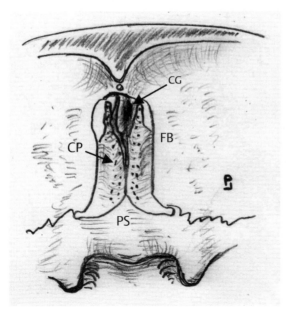

Figure 19–1 This diagram illustrates the view of the anterior skull base from above (intracranial side). The crista galli (CG), cribriform plate (CP), orbital plate of the frontal bone (FB), and planum sphenoidale (PS) of the lesser wing of the sphenoid bone are visible.

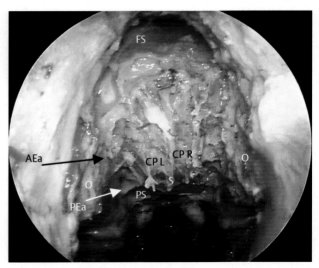

Figure 19–3 This cadaver dissection illustrates the anatomy of the anterior skull base after resection of both middle turbinates and septum (S) with exposure of cribriform plate left (CP L) and right (CP R). The communal frontal sinus (FS) ostium can be seen anteriorly with the exposed orbits (O) forming the lateral borders of the dissection. Posteriorly, the planum sphenoidale (PS) can be seen in the sphenoid sinus.

lamella, which is the upward continuation of the anterior face of the bulla ethmoidalis.

Resection of the skull base is only possible once the entire skull base has been exposed. This requires as a first step bilateral sphenoethmoidectomies with exposure of the skull base within the sphenoids, anterior and posterior ethmoids, and visualization of the frontal ostia. If the entire anterior skull base is to be resected, the frontal sinuses need to be drilled out with an endoscopic modified Lothrop procedure.

Once this has been done, the septum is detached from the anterior skull base and the anatomy of the skull base can be viewed (**Fig. 19–3**).

Once the skull base has been dropped down and removed, the anterior cranial fossa can be viewed. The two olfactory bulbs and olfactory tracts are seen on the undersurface of the anterior cerebral hemispheres. The major vascular structures are the anterior cerebral arteries and branches from these arteries. The venous drainage of the anterior cranial fossa is

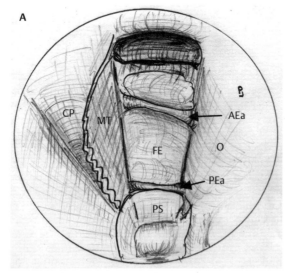

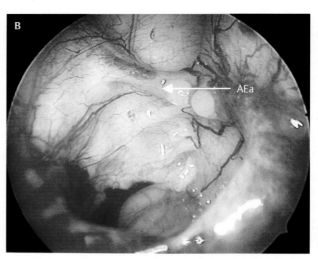

Figure 19–2 (A) A diagram of the entire left anterior skull base with the planum sphenoidale, posterior ethmoidal artery (PEa), fovea ethmoidalis (FE), anterior ethmoidal artery (AEa), frontal ostium (FS), orbit (O), and cribriform plate (CP) visible medial to the middle turbinate (MT). **(B)** An endoscopic photograph of the left anterior ethmoidal artery (AEa) on the skull base.

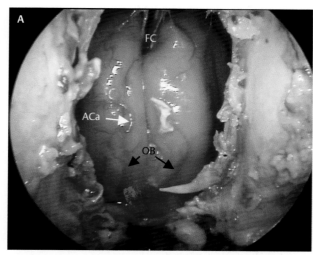

Figure 19–4 In dissection (**A**), the skull base has been removed affording a view of the inferior aspect of both anterior cerebral lobes. The olfactory bulbs (OB), anterior cerebral artery (ACa), and cut inferior aspect of the falx cerebri (FC) can be seen. In diagram (**B**), the anterior attachment of the falx cerebri (FC) to

crista galli (CG) is seen. Note the superior sagittal sinus (SSS) running in the superior aspect of the falx cerebri within the inferior sagittal sinus (ISS) in the lower margin of the falx cerebri. The inferior sagittal sinus becomes the straight sinus (SS) after it joins with the great cerebral vein.

via the superior and inferior sagittal sinuses. The superior sagittal sinus runs in the upper border of the falx cerebri, and the inferior sagittal sinus runs in the lower border of the falx cerebri (**Fig. 19–4**). Large anterior skull base tumors may have large veins draining into the inferior sagittal sinus, which if disrupted can bleed significantly.

◆ SURGICAL TECHNIQUE

The surgical removal of anterior skull base tumors requires a team consisting of an endoscopic sinus surgeon and a neurosurgeon. It is vitally important that both members of this skull base team have endoscopic skills. These are best learned doing pituitary tumor resections as a team. Here the neurosurgeon learns how to manage the endoscope and how to work from the video monitor in two dimensions rather than with the microscope in three dimensions. The sinus surgeon learns how to manipulate intracranial tumors and surrounding neural and vascular structures. These hours spent on pituitary tumor resection build confidence within the skull base team enabling benign or malignant nasal tumors with intracranial extension to be tackled.

The first steps for access are complete sphenoethmoidectomy with exposure of the entire skull base. If the tumor is relatively posteriorly situated with a relatively small intracranial extension, skull base resection can be performed without a modified Lothrop procedure. In such cases, the intracranial extension of tumor must be small and the resection of this extension should be possible without it being necessary to resect across the midline. Surgically, the skull base defect should be clearly delineated and then enlarged to expose uninvolved dura on all sides of the defect. The dura is then excised with a combination of endoscopic skull base scissors* (Medtronic ENT) or scalpel with a normal margin of dura and the tumor extension and dura delivered into the nose.

However, if a complete resection of the anterior skull base is required, then the next step is to perform an endoscopic modified Lothrop procedure allowing the anterior aspect of the skull base to be delineated (**Fig. 19–3**). The nasal septum is separated from the skull base allowing visualization of the entire skull base from the frontal sinuses anteriorly to the anterior face of the pituitary fossa. Both laminae papyracea should be on view forming the lateral limits of the resection. Before the skull base can be resected, the anterior and posterior ethmoidal arteries need to be identified and ligated or cauterized and divided. There are two ways to identify and ligate the anterior ethmoidal arteries. They can be exposed by removing a small amount of lamina papyracea adjacent to the artery and then mobilizing the orbital periosteum. Pushing this laterally tents the anterior ethmoidal artery and allows ligation or cautery before it is divided with the endoscopic skull base scissors (Skull Base Set, Medtronic ENT) (**Fig. 19–5**). However, this technique does risk rupture of the orbital periosteum with fat prolapse, which can then make identification of the artery very difficult. An easier and safer technique is to run the diamond burr over the region of the anterior ethmoidal artery, removing the bone until the artery is exposed in its canal. The bone is removed laterally and the artery identified and exposed where it enters the skull base at which point it is ligated, cauterized, and divided. This is done bilaterally before the posterior ethmoidal arteries are also identified using the diamond drill on the skull base. The arteries usually enter the skull base at the junction of the posterior ethmoids and sphenoid, and the drill is run over this region of the skull base until the artery is clearly identified, cauterized, and cut on both sides (**Fig. 19–5**).

The next step is to perform an endoscopic modified Lothrop procedure as set out in Chapter 9. A septal perforation is performed and the frontal sinus opened bilaterally and communicated by removal of the intersinus septum (**Fig. 19–6**).

229

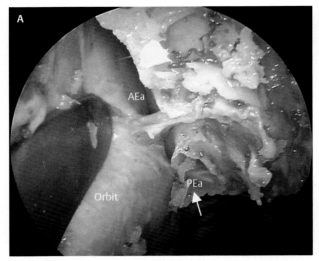

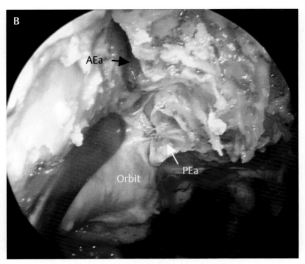

Figure 19–5 On the right side in dissection (**A**), the anterior ethmoidal artery (AEa) is tented by the Freer elevator pushing on the orbital periosteum. The posterior ethmoidal artery (PEa) can also be seen in the skull base just anterior to the anterior wall of the sphenoid sinus. In dissection (**B**), the anterior ethmoidal artery (AEa) has been divided, and the posterior ethmoidal artery (PEa) is identified on the skull base.

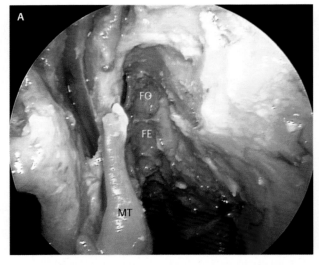

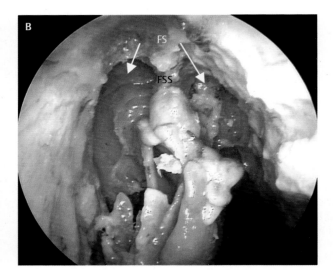

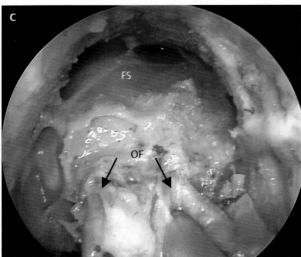

Figure 19–6 In dissection (**A**), the left frontal ostium (FO) has been exposed with the fovea ethmoidalis (FE) visible lateral to the middle turbinate (MT). In (**B**), both frontal sinuses (FS) have been opened with the frontal sinus septum (FSS) between them. After removal of this septum, the communal frontal sinus (FS) is seen as well as both olfactory fossae (OF).

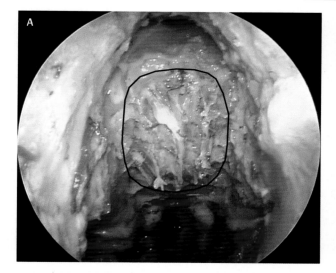

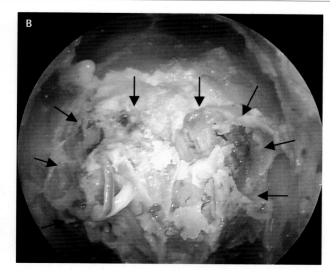

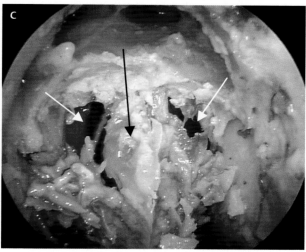

Figure 19–7 In dissection (**A**), the septum has been separated from the skull base, and the osteotomies are outlined in black. In (**B**), the osteotomy in the posterior wall of the frontal sinus is indicated with black arrows. Note that the underlying dura is intact. In (**C**), the dura has been incised with exposure of the intracranial cavity (*white arrows*) with the skull base attached to the crista galli (*black arrow*).

The final preparation step is to disconnect the nasal septum from the skull base. A straight though-cutting Blakesley is used to cut the nasal septum at its insertion on the skull base. This isolates the skull base and allows the osteotomies to be made so that the skull base can be dropped into the nasal cavity. In **Fig. 19–7**, these osteotomes are outlined in black. A rough dacryocystorhinostomy (DCR) diamond or skull base diamond burr (Medtronic ENT) is used to create the osteotomies along the lines shown in **Fig. 19–7A**. The dura is exposed but can largely be preserved. A 2-mm, 40-degree, forward-biting Kerrison punch can also be used to remove the bone in the fovea ethmoidalis region. However, the osteotomies in the planum sphenoidale usually require the drill to complete as they cross the midline. Next, the dura needs to be incised with a scalpel. The only residual attachment holding the skull base is the attachment of the falx cerebri to the crista galli.

An endoscopic skull base scissors* (Medtronic ENT) is used to cut the falx cerebri, and the skull base is dropped into the nasal cavity and removed (**Fig. 19–8**). To perform this maneuver, both surgeons need to mobilize the skull base, and the simultaneous use of the suction and scalpel will allow small residual attachments to be precisely severed. If the posterior osteotomy is not complete, this attachment can be gently fractured through the osteotomy lines but the dura will need to be cut under direct vision. In most cases, limited extension of tumor through the skull base will be removed en bloc with this technique in a similar fashion to a craniofacial resection performed through a craniotomy. Removal of the entire skull base in this fashion exposes the anterior cranial fossa, and tumor that remains can now be dissected free. Such a dissection is again very delicate requiring great endoscopic skill from both surgeons. The arachnoid plane needs to be developed and the tumor dissected from the arachnoid. Vessels that can be preserved are carefully dissected free from the tumor, but vessels supplying the tumor are cauterized with bipolar forceps and divided.

Skull Base Closure

To repair this large skull base defect, two large pieces of fascia lata are harvested from the thigh. Each piece needs to overlap the defect circumferentially by at least 2 cm (**Fig. 19–9**). The

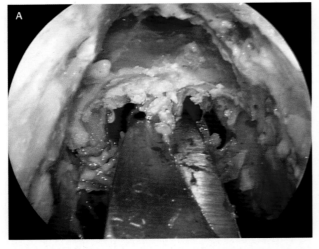

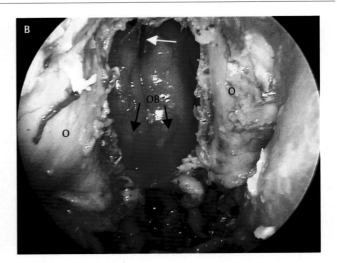

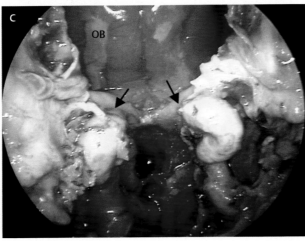

Figure 19–8 In dissection (**A**), scissors are used to cut the falx cerebri where it attaches to the crista galli allowing the skull base to be dropped into the nasal cavity. In (**B**), the cut edge of the falx cerebri (*white arrow*) can be seen with the olfactory bulbs and anterior cerebral hemispheres. The adjacent orbits (O) are noted. In (**C**), the planum sphenoidale has been completely removed with exposure of both optic nerves (*black arrows*). This is usually not necessary, but the position of these nerves needs to be identified before the planum sphenoidale osteotomies are made so that they may be protected.

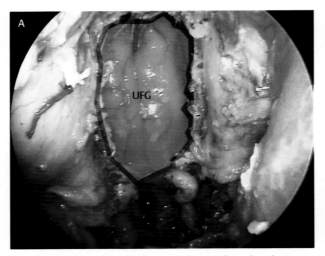

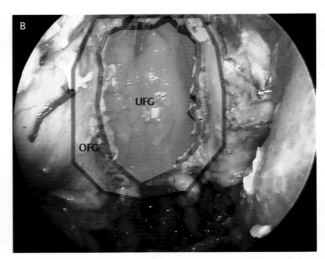

Figure 19–9 In dissection (**A**), the fascia lata graft is placed as an underlay (UFG) on the inside of the cranial cavity and the edges smoothed out. In dissection (**B**), the second fascia lata graft is placed on the nasal surface of the defect as on overlay graft (OFG) again smoothing out the edges to ensure that the graft fits snugly around the entire defect.

first layer is placed in the intracranial surface and if possible attached to the intracranial surface of the dura with 2/0 Vicryl sutures in the region of the planum sphenoidale. In some patients, there is not sufficient dura to place these sutures, and in these patients the dura is tucked into the intracranial cavity as an underlay graft. The malleable skull base probe is used to ensure that the graft is properly tucked intracranially without any folds and is smoothly adherent to the inner surface of the skull base. The second layer of fascia lata is placed as an overlay on the skull base again ensuring that there are no folds and that it lies closely approximated to the skull base (**Fig. 19–9**). Fibrin glue is applied to this second layer followed by large sheets of Gelfoam. The Gelfoam ensures that the nasal pack does not stick to the grafts. The nasal cavity is packed with ribbon gauze soaked in the antiseptic bismuth iodoform paraffin paste (BIPP). Be aware that there may be loss of lamina papyracea from both orbits, and if the pack is placed too tightly, this can cause proptosis. In two of our patients, the nasal pack needed to be removed and replaced due to proptosis from a too tightly placed pack. The anesthetist needs to be aware that as the patient is recovering from the anesthesia, the patient

should be extubated while under relatively deep anesthesia and a laryngeal mask inserted. This allows the patient to be ventilated without the need to use a face mask and also helps to ensure that the patient does not cough or strain during extubation, which may precipitate intracranial bleeding. The nasal pack is left in place for 1 week and the patient is usually discharged with the pack in place. The pack is removed after 1 week at the first postoperative visit to the outpatient department.

◆ CASE EXAMPLES

Anterior skull base midline meningiomas are one of the tumors that are suitable for a wholly endoscopic approach. These tumors arise from the dura and bone of the anterior skull base and may present late due to lack of symptoms. Often, typical frontal lobe symptoms such as a subtle change in personality or inappropriate uncharacteristic behavior may be the only presenting feature. The intracranial pressure may be raised, and the patient may complain of headaches. Meningiomas do have

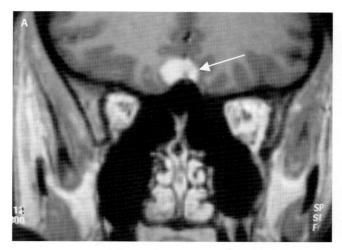

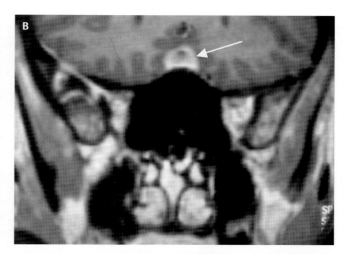

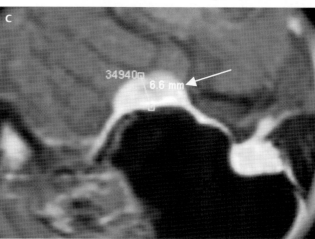

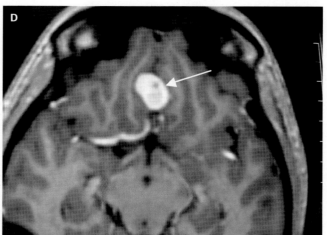

Figure 19–10 **(A, B)** In coronal MRI scans, the meningioma is indicated with a *white arrow*. **(C)** In the parasagittal MRI scan, the roof of the sphenoid is arched upward with the meningioma (*white arrow*) on its roof. **(D)** In the axial MRI scan, the meningioma is seen to push between the two cerebral hemispheres.

a tendency to recur after removal, and recent papers discussing the high recurrence rate of sphenoid wing meningiomas concluded that tumor remnants left in the underlying bone were responsible for the recurrences.[11] The transnasal endoscopic approach overcomes this problem by removal of both the dura and underlying bone from which the tumor has arisen, potentially lessening the possibility of recurrence after surgery.

Example 1

The first case example is of a young woman who presented with headache. A midline meningioma was diagnosed and initially was monitored with serial magnetic resonance imaging (MRI) scans but the tumor continued to grow (**Fig. 19–10**). She was offered both endoscopic and traditional external approach but chose to have an endoscopic resection.

The surgical plan for this patient was to do a bilateral complete sphenoethmoidectomy with exposure of the frontal ostia. It was not necessary to perform a modified Lothrop procedure as the tumor was located in the posterior region of the anterior skull base. The posterior half of the septum

was removed. The next step was to establish the extent of the tumor. With the aid of the computer-aided surgical (CAS) navigation system, the skull base osteotomies were marked out. The osteotomies were performed around the outside of the tumor using diamond burrs and Kerrison punches. A combination of scalpel and endoscopic scissors were used to incise the dura allowing the tumor to drop into the nasal cavity. Arachnoid attachments were carefully dissected free of the tumor and the supplying blood vessels cauterized and divided. The entire tumor and attached dura were removed. The skull base was repaired using the previously described underlay and onlay layers of fascia lata, fibrin glue, and nasal pack. The patient was discharged the following day. Postoperative endoscopy shows a well-healed nasal cavity and skull base, and follow-up MRI scans over the past 3 years have not shown any recurrence or residual tumor (**Fig. 19–11**).

Example 2

This elderly lady presented with memory loss and headaches. The large anterior cranial fossa meningioma had

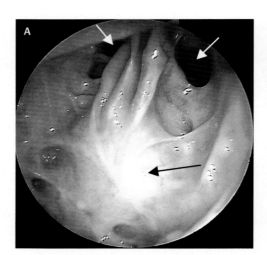

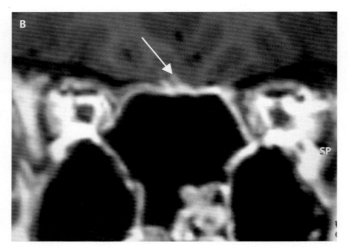

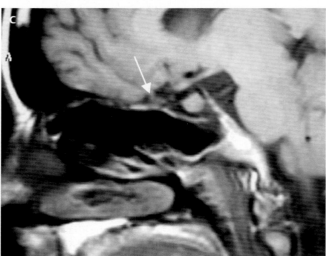

Figure 19–11 In endoscopic picture (**A**), the region of skull base reconstruction is indicated with a black arrow. Note the two frontal ostia anteriorly (*white arrows*). In coronal MRI scan (**B**) and parasagittal MRI (**C**), the region of skull base reconstruction and previous tumor is indicated with a *white arrow*.

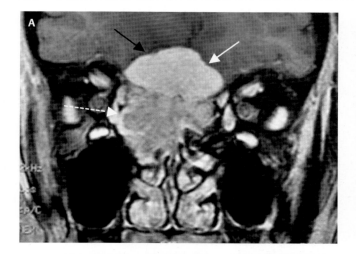

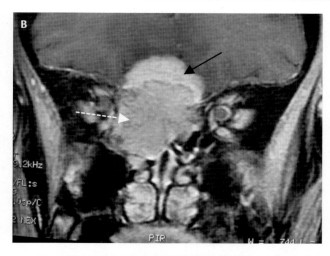

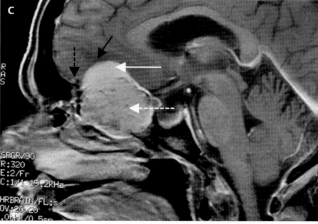

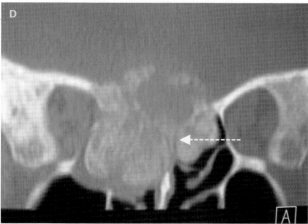

Figure 19–12 In coronal MRI scans (**A, B**) and parasagittal MRI (**C**), the two consistencies of tumor are visible. The soft tumor is marked with a *solid white arrow*, and the calcified tumor is marked with a *broken white arrow*. In coronal CT scan (**D**), the calcified part of the tumor is clearly seen (*broken white arrow*). Brain edema is indicated with a *solid black arrow* in (**A, C**). The other important feature seen in (**C**) is the close approximation of the tumor to the posterior wall of the frontal sinus (*broken black arrow*). This means that the anterior osteotomy should be through the posterior wall of the frontal sinus.

significant extension intranasally (**Fig. 19–12**). Note the calcification within the tumor and the different consistencies of the tumor in the nose and in the intracranial cavity. Also note that there was substantial brain edema around the intracranial tumor.

The surgical approach for this patient is to perform bilateral maxillary antrostomies and complete sphenoethmoidectomies debulking the tumor during exposure of the sinuses. This debulking should be continued to where the skull base normally would be. An endoscopic modified Lothrop procedure is performed to expose the posterior wall of the frontal sinuses, and the bone directly anterior to the tumor edge is removed. The inside of the tumor is carefully debulked removing most of the inside of the tumor but retaining the outer shell. Once this has been completed, the surgical plane between the tumor and the anterior cerebral lobes is identified and the tumor carefully dissected away from the arachnoid. Neuropatties are placed where this dissection has been performed to maintain this plane and allow adjacent dissection to continue in the same

plane. It also protects the underlying brain tissue from inadvertent damage. Any feeding vessels or veins draining from the tumor are cauterized with the suction bipolar forceps* (Medtronic ENT) and divided. In this way, the tumor is progressively delivered into the nasal cavity until complete removal is achieved. The cavity is irrigated with warm lactated Ringer's solution and any bleeding vessels cauterized. The skull base is repaired in the manner previously described with two layers of fascia lata: the first placed as an underlay and the second as an overlay, followed by fibrin glue, Gelfoam, and a BIPP ribbon gauze nasal pack. The pack is removed after 7 days. No lumbar drains are used during the first week, but one may be inserted if there is a small leak after the pack has been removed.

Example 3

The third patient is a middle-aged man who presented with visual symptoms, headaches, and inappropriate euphoria.

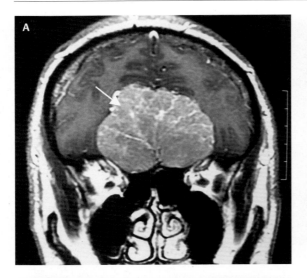

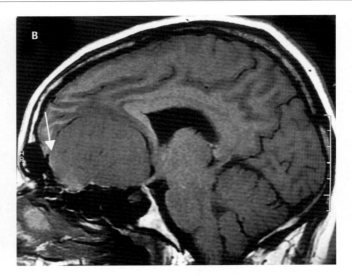

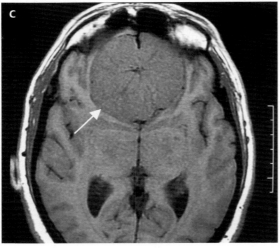

Figure 19–13 In the following MRI scans ([**A**] coronal, [**B**] parasagittal, [**C**] axial), the tumor is indicated with a *white arrow*. Note in (**B**) how the tumor closely approximates the posterior wall of the frontal sinus.

This midline olfactory groove meningioma was similar to the second case example but significantly larger, and there was no nasal or sinus involvement (**Fig. 19–13**).

There are several ways that this meningioma could be tackled. The most common would be the bifrontal and pterional approaches.[7,8] The bifrontal approach gives good access to both sides but results in significant frontal lobe retraction, and the important vascular structures are only approached late in the dissection.[7,8] The pterional approach[9,10] is rapid and requires ipsilateral frontal lobe retraction, but the opposite frontal lobe does not need retraction, and this has an advantage over the bifrontal approach. However, controversy exists as to whether it gives sufficient exposure to the contralateral side in patients with significant bilateral tumor extension.[9,10] In addition, it allows access to the skull base vasculature relatively late in the dissection. The attraction of the transnasal approach is that the major arterial supply of the tumor, the anterior and posterior ethmoidal arteries, are ligated before the tumor resection begins. In addition, this approach removes the dura and underlying bone of the tumor therefore theoretically lessen-

ing the chances of recurrence.[11] A significant advantage of this approach is the complete lack of brain retraction. The downside of the endoscopic approach is the inability of the surgeons to control significant bleeding from the arterial and venous bleeders. It is therefore important to evaluate the arterial blood supply of the tumor preoperatively with an angiogram and assess the arterial supply to the outer surface of the tumor—the so-called peel supply. If this is significant, then the endoscopic approach may not be suitable. In addition, during this procedure any major feeding vessels from the external carotid artery such as the middle meningeal artery can be embolized.

Image guidance is essential for a patient such as this, as it allows the tumor to be "seen" through the skull base so that the anterior osteotomy can be placed through bone directly adjacent to the tumor. Correct placement of the osteotomies allows the surgeon to identify the surgical plane between the outer surface of the tumor and normal brain tissue. This helps both with the removal of the core of the tumor while preserving the outer layer as well as when this outer layer is dissected from the arachnoid and brain.

The standard preparation for resection of this tumor is bilateral maxillary antrostomies, complete sphenoethmoidectomies, and the endoscopic modified Lothrop procedure on the frontal sinuses. Once this is complete, the anterior and posterior ethmoidal arteries are identified and ligated or cauterized and divided. The posterior osteotomies are performed with the diamond burr and the lateral osteotomies in the fovea ethmoidalis with either a diamond burr or Kerrison punch. The skull base is dropped into the nasal cavity after the fibrous attachment between the crista galli and falx is cut. It can then be removed from the nose and the base of the tumor exposed. In a tumor such as this, it is crucial that the tumor should be for the most part removed from the inside out, thereby allowing the tumor to be collapsed inward on itself. If the tumor is soft, this can be done with the skull base suction dissection instruments* (Medtronic ENT) or with the 2.7-mm microdebrider blade. Great care must be taken when using the microdebrider blade within the intracranial cavity as it can be very aggressive when removing soft tissue. The suction should be placed on a suction regulator to minimize the amount of tissue sucked into the cutting region. In addition, the oscillating speed of the blade should be below 1000 rpm and the entire extent of the blade should be visible during use. The blade is generally used facing superiorly so that the endoscope is looking at the opening when in use, and the blade can be stopped if too much tissue is sucked into the opening or the tumor that is being resected is thought to contain a vessel.

The second technique for removing the core of the tumor involves using the blades of the suction bipolar forceps to grasp the fibrous threads within the tumor, and while gentle traction is placed on these, the bipolar is activated further shrinking the tumor and causing the tumor to collapse inward. Once it is felt that only a relatively thin shell of tumor remains, the surgical plane between the arachnoid and the brain is established and developed. A combination of malleable probes, suction Freer elevator, and neuropatties are used to mobilize the tumor from the brain. Vessels that are seen are cauterized with the bipolar forceps before being divided. In this patient, the surgery went relatively uneventfully until a relatively large vein draining the tumor

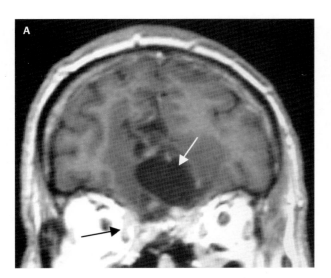

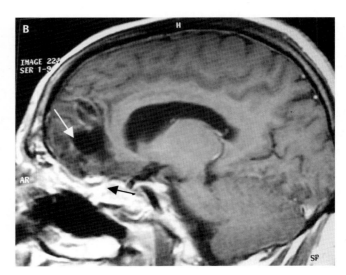

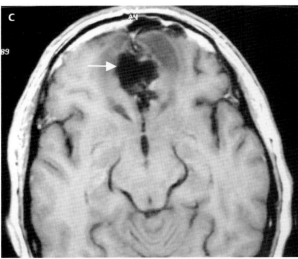

Figure 19–14 In the following postoperative MRI scans ([**A**] coronal, [**B**] parasagittal, [**C**] axial), the region where the tumor was resected is indicated with a *white arrow* and the reconstructed skull base with a *black arrow*.

into in the inferior sagittal sinus was avulsed from the sinus. Ligar clips controlled the bleeding from the sinus, and the remaining surgery was uneventful. This would not have been possible without two surgeons working simultaneously in the intracranial cavity. Skull base reconstruction was performed with an underlay and onlay fascia lata graft, fibrin glue, Gelfoam, and a BIPP nasal pack. The pack was removed after 1 week. Postoperative MRI shows complete removal of the tumor (**Fig. 19–14**).

◆ KEY POINTS

Endoscopic transnasal intracranial surgery is a new and exciting development in sinus surgery. However, this surgery requires a high level of training and skill from both the sinus surgeon and the neurosurgeon. To perform such surgeries, sinus surgeons and neurosurgeons need to form a skull base team. Such a team should develop their endoscopic skills by doing numerous endoscopic pituitary tumor dissections. As the level of expertise develops, the team can tackle smaller selected intracranial tumors. Case selection and preparation are vitally important to the success of the surgery, and the team should always be mindful that surgery with the highest likelihood of success and least morbidity should be chosen. One of the most important aspects of this surgery is the two-surgeon approach. Having two surgeons operating at the same time has huge advantages for both the ability of the surgeons to remove the tumor by placing traction on it and for the management of complications especially if significant hemorrhage occurs. The exact role of endoscopic cranial base resection in the management of malignancies is still not clear, but it is likely that endoscopic techniques will increasingly play a role in the management of these patients. Finally, there is no substitute for a sound knowledge of anatomy, and this chapter (and book) focuses on presenting the surgical anatomy in detail. This should be augmented with multiple cadaver dissections until the surgeon has extensive and detailed knowledge of the anatomy in this region.

References

1. Howard DJ, Lund VJ, Wei WI. Craniofacial resection for tumors of the nasal cavity and paranasal sinuses: a 25-year experience. Head Neck 2006;28:867–873
2. Batra PS, Citardi MJ, Worley S, Lee J, Lanza DC. Resection of anterior skull base tumors: comparison of combined traditional and endoscopic techniques. Am J Rhinol 2005;19:521–528
3. Castelnuovo PG, Belli E, Bignami M, Battaglia P, Sberze F, Tomei G. Endoscopic nasal and anterior craniotomy resection for malignant nasoethmoid tumors involving the anterior skull base. Skull Base 2006;16:15–18
4. Leong JL, Citardi MJ, Batra PS. Reconstruction of skull base defects after minimally invasive endoscopic resection of anterior skull base neoplasms. Am J Rhinol 2006;20:476–482
5. Buchmann L, Larsen C, Pollack A, Tawfik O. Endoscopic techniques in resection of anterior skull base/paranasal sinus malignancies. Laryngoscope 2006;116:1749–1754
6. Snyderman CH, Kassam AB. Endoscopic techniques for pathology of the anterior cranial fossa and ventral skull base. J Am Coll Surg 2006;202:563
7. Hentschel SJ, DeMonte F. Olfactory groove meningiomas. Neurosurg Focus 2003;14(6):e4
8. Spektor S, Valarezo J, Fliss D. Olfactory groove meningiomas from neurosurgical and ear, nose and throat perspectives; approaches, techniques and outcomes. Neurosurgery 2005;57(4 Suppl)268–280
9. Turazzi S, Cristofori L, Gambin R, Bricolo A. The pterional approach for the microsurgical removal of olfactory groove meningiomas. Neurosurgery 1999;45(4):821–826
10. Babu R, Barton A, Kasoff S. Resection of olfactory groove meningiomas: technical note revisited. Surg Neurol 1995;44:567–572
11. Pieper DR, Al-Mefty O, Hanada Y, Buechner D. Hyperostosis associated with meningioma of the cranial base: secondary changes or tumour invasion. Neurosurgery 1999;44(4):742–746

Index

Note: Page numbers followed by *f* and *t* indicate figures and tables, respectively.